MIRACLE FOOD CURES FROM THE BIBLE

REESE DUBIN

REWARD BOOKS

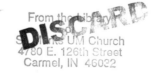

Library of Congress Cataloging in Publication Data

Dubin, Reese P.
    Miracle food cures from the Bible / Reese Dubin.
       p. cm.
    Includes index.
    ISBN 0-13-621269-7
    1. Diet therapy. 2. Food in the Bible. I. Title.
    RM 217.D78 1999
    615.8'54—dc21   99-19393
                                              CIP

© 1999 by Prentice Hall

Printed in the United States of America

This book is intended as a reference volume only, not as a medical guide. The information provided is intended to help the reader make informed decisions about his or her health, but is in no way intended as a substitute for any professional medical treatments.

10 9 8 7 6 5

ISBN 0-13-621269-7

REWARD BOOKS
Paramus, NJ 07652

On the World Wide Web at http://www.phdirect.com

This book is dedicated to my mother,
Pauline N. Dubin

To my late maternal grandparents,
Bertha Sachs and Morris Nicenholtz

To my beloved uncle,
Sam M. Nicenholtz (1915-1979)
and my father David J. Dubin (1909-1956)

To Wayne Carson, Esq.
(but for whom)

To the late George L. Costello
Executive Vice President
Prentice-Hall

To Stewart C. Sloan, V.P. (retired)
Editor-in-Chief, Advertising Manager
Parker Publishing Co., Prentice-Hall
(sorry SS, late again)

To Joseph Schaumburger, V.P. (retired)
Parker publishing Co., Prentice-Hall
(my lifetime mentor)

To Vincent Wilhelm, V.P.
Prentice-Hall Direct
(but for whom)

To Douglas Corcoran, Senior Editor
Prentice-Hall Direct
(my greatest ally and sponsor)

Special thanks to:
Phyllis Rosenthal Palley, Director,
and the staff of the New Milford Public Library;
the Inter-Library Loan System;
Ruth Holz of the Bracebridge Ontario Public Library;
and the National Library of Canada

CONTENTS

CHAPTER 4

The Healing Powers of *Charoset*   39

CHAPTER 5

A Miracle Leaf from the Last Supper:
Thousands Claimed It Saved Their Lives   61

CHAPTER 6

A Miracle Berry from the Crown of Thorns   95

CHAPTER 7

"The Hand of God," a Household Plant That Saves Lives   107

CHAPTER 8

The Amazing Healing Power of a Grain Blessed by Jesus   125

CHAPTER 9

Miracle Cures from an Omega-3 Food Blessed by Jesus   135

CHAPTER 10

A Bible Food That Wipes Out Arthritis Pain 171

CHAPTER 11

Strange Juice Medicine Revealed by the Bible Claimed by Many to Heal Ailments Quickly 189

CHAPTER 12

The Sacred Medicinal Drink
That Saved Thousands, Prevents Blood Clots, Relieves Pain, and Melts Fat Off Artery Walls   209

CHAPTER 13
The "Methuselah" Plant:
He Used It and Lived
in Three Centuries 227

CHAPTER 14

How Some of the Most Famous Bible Foods Fight AIDS, Alzheimer's, Parkinson's and More   247

CHAPTER 15
Direct from the Bible:
The World's Most Powerful Natural Antibiotic   309

CHAPTER 16

The Nectar of Heaven That Works Healing Miracles on Earth 343

CHAPTER 17

Abraham's Oak 357

CHAPTER 18

The Lowly Outcast Plant with Miracle Healing Power 363

CHAPTER · I
MIRACLE FOOD CURES FROM THE BIBLE

... a healing for your flesh and a refreshment for your body.

Proverbs 3:8

What is the Bible telling us when it mentions certain foods again and again? I believe the message is clear: *These are Bible healing foods— use them, and many of your problems will vanish.* What's more, in these pages I present strong scientific evidence that—

The Bible does indeed contain Miracle Food Cures for every ailment imaginable: for cataracts, gallstones, bleeding gums, pleurisy, epilepsy, sciatica, stomach and intestinal problems, skin problems, vaginal infection, arthritis, infertility, herpes, even medicines that— thousands of years later—fight AIDS!

I'll show you exactly which foods are Bible healing foods, and I'll show you step-by-step how each and every one may be used quickly and easily, to relieve almost any health problem or condition you can think of. In almost every case, these foods are available from your garden, corner grocery, or health-food store. And in the few instances where this may not be so, I tell you exactly where and how they may be obtained.

I

⌐ewsbreaking Discoveries Are in Scriptures Written 3,000 Years Ago!

The Bible is amazingly up-to-date. For example, Viagra may be making headlines now, but the Book of Daniel reveals a Bible food that reportedly has the same effect. In addition, 16 oz. of this Bible food contain enough of the chemical used to treat Parkinson's disease to be therapeutically active in early cases. (For more details, see page 258.)

Here are more fascinating examples—

+ A plant that gave shelter to the Virgin Mary in the flight to Egypt contains six chemical compounds known to fight cataracts, that can help protect your vision as you grow older. (See page 15.)

+ This same Bible healing plant has a long history as a memory enhancer and contains a half dozen chemical compounds that fight Alzheimer's disease in the same way that certain drugs do. (See page 16.)

+ So powerful is this Bible healing plant that merely soaking it in wine and then applying it to the legs is said to have cured the Queen of Hungary of rheumatism and gout, at age 72. (See page 15)

+ The plant chosen by Jesus as His symbol of salvation—which He carried when He entered Jerusalem—contains a substance that seems to prevent bone loss in menopausal women . . . it literally holds your bones together. (See page 47.)

+ One of the bitter herbs of the Last Supper contains an oil that can relieve a terrible headache in minutes—*merely by wiping it across your forehead!* (See page 12.)

+ A miracle berry from the Crown of Thorns is said to be the finest heart tonic ever discovered, able to relieve both high and low blood pressure; rapid, feeble, or irregular heartbeat; cardiac edema; labored breathing; and insomnia. Experts have said it improves circulation, opens clogged arteries, and strengthens the heart muscle. Sufferers barely able to shuffle a few feet were transformed from hopeless invalids to hearty men and women with this Bible healing food. (See page 95.)

+ One of these Bible healing plants—said to have cured arthritis, stomach ulcers, diabetes, high blood pressure, tooth and gum decay, and more—is one of the plants used to preserve the body of Jesus. It is now being tested for its ability to relieve AIDS symptoms. ("Symptoms disappear almost completely," says one doctor, although no cure can be confirmed.) (See page 107.)

+ An overactive thyroid—known as Grave's disease—may be helped with a Bible healing food said to suppress the thyroid hormone. (See page 17.)

+ An underactive thyroid—known as hypothyroidism—may be helped by a miracle food from the Last Supper, said to increase the thyroid hormone (thyroxin) by as much as 100 percent. (See page 42.)

+ This Bible food—often found in candy bars and ice cream—contains a pain-relieving substance similar to powerful drugs, without the side effects, for ailments such as arthritis, rheumatism, and heart disease. It is also a powerful sedative that can give you a good night's sleep. (See page 14.)

+ This same healing food from the Bible is one of the few effective treatments for curing herpes, eczema, skin ulcers, acne, psoriasis, ringworm, warts, and age spots. Skin blemishes seem to disappear as if by magic, claims one expert. It also destroys yeast infections, such as Candida, better than a commonly prescribed antifungal drug, according to another expert. (See page 43.)

+ The Seven-Candle Plant—a Bible plant with seven branches symbolizing the seven days of creation—is saving lives in China, where it is used to restore circulation in cases of heart blockage and heart pains. (See page 292.)

+ The Seven-Candle Plant was said to relieve shaking palsy as far back as the eighteenth century, has recently been found to help prevent and treat Alzheimer's, and has a long-standing reputation for darkening gray hair and growing new hair. (See page 294.)

+ While doctors search for a cure for arthritis—a Bible food blessed by Jesus is wiping out pain, stiffness, and swelling in hundreds of cases. X-rays show fused joints unlocking, compressed vertebrae regenerating, and normal movement restored in almost all cases, starting in 3 to 10 days, according to one doctor. (See page 171.)

+ Is there a Bible food so powerful that it can protect you from bubonic plague? So powerful that scientists are testing it against AIDS? So powerful that even a milder version of this plant could heal a short, withered, paralyzed arm? Incredibly, there *is,* and you'll find it—not in your medicine chest—but in your vegetable garden. (See page 309.)

+ During a gallstone attack, if I didn't have access to a doctor, I'd drink some strong tea made from one of the miracle herbs of the Last Supper. This Bible healing plant may actually dissolve gallstones safely and nonsurgically, say researchers. (See page 25.)

+ Another miracle healing food from the Bible whose name in Hebrew means "a gift from God" is said to be the only successful medicine for eliminating wrinkles, outside of plastic surgery. It was used by a great French beauty who, at 90, was still so attractive that young men fell hopelessly in love with her. Her face was as smooth and free of wrinkles as it had been when she was 20. (See page 248.)

+ A Bible healing food blessed by Jesus has been found to double the life expectancies of people who were HIV positive. This food is packed with a substance that seems to ward off postmenopausal breast cancer in women over 50. (See pages 138, 139.)

+ This same Bible food seems to ward off asthma, bronchitis, emphysema, type II diabetes, glaucoma, lupus, eczema, psoriasis, multiple-sclerosis symptoms, heart attack, blood clots, stroke, high blood pressure, ulcerative colitis, colon polyps, Crohn's disease, and Raynaud's disease. (See pages 135, 288.)

+ This miracle food—available at every supermarket—contains a substance that seemed to help 50 cystic fibrosis patients, aged

3 months to 37 years (bowels normalized, lung mucus reduced, increased energy, weight gain, increased resistance to infections). (See page 155.)

+ A patient with late-stage muscular dystrophy, told nothing could be done for him, tried this Bible food and other foods containing this substance. His triglyceride, cholesterol, and CPK scores improved dramatically. (See page 156.)

+ Scientists have found substances in a grain blessed by Jesus that suppress the liver's ability to make bad (LDL) cholesterol. *This is the very idea behind a popular pill called Mevacor.* (See page 132.)

+ This same Bible food was part of a gallstone remedy that the Jews of antiquity called "spear water" because it "spears" or breaks up gall and can be made merely by boiling the grain in water and drinking it. (See page 127.)

+ One of these Bible plants has been used to successfully treat benign prostate enlargement. Its action is similar to a popular prescription drug, Proscar. (See page 371.)

+ This plant has been hailed as a goiter cure, an amazing weight reducer, and is famous for relieving arthritis, rheumatism, gout, sciatica, and hay fever. (See page 363.)

+ On the Mount from which Jesus is said to have ascended to heaven grows the very plant that many scientists believe is responsible for the incredibly long lifespans of the Jews of antiquity—the Methuselah plant that one man, in failing health at 65, used to become hale and hearty again, able to do somersaults at 100, ride a bicycle at 108, dance all evening with a teenaged girl at 110, ultimately living to the same age as Moses, in a life spanning three centuries. (See page 227.)

One of the biggest news stories in recent years was that scientists have discovered drugs that dry up the blood supply around a tumor, thereby starving it down to the size of a pinhead in lab animals. Human tests are about to begin. But 2,000 years ago, Jesus blessed a certain type of food said to work the same way. No one really knows if this can work—or how the food would compare to the drugs being tested—but the basic idea is very similar. (See page 164 for details.)

Here Are Fully Documented Facts . . .

Startling evidence pro and con—some of it overwhelmingly convincing—is presented. As in most health-related matters, use of ordinary non-prescription foods as medicine is controversial. Some doctors praise them to the sky, use them themselves, and recommend them to all their friends. They are considered minority unorthodox practitioners. Most violently disagree and say that such things are totally worthless, or should not be used by lay practitioners.

. . . And a Word of Advice!

This book is not a substitute for the clear identification, diagnosis, and treatment of your problem that only a licensed medical doctor can give you. He can also tell if you're allergic to any specific food mentioned, or if it would interfere or interact in some harmful way with some medication or treatment you may already be taking—which are obviously things this book can't do. And *cures* is used only in the sense of folk remedies or treatments. But each and every Bible healing food revealed here does have a long history of reputed healings—in many cases, so-called miracle healings—behind it. And since they are foods, rather than prescription drugs, all available for purchase in the United States, Canada, South America, Europe, and throughout the world, they may be regarded as harmless supplements to existing therapy, if your doctor approves. Unless your doctor gives his approval, they should never be used as the sole means of treating your condition.

". . . And the Years of Your Life Shall Be Multiplied"

"Take my words to heart, and the years of your life shall be multiplied," says Proverbs 4:10. Disobey and suffer illness, it seems to say. In these pages, you'll see how Miracle Food Cures from the Bible have saved countless lives down through the ages.

CHAPTER 2
CURATIVE PLANT OILS THAT POWERED THE BURNING BUSH

And the angel of the Lord appeared unto him in a flame of fire
out of the midst of a bush: and he looked, and behold, the bush
burned with fire, and the bush was not consumed. And Moses
said, I will now turn aside, and see this great sight, why the
bush is not burnt. And . . . God called unto him out of the
midst of the bush. *Exodus 3:2–4*

The phenomenon of the bush that "burned with fire" yet "was not
consumed" was, in all likelihood, white dittany (*Dictamnus albus*)—
a plant covered with thousands of oil glands, the oil of which is so
volatile that it escapes continually into the atmosphere, giving off a
lemon-peel odor.

During hot, dry, or cloudy weather, this vapor is so inflammable that the slightest spark, as from a candle or a bolt of lightning,
will cause the air around the plant to burst into flames without
destroying the plant itself!

Scientists say it could not have burned long enough for the
incidents in the Bible to have taken place, that Moses probably mis-
took bright blossoming mistletoe for fire. But Moses was well edu-
cated and knew this countryside well. To me, the power of God
could well have caused the bush to continue burning.

Oils from the Burning Bush that Heal

Think of white dittany—the burning bush—as the first of the aromatic plant medicines, whose essential oils are used to ward off disease.

In natural form, as part of a plant itself, essential oils can help relieve pain, swelling, stiffness, seizures, fever, and many other symptoms safely when the plant is consumed as a kind of tea.

But in bottled form, as a bath oil, body rub, or inhalant, essential oils should be used only externally. As sold in pure concentrated bottled form they are poisonous.

The roots of white dittany, when powdered and steeped in boiling water, have been used medicinally for:

+ tuberculosis
+ nerve disorders
+ epilepsy
+ intermittent fevers
+ spongy gums
+ loose teeth
+ stomach and digestive disorders

According to famed herbalist Maude Grieve, the powdered form, combined with that of peppermint, has been used in cases of epilepsy: "Dosage: of the powdered root, 4 to 8 grams [1/4 to 1/2 ounce] as an infusion." (Unlike tea, an infusion is steeped in hot water for 10–15 minutes, then strained and sweetened.)

Dittany strongly stimulates the muscles of the uterus, inducing menstruation. A pregnant woman should not use it, since this can cause miscarriage.

More Powerful Plant Oils that Can Be Used Medicinally

The same type of oils that powered the burning bush are present in many other plants and have strong medicinal powers.

Some are even volatile (inflammable) like the burning bush, but on a smaller scale. You can easily see this for yourself. For example, get a candle and some fresh orange peel. Light the candle and squeeze the peel between your fingers so the oil is released in a fine spray toward the flame. Watch the fireworks.

Essential or volatile oils provide the rich smells of plants. When a plant is squeezed, its aroma or essence easily escapes into the atmosphere. When plant oils are rubbed onto the skin, they are quickly absorbed by the bloodstream and carried to all parts of the body.

Medicated Air

For example, white dittany—the burning bush—has long had a medical reputation similar to peppermint, spearmint, and other members of the mint family. Mints are common in Palestine. In fact, it is believed that mint was one of the bitter herbs of the Last Supper.

The Jews of antiquity strewed synagogue floors with mint leaves so that their fragrance scented the air with each footstep. The aromatic fumes that issued forth were supposed to have a sort of sanitary effect upon the crowded temple gatherings by penetrating to the lungs and thence the bloodstream, like an airborne antiseptic to ward off disease.

The inhalation of mint and other aromatic plants such as frankincense and myrrh helped to preserve the health of the Jews in thickly populated camps during their Exodus from Egypt. The holy incense, which was kept burning morning and evening upon the altar of the Sanctuary, also acted as a deodorant and fumigator to purify the air and so act as a disinfectant in contagious epidemics.

"... And the Plague Was Stayed"

Acron of Agrigentum was said to have conquered the plague in Athens in 430 B.C. by causing fires to be made and aromatics thrown into them to purify the air. Yet, almost a thousand years before him, according to Numbers 17:11–13:

Moses ordered Aaron to take his censer, put fire thereon and pour in the holy incense, and to go quickly among the people . . . And he stood between the dead and living, and the plague was stayed.

This was altogether in keeping with the Mosaic Laws—the first, and surprisingly modern system of public sanitation ever recorded—dictated to Moses by God, and if not by God then certainly by some extraordinary being with knowledge far beyond what Moses or anyone else at that time, *without microscopes or any knowledge of germs,* possessed.

The Secret Healing Power of Mint Leaves

Plants of the mint family owe their healing power to their aromatic oils. To take one of the best known mints as an example, peppermint oil is mostly *menthol.* The writers of the Bible were definitely on the right track, because peppermint oil, like most mint oils, is actively germicidal.

Peppermint oil, in the test tube, kills:

+ Influenza A viruses, the cause of much Asian flu
+ Herpes simplex, the source of cold sores and genital herpes
+ Mumps virus
+ Streptococcus aureus, from which we acquire pneumonia, sinusitis, impetigo, and endocarditis
+ Pseudomonas acruginosa, which produces a great variety of infections with running pus
+ Candida albicans, the cause of vaginal yeast infection

. . . altogether more than 30 dangerous microorganisms stopped dead in their tracks by peppermint.

The major ingredient of peppermint is menthol (50–78 percent), a powerful anesthetic when applied to wounds, burns, scalds, stings, and toothache. Its vapors can relieve asthma, hay fever, colds, cough, flu, nasal, sinus and chest congestion. It's an ingredient in Mentholatum, Vicks VapoRub, Solarcaine, Unguentine, Ben-Gay, and Noxema.

Relieves Spasms

Well-known to herbalists everywhere is the ability of peppermint to calm upset stomach and soothe the gastrointestinal tract.

Peppermint relieves cramps and spasms just as effectively as many anti-spasmodic drugs, such as Bentyl, Librax, and Donnatal.

Peppermint has been found to relax the lower esophageal sphincter muscle so that trapped gas—the culprit in many a case of painful indigestion—is able to escape more easily.

Digestive Aid—Because it soothes digestion, relieves gas, nausea, and colic, peppermint is an ingredient in Tums, Gelusil, BiSoDol, and Phillips' Milk of Magnesia. German and Russian studies show that it may also help to prevent stomach ulcers and that it stimulates the flow of bile to the stomach, which promotes digestion. It can also reduce hunger pangs.

A California woman says a quarter cup of lukewarm peppermint tea is usually enough to quell the crankiness in the most colicky kid. "It really calms them down," she says. "Within 20 minutes, they're asleep."

To soothe your stomach, try peppermint tea, which is widely available in powdered form (1–2 teaspoonfuls in a cup of boiling water, steeped for 10 minutes, and strained), or use peppermint tea bags and sweeten to taste. Drink it up to three times a day. Or try peppermint candy. Some experts say peppermint should not be given to infants and young children because they gag on the menthol in it. If so, try something else. Stay away from peppermint if you have a tendency toward heartburn, for reasons explained below.

Irritable Bowel Syndrome—Peppermint oil can relieve irritable bowel syndrome. The oil is given in capsules or enteric-coated pills to prevent it from being released in the stomach. Instead, the oil travels to the small and large intestines where it relaxes intestinal muscles, thereby relieving symptoms. Two drops of peppermint oil are placed in an empty coated gelatin capsule. One capsule is swallowed with a glass of water 10 minutes before meals, three times a day. Or you can also buy such capsules ready-made at most health-food stores. One typical brand is Peppermint Plus, made by Enzymatic Therapy.

In the stomach, peppermint can cause heartburn by relaxing the sphincter muscle that separates the stomach from the esophagus, allowing an upsurge (reflux) of acid from the stomach into the esophagus, which is why the capsules are coated to prevent them from melting in the stomach.

Gallstones—Peppermint may actually dissolve gallstones. Its essential oils stimulate contractions of the gallbladder and encourage secretion of bile. Mints have traditionally been used to treat gallstones. A British over-the-counter "gallstone" tea, called Rowachol, contains peppermint oil and several other mint oils.

During a gallbladder attack, if I didn't have access to a doctor, I'd drink some strong peppermint tea for its medicinal effect in relieving gallstone colic. I no longer have gallstones, but for many years I did, and this tea never failed to bring relief.

Menthol has been shown to help dissolve gallstones safely over a period of time (up to 4 years). It does this by reducing bile cholesterol levels while increasing bile acids in the gallbladder. Since peppermint is mostly menthol, its oil may have the same effect. See "Irritable Bowel Syndrome" for suggested dosage.

Arthritis—The menthol in peppermint leaves can be used as a counterirritant in the treatment of arthritis, fibromyositis, tendonitis, and other inflammatory conditions. Bruised fresh peppermint leaf will relieve pains if applied to the skin locally. For neuralgia, rheumatism and lumbago, simply paint the skin over the affected area with peppermint oil. Discontinue if a rash develops.

Miracle Headache Relief—Peppermint oil is a miracle cure for headaches—fast-acting and safer than aspirin or even 1,000 mg. of Extra Strength Tylenol—*and all you do is rub it on your forehead.* Used this way, it has no side effects, whereas aspirin has been linked to stomach ulcers and tinnitus (ringing in the ears), and Tylenol to severe kidney and liver damage.

In tests in Germany on 41 patients ages 18–65, who suffered up to 22 tension headache attacks per month, a little peppermint oil spread across their foreheads brought relief in 15 minutes to most sufferers, regardless of age or sex, with no side effects.

For ordinary headaches, the oil is simply spread lightly across the forehead from temple to temple, or on the neck for pain at the back of the head, using your fingertips or a cotton swab. If any gets in your eye, rinse it out with water; it may burn but is not harmful. Bruised fresh peppermint leaf will also relieve headache if applied to the forehead or temples. Only a doctor can determine whether a headache is simple, or of a more serious nature requiring other treatment.

Toothache Relief—The local anesthetic action of peppermint oil is exceptionally strong. It is also powerfully antiseptic, the two properties making it valuable in the relief of toothache and in the treatment of cavities in the teeth. For emergency relief, until you can get to a dentist, you can apply a few drops of peppermint oil to the sore tooth or gum. Clove oil gives similar relief.

A very useful and harmless preparation for children during teething is prepared as follows: 1/2 ounce peppermint herb, 1/2 ounce skullcap herb, 1/2 ounce pennyroyal herb. Pour on 1 pint of boiling water, cover and let stand in a warm place 30 minutes. Strain and sweeten to taste and give frequently in teaspoonful doses, warm.

Mental Alertness, Senility—Peppermint can increase mental alertness, powers of recall and concentration by improving blood circulation to the brain. It strengthens and calms the nerves as well. This is due to the presence of several essential oils in peppermint that prevent blood congestion in the brain. When university students were given peppermint tea, their test-taking skills and examination scores all improved.

Sudden Pains and Cramp in Abdomen—Maude Grieve says: "Boiled in milk and drunk hot, peppermint herb is good for abdominal pains." The essential oil that the herb contains is antispasmodic. That means it soothes abdominal muscles and reduces muscular contractions, thereby relieving spasms, sudden pains, and cramps in the abdomen. (Author's note: Ingestion of pure peppermint oil is dangerous without a doctor's supervision. Peppermint tea, which is widely available in supermarkets and health-food stores, is safer and preferable.)

Women's Problems—Peppermint, like most mints, promotes menstruation by stimulating uterine contractions. It is also said to relieve morning sickness. Pregnant women who want to try it should use it in weak tea solutions rather than stronger, more medicinal concentrations, which can cause miscarriage.

Nausea and Sea Sickness—"Peppermint oil allays sickness and nausea," says Mrs. Grieve. "On account of its anesthetic effect on the nerve endings of the stomach, it is of use to prevent sea-sickness."

If you get carsick or airsick, or simply feel queasy after a meal, put a few drops of tincture of peppermint under your tongue. It will calm your stomach in minutes.

Or try peppermint tea or peppermint candies. They work well, too. Avoid peppermint if you have a tendency to heartburn.

Insomnia Relief—The following simple preparation has been found useful in insomnia: 1 ounce peppermint herb, cut fine, 1/2 ounce rue herb, 1/2 ounce wood betony. Mix well and place a large tablespoonful in a teacup, fill with boiling water, stir, and cover for 20 minutes, strain and sweeten, and drink the warm infusion at bedtime.

Shingles, Cold Sores, Burns, Wounds—Oil of peppermint, which should never be taken internally, has been applied to the skin to relieve the pain of shingles and is often included in analgesic massage oils and liniments. To relieve pain, apply a few drops of peppermint oil directly to the affected area. Discontinue if a rash develops.

Colds, Flu, and Sinusitis—For respiratory problems and general infections, inhalations are a way of introducing the essential oil into the bloodstream to help destroy invading bacteria. Inhaling the medicinal vapors also helps fight viruses and bacteria in the nose, throat, and respiratory system. (Peppermint oil is for external use only; do not ingest it.)

You can make your own inhalant by placing two or three drops of peppermint oil in a bowl of hot water and then inhaling the vapors. At the onset of a cold, free use of peppermint tea will, in many cases, cure it, says one expert. The menthol in the tea acts as a nasal and bronchial decongestant as well.

Bronchitis and Emphysema—Peppermint contains nine expectorant compounds to thin mucus and help propel it out of the lungs. Also, its main component—menthol—has mucus-thinning abilities, which makes it useful for bronchitis, in which the tiny hairs (cilia) that line the respiratory tract lose their ability to sweep out mucus; this condition usually goes hand in hand with emphysema, in which the tiny air sacs in the lungs turn leathery and lose their ability to transfer oxygen into, and carbon dioxide out of, the bloodstream.

More Mint Surprises

Some unsung heroes of the mint family, with miracle healing power, include rosemary and lemon balm. Lemon balm is associated with long life and a clear mind. Englishman John Hussey, who lived to age 116, drank balm tea every morning for 50 years, as did Llewelyn, Prince of Glamorgan, who lived to 108.

Rosemary, another mint, is revered in Spain as one of the bushes that gave shelter to the Virgin Mary in the flight into Egypt. (They call it *Romero,* the Pilgrim's Flower.) In 1235, Queen Elizabeth of Hungary fell in love with it when she was 72, crippled with rheumatism and gout. Rosemary, soaked in wine for 4 days and applied to her legs, cured her, gave her back her youth to such an extent that the King of Poland asked her to marry him.

There are some 60 varieties of mint—all very similar to peppermint—that are useful in ailments ranging from arthritis, asthma, and emphysema, to baldness, depression, and wrinkles, from cataract, glaucoma, and hypertension, to HIV and more. For example:

+ *Can This Simple Tea Prevent Cataracts?* Rosemary contains six chemical compounds known to fight cataracts, that can help protect your vision as you grow older. Patients with cerebral arteriosclerosis respond surprisingly well to rosemary. To make a tea for these purposes, add 1/2 ounce of rosemary to a pint of boiled water and steep for 10 minutes in a covered vessel. Strain and sweeten to taste. This will also relieve headaches as well as aspirin.

+ *For Heart Palpitations*   Rosemary wine is said to quiet palpitations of the heart, and relieve swelling or edema of the limbs. It is made by chopping up sprigs of green rosemary and pouring white wine on them. This is allowed to steep for 3–4 days; then the wine is strained and ready to use, one small glass between meals.

+ *To Stimulate Hair Growth*   Rosemary is employed externally for its effect in stimulating the hair bulbs to renewed activity to prevent baldness. Use strong cooled rosemary tea for this purpose (see instructions above for making it) as a rinse after shampoo.

+ *For Renewed Energy*   For renewed energy, and to get rid of that "tired" feeling, put a good handful of rosemary petals and leaves into 1-3/4 pints of boiled water. Allow to steep for 10 minutes in a covered vessel. Then stir into bath water. Rosemary baths are so energizing they should never be taken at night, as they may prevent sleep.

+ *A Memory-Enhancing Herb Fights Alzheimers*   Rosemary has a long history as a memory-enhancing herb. It contains compounds that prevent the loss of a chemical (acetylcholine) vital to thinking and reasoning. People with Alzheimers are often low on this chemical. An old herbal states:

As one of the herbs of old age with failing memory and stiff joints, Rosemary brings added mobility and lively intellect. Grecians drank it to clear the head and to facilitate mental labor. An infusion delighteth the head and is wonderfully refreshing to tired businessmen and students. It is a natural antidote to mental fatigue and it also strengthens sight. It is known to restore speech after a stroke.

When asked how she managed to retain such a keen, alert memory at 88 years of age, Mrs. D. B. replied: "I don't know what all the fuss is about—so many people asking about my memory. In the little village where I grew up, everyone young and old drank rosemary tea every day. Why, I thought folks everywhere in the world knew that rosemary was good for the memory." With that she pointed toward a row of bushes in her yard. "That's all rosemary," she said. "I planted that myself years ago when I moved here. I wouldn't dream of being without my rosemary tea!"[1]

Grave's Disease (Overactive Thyroid) Symptoms of an overactive thyroid, known as hyperthyroidism or Grave's disease—such as a lump in the front of the throat, bulging eyes, rapid pulse, profuse sweating, fatigue, unwanted weight loss, restlessness, irritability, fine-muscle tremors—should be brought to a doctor's attention and never self-treated. Information about herbs that may help in this condition should be discussed with your doctor and used only with his permission. Doctors treat an overactive thyroid by trying to suppress thyroid-hormone production, with drugs or by using nuclear medicine to destroy part of the gland.

Herbs that do the same thing—suppress an overactive thyroid—include two mints: bugleweed and motherwort, and another Bible plant (see page 265), common cabbage!

Bugleweed and motherwort contain substances that inhibit or altogether block thyroid hormone production. Their actions are less powerful than those of synthetic drugs, but they are usually quite adequate in less severe cases, according to Fritz Weiss, M.D. The advantage, he says, is that like many herbal drugs they are safe and therefore suitable for long-term treatment.

Very small quantities are all that are required. Leaf extracts have proved to be much more active than root extracts, says Weiss.

To prepare bugleweed, says herbalist Maude Grieve, an infusion (see page 0) is made from 1 ounce of the dried herb to 1 pint of boiling water, taken in wineglassful doses, once or twice a day.

You will not notice any effect for at least a couple of weeks. It takes 3 or 4 weeks to kick in. At that point, symptoms of an over-

---

[1]From *The Magic of Herbs in Daily Living* by Richard Lucas, West Nyack, NY: Parker Publishing Company, Inc., 1972.

active thyroid should subside. It has been confirmed in tests on humans that bugleweed extracts inhibit iodine metabolism and thyroxine release in the thyroid.

Motherwort, says Dr. Weiss, is best prescribed as a tea made from the herb, 2 teaspoons to a cup of boiling water, one cup to be taken morning and night. It is used for relief of palpitation and tachycardia, symptoms frequently complained of by patients with hyperthyroidism.

Interestingly, the idea of using plants to suppress thyroid hormones began with ordinary white cabbage. Doctors noticed that people who ate large amounts of cabbage, notably in wartime, developed goiters, due to a decrease in iodine levels in the thyroid.

All members of the cabbage family gently suppress thyroid production. Cabbage's cousins include broccoli, brussels sprouts, cauliflower, kale, mustard greens, radishes, rutabagas, and turnips.

CHAPTER 3
MIRACLE FOOD CURES FROM THE LAST SUPPER

The Last Supper took place on the night before Jesus' death. It consisted of Passover and the Lord's Supper. Passover commemorates the passing over of Jewish homes by the Angel of Death sent by God to punish the Pharaoh for refusing to release them from bondage:

> For I will pass through the land of Egypt this night, and will
>
> smite all the firstborn in the land . . . take to them every man a
>
> lamb . . . kill it . . . take of the blood, and strike it on the [door
>
> posts] of the houses . . . and when I see the blood, I will pass
>
> over you, and the plague shall not be upon you . . . *Exodus*
>
> *23:2–13*

Jesus celebrated Passover on his last night on earth by partaking of lamb with bitter herbs, as instructed in the Old Testament . . .

> And they shall eat the flesh . . . roast with fire, and unleavened
>
> bread; and *with bitter herbs* shall they eat it. *Exodus 12:8*

. . . with 4 cups of wine during the meal, to commemorate the four promises of God ("I will bring you out"; "I will deliver you"; "I will redeem you"; "I will take you to me for a people"—Exodus 6:6), and an egg to symbolize rebirth and spring.

At the close of the Passover Supper, Jesus instituted the Lord's Supper, with Himself as the sacrificial lamb:

> And as they were eating, Jesus took bread, and blessed it, and brake it, and gave it to the disciples, and said, Take, eat; this is my body. And he took the cup, and gave thanks, and gave it to them, saying, Drink ye all of it; for this is my blood . . . which is shed for many . . . *Matthew 26:26–30*

Jesus expired on the Cross on the same day in which sacrificial lambs were being slain in the Temple for Passover.

What Strange Powers Do These Bitter Herbs Possess?

If you look at what was on the table during the Last Supper, you'll find some unusual plant medicines. You'll discover the Sacred Medicinal Drink, part of . . .

A special medicine revealed by angels—a mixture of four Bible foods said to make all heart pain disappear. "All my complaints have vanished," says a heart patient on page 211. You'll discover how an oil from one of the miracle plants of the Last Supper can relieve a terrible headache in minutes, merely by wiping it across your forehead (page 12) . . .

. . . how it wipes out the germs that cause influenza, herpes, mumps, pneumonia, and more. The bitter herbs of the Last Supper, God's legacy to the world, all possess special and specific medicinal powers . . .

+ Did you know, for example, that one of the herbs served at the Last Supper is a safe, legal garden vegetable with opiate-like power to relieve pain similar to codeine and morphine, but non-habit forming? (See page 22.)

+ That another herb on that table is one of the finest diuretics known, able to drain pounds of excess fluid, and is used by drugless doctors to relieve swelling . . . cystitis . . . nephritis . . . and hepatitis? (See page 26.)

+ That this herb can be used as a simple remedy for varicose veins . . . breast pain (mastitis) . . . eye diseases . . . gallstones . . . kidney stones . . . and the rapid cure of even the most serious cases of hepatitis, according to one researcher! (See page 29.)

+ That an arthritic cripple went dancing after using this and another bitter herb from the Last Supper! (See page 28.)

+ That another bitter herb from the Last Supper is not only a remedy for stones and gravel, but acts like a male birth control pill? (See page 34.)

+ Did you know that another herb from the Last Supper is a remedy for sexually transmitted diseases, tuberculosis, shingles, and gingivitis, and is one of three Bible foods that kept a hopeless diabetic alive for 30 years after he'd been sent home to die? (See page 35.)

+ That another herb on that table is said in many cases to make menopausal joint pain disappear? An elderly man who could barely hobble around on two canes used this herb and was able to throw his canes away. It helps prevent hernias . . . relieve prostate pressure . . . and can bring instant allergy relief. (See page 52.)

+ That a vegetable that Jesus ate at the Last Supper contains natural calcium blockers that help prevent and treat irregular heartbeat, lower blood pressure and cholesterol? (See page 59.)

+ That this vegetable is a natural alternative to prescription drugs for gout, also said to prevent bursitis, rheumatism, facial neuralgia, and cataracts?

+ Did you know that another herb from the Last Supper is part of a famous, though unproven, anticancer treatment—a simple herbal tea—claimed by many to relieve pain, restore strength, and to have saved their lives when all else failed. Most medical authorities warn that it is not a cure, and should never be used as the sole means of treating this disease. Three of the four herbs in this tea are from the Bible. (See Chapter 5.)

What were the bitter herbs of the Last Supper? Today these forgotten herbs—there were 7—are sometimes symbolized by a single food at Passover: horseradish. In Jesus' time, the original bitter herbs were used. Here they are, and the astonishing discoveries that have been made about them:

Lettuce Opium:
A Safe Non-prescription Pain Reliever

Lettuce tea has long been known as a soother of pain and a sleep inducer when opium was not available. Its opiate-like action is due to a bitter white juice, which exudes from the plant when it is wounded. This juice, when dried, is called lettuce-opium, *lactucarium,* and gives off a characteristic opium-like odor.

Lettuce opium is like a mild dose of opium—without opium's tendency to upset the digestive system. Pharmacological studies have shown this substance to have sedative and cough suppressant properties similar to morphine and codeine but much weaker, without any risk of addiction.

All lettuces possess some of this narcotic juice, wild lettuce having the most, followed by prickly lettuce, and garden lettuce. The narcotic is obtained by wounding the plant in its flowering season, when the stem and stalks are so full of juice that they often rupture from the slightest touch or injury. A cut is made, allowing the juice to exude. This is collected on small pieces of cotton which are thrown into a vessel full of water, in which the lettuce opium dissolves. The water is then boiled off, leaving a brownish gumlike resin. An easier way to collect it is to steep or soak the newly mature stems and leaves for 24 hours (this is called a maceration). The water is then boiled for 3 hours and allowed to evaporate in a shallow bowl, leaving a medicinal gumlike residue.

Dissolved in wine, it is said to soothe, calm, comfort, and relieve pain. In France, water distilled from lettuce is used as a mild sedative in doses of 2–4 ounces, and the fresh leaves boiled in water are sometimes used as a poultice. An old-fashioned remedy for sleeplessness is lettuce tea. Two or three of the outer leaves, which contain 30 percent more nutrients than the inner leaves, are washed thoroughly, then simmered for 20 minutes in one-half pint of water. This is strained and drunk hot just before bedtime.

The simplest way to obtain lettuce's opiate-like action for those troubled with insomnia is to eat some lettuce last thing at night, just before bed. It helped soldiers in battle to sleep better. There's no better recommendation than that.

Reported uses:

People use an infusion of lettuce for gastric spasms, fevers, and insomnia, and they apply the sap to rashes, warts, and acne. An infusion is like tea but somewhat stronger. A pint of boiling water is poured over the plant, the container is covered, and the solution is allowed to stand for 15 minutes before drinking. It is then strained and sweetened to taste.

English herbalist Nicholas Culpepper (1616–1654), whose books and pamphlets on herbal remedies were condemned by the medical profession but enjoyed huge sales among the common people, suffered recurring headaches and insomnia after being wounded in battle. His wounds healed, but the headaches continued. After trying various plant remedies, he took some common garden lettuce, pounded the juice out of the leaves, mixed it with the juice of rose petal leaves, and rubbed this on his forehead and temples. To his astonishment, his headaches quickly vanished, and he was able to sleep comfortably once more.

Some years ago, a correspondent to the London *Times* wrote that her great-great-grandfather, Dr. James Murdoch, was a medical officer at the penal colony in Van Dieman's Land for 26 years, until it closed in 1849. According to his memoir, when supplies of opium were not available, he "sent to the garden for some lettuces, crushed them with a pestle, and extracted an opiate from them."

During World War II, when codeine was in short supply, doctors turned to the bitter juice in lettuce—called lettuce opium—for its sedative and cough suppressant properties similar to codeine and morphine, only milder. Extracts of lettuce juice were given to soldiers who had respiratory problems, or were in need of sleep and pain relief, and it worked quite well.

In one study, 23 out of 24 cases of edema (fluid retention) were cured by taking doses of 18 grains (3/10 of a teaspoon) to 3 drachms (3 teaspoonfuls) of wild lettuce extract in 24 hours.

Several vegetables and fruits have been found quite consistently associated with lower risk of stomach cancer, fruit and *lettuce in particular.*

"Even the Most Serious Cases . . . Have Been Rapidly Cured" with This Bible Food

The next bitter herb of the Last Supper is dandelion. The main benefits of this great herb are its healing effects on the liver and gallbladder. It clears obstructions and helps the liver get rid of toxins from the blood. This is primarily due to a bitter substance it contains called taraxacin. "Even the most serious cases of hepatitis have rapidly been cured, sometimes within a week," says Dr. Tierra, "with dandelion root tea taken in cupful doses four to six times daily and a light, easily digested diet of vegetable broths, and rice and mung bean porridge."[1]

In one study, dandelion extract was used to successfully treat hepatitis, swelling of the liver, jaundice, and dyspepsia with deficient bile secretion. In another study, patients with severe liver imbalance and such symptoms as jaundice, low energy, and lack of appetite were treated with dandelion extract (one injection daily, 5 ml for 20 days). Nearly all of them showed a dramatic decrease in blood cholesterol.

---

[1]Reprinted with permission of Pocket Books, a Division of Simon & Schuster, from *The Way of Herbs* by Michael Tierra. Copyright © 1980, 1983, 1990 by Michael Tierra.

Reported cases:

Around the turn of the century, a doctor wrote: "Fifteen years ago I was afflicted with the liver complaint. I used all my skill trying to cure it, but failed." Then an old nurse told him that dandelion root was a good liver remedy. He tried it, "taking a teacupful of a strong decoction of it twice a day." He claimed: "In almost every instance I have succeeded in restoring those who have used this plant," including himself.

"While chatting with a retired doctor, I mentioned that my son had hepatitis and had been forced to take a leave of absence from college on account of it. He was about to miss a second semester. The doctor said that that dandelion tea was an old-time liver remedy that was very reliable. I relayed this information to my son, who began drinking several strong cups of it every day. In a little over a month, he was cured."—Mrs. S. W.

"A few years ago some friends of mine came down with hepatitis after eating clams during their vacation in New Orleans. The man's wife, a strong believer in herbal medicine, drank dandelion root tea 3–4 times a day for nearly a month and felt 100% recovered. Her husband, who had taken a prescription medicine, has never fully recovered."—Mrs. N. D.

An infusion of 1 teaspoon of the root to a cup of water may be prepared and taken freely, according to one expert. Or a decoction may be made by boiling the solution for 15 minutes. Several cupfuls of this stronger medicine may be taken each day, he says, and can be sweetened to taste with honey.

A Bible Food Remedy for Gallstone Distress

Dandelion tea is a good remedy for gallbladder complaints, says one medical doctor. Recent research shows that this is especially true for people with a tendency to form gallstones, he says, adding that it should be given over a period of 4 to 6 weeks in such cases. "Patients feel refreshed after the course of treatment, symptoms in the upper epigastrium disappear, and there are no further relapses, or at least far fewer ones," says this doctor.

Dandelion tea is completely harmless even if taken for extended periods, he says.

A tea is made from the dried chopped root or herb, 1–2 teaspoons to a cup of water, boiled briefly, and left to draw for 15 minutes. One cup of this is taken morning and evening for 4 to 6 weeks. Fresh dandelion juice is also available, and a tablespoonful of this is taken morning and evening in half a glass of water, according to this doctor.

"One of the Finest Diuretics Known . . . for Fluid Retention, Cystitis, Nephritis, Weight-Loss, Hepatitis"

Although dandelion's specific action is on the liver, it benefits the whole body. According to Dr. Tierra, "The root is also useful for clearing up obstructions of the spleen, pancreas, gallbladder, bladder, and kidneys. It is of tremendous benefit to the stomach and intestines. . . ."[2]

In ridding the body of excess fluid (edema): "Dandelion leaf tea is one of the finest diuretics known, at least equal to any known drug medicine," says Dr. Tierra. "Thus dandelion leaf tea can be taken for fluid retention, cystitis, nephritis, weight-loss and hepatitis. . . ."[3]

Dandelion root helps decrease high blood pressure, thus aiding the action of the heart. It can also be helpful in treating anemia by supplying necessary nutritive minerals.

---

[2]*The Way of Herbs* by Michael Tierra, *op. cit.*
[3]Tierra, *op. cit.*

A Bible Food for Low Blood Sugar, Recent-Onset Diabetes

"I consider dandelion root a specific for hypoglycemia," says Dr. Tierra, "but it may need to be combined with other tonic herbs such as ginseng and a little ginger for maximum benefit. A cup of dandelion-root tea is taken three times daily along with the recommended balanced diet. Similarly it can be used to remedy recent-onset diabetes, especially when combined with huckleberry leaf in tea."[4]

Bible Food Helps Kidney Stones Pass

Kidney stone pain is the most excruciating pain the body can suffer, with sudden grating pain in the back that won't go away. Fortunately, this condition resolves itself spontaneously in many cases. To ease the pain, some doctors recommend a really hot bath or hot compresses to the kidney region. This will sometimes prove sufficient. Often, powerful painkillers are needed. When the acute stage of pain has passed, sipping hot chamomile tea slowly, for its antispasmodic effect, can help.

When calm has been restored, large quantities of dandelion tea often cause a kidney stone to dissolve or pass. Herbalist Michael Moore recommends up to an ounce of the chopped root, boiled and drunk several times a day, for at least 10 days. Rudolph Fritz Weiss, M.D., recommends up to 10 cups of dandelion tea every morning upon arising, until the stone passes.

To make sure a stone has passed, urine must be voided into a container. There will be a definite click when it leaves the urethra and strikes the bottom of the vessel. The battle is then over and there will be no more pain.

---

[4]Tierra, *op. cit.*

Bible Foods that Fight Osteoporosis

Medical writer Carlson Wade once told me that dandelion shoots contain 130 parts per million of boron—running a close second to cabbage (see page 265) which contains 150. Boron, he pointed out, helps raise estrogen levels in the blood, and estrogen helps preserve bone, and prevents osteoporosis.

Dandelion, said Wade, is also a fair source of silicon, which some studies suggest also helps strengthen bone.

Arthritic Cripple Goes Dancing After Using 2 Bitter Herbs from Last Supper

Dandelion, says Dr. Weiss, is one of the best remedies to use in chronic rheumatic complaints. He regarded it as specific for chronic degenerative joint disease. He gave dandelion juice to his arthritic patients, and told them to take one-half cup of it morning and evening on an empty stomach. In more severe cases—where patients were crippled or bedridden, unable to move around—he'd prescribe a mixture of equal parts of dandelion and watercress, another bitter herb from the Last Supper (see page 38).

Reported case:

In one case, Mrs. F. M., age 61, had nodular rheumatism, with painful swelling in the joints of her hands and feet, mild fever, weight loss, and a constant feeling of illness, weakness, and tiredness. Her doctors had prescribed aspirin, salicylates, various NSAID drugs such as Motrin, Voltarin, and Naproxyn, finally gold injections, then steroids injected directly into the joints. Each of these brought side effects, such as gastric irritation, intestinal bleeding, ringing in the ears, liver and kidney dysfunction. Then she went to Dr. Weiss, who put her on a simple dandelion-watercress-juice program and a restricted diet. Within 2 weeks she was able to move her misshapen fingers and toes. Within a month, her pain and joint swelling were almost gone and she was able to hold a pencil and grasp kitchen utensils. In 2 months she was walking up to a mile a day and climbing stairs, and when last heard from was able to go dancing with her husband.

Dr. Weiss regarded dandelion as God's special gift for relief of liver and kidney problems, Bright's disease, gallstones and kidney stones, arteriosclerosis, obesity, and high blood pressure—and had many success stories to prove it.

Bible-Food Remedy for Varicose Veins

A woman with varicose-vein problems was told about an herbal tea that could heal them, made with dandelion, marjoram, and oregano, as follows:

1 quart water
2 tablespoons dandelion root
1 teaspoon each marjoram and oregano

Allow the dandelion root to simmer in a covered pot for 10 minutes. Add spices, stir, cover again, and simmer another 2–3 minutes. Then remove from heat and allow to sit another 20 minutes. Strain, sweeten to taste, and drink 1 cup three times daily, between meals.

"In a little over a month," she said, "all my varicose veins had faded away, and my legs looked and felt fresher and years younger."

A Bible Food for Night Blindness

Dandelion-juice extract was routinely prescribed for night blindness, with remarkable success, by a Dr. Niedermeier, as reported in *Deutsche medizinische Wochenschrift* (76:210, February 16, 1951). He attributed this success to a substance in dandelion called helenin, which produces visual purple for the eye in the presence of vitamins A and B, which dandelion also contains in abundance. It seemed to work as well for the night blindness that accompanies retinitis pigmentosa—a chronic inflammation of the retina at the back of the eye.

Incredible Energy Boost Linked to 2 Bitter Herbs from Last Supper

"Drinking one cup of dandelion juice by itself," says John Heinerman, "or in combination with an equal amount of watercress [also from the Last Supper], will give the body a 'natural high' or incredible sensation of energy when the juice hits the liver. In some cases, this may be somewhat overpowering for older people or those with delicate digestive tracts. In the event this proves to be so, simply dilute the dandelion juice with a little carrot juice."[5]

How This Bible Food Remedy Is Used to Heal Breast Pain, Eye Diseases and More in China

In China, dandelion has been used to treat breast problems (cancer, inflammation, lack of milk flow, and so forth). In his book *Chinese Herbal Cures,* Dr. Henry C. Lu tells the following story:

The 16-year-old daughter of a government official in ancient China was suffering from mastitis with a triangular lump underneath her left breast. She was in pain and became suicidal. She tried to drown herself, but was saved by a fisherman and his daughter. In changing the girl's clothes, the fisherman's daughter noticed the swelling in her left breast. She told her father, who said, "We will go dig some plants for her breast first thing in the morning." The plants turned out to be dandelions, found on a roadside not far from the river. They dug out a few plants totaling about one-quarter pound, washed them clean, and boiled them in water. They told the girl to drink the liquid. Meanwhile, they crushed some of the plants and applied them to her breast externally.

The girl returned home to her parents, bringing a bunch of dandelions with her, and continued using the plants as the fish-

---

[5]*Heinerman's Encyclopedia of Healing Juices,* 1994.

erman had instructed. After recovering from her illness, she had dandelions planted in her garden, and called them Fisherman's Herb—*pugongying*.[6]

According to Dr. Lu: "Asian dandelion is now being used to treat many inflammatory diseases, including mumps, tonsillitis, and mastitis. Although this herb tastes bitter, the Chinese in the rural areas are in the habit of making tea out of it and then drinking it as a remedy for eye diseases, redness in the eyes, nose diseases, and urination disturbances.

"The Chinese use Asian dandelion to treat such symptoms by decocting 50 g [about 2 ounces or 1/4 cup] dandelion in two glasses of water until the water is reduced by half, then they strain it and drink the liquid once daily. In the treatment of eye disorders, they also take a cotton ball soaked in the fluid and press it over the closed eyes for about a half hour daily. Unlike most Chinese herbs, when Asian dandelion is used to treat inflammatory diseases, both internal and external methods should be applied, whether in treating mastitis, tonsillitis, or mumps."[7]

How to Use This Bible Healing Food

All parts of the plant contain a somewhat bitter, milky juice, but the juice of the root, being the most potent, is the part of the plant most used for medicinal purposes.

+ To remove warts, an old folk remedy that seems to work for many people is to break off a dandelion stem and squeeze the milk out several times a day onto the wart. Within a week or so, the wart shrivels and disappears.

+ A broth of dandelion roots, sliced and stewed in boiling water with some leaves of sorrel and the yolk of an egg,

---

[6]From *Chinese Herbal Cures* by Henry C. Lu © 1991. Published by Sterling Publishing Co., Inc., NY. Reprinted with permission.

[7]Lu, *op. cit.*

taken daily for some months, has been known to cure seemingly intractable cases of chronic liver congestion.

✛ In cases of stone or gravel, a decoction is made by boiling a pint of the sliced root in 20 parts of water for 15 minutes, straining this when cold, and sweetening with brown sugar or honey. A small teacupful may be taken once or twice a day.

✛ When the stomach is irritated, a decoction or extract of dandelion administered three or four times a day will often prove a valuable remedy, increasing the appetite and improving digestion.

✛ Numerous clinical trials have demonstrated dandelion's effectiveness against pneumonia, bronchitis, and upper-respiratory infections, according to Albert Leung, Ph.D. My friend Carlson Wade suggested cooking the greens and roots, and then drinking the pot liquor, the juice that remains after the greens are cooked. Dandelion tea or dandelion capsules are also good, he said.

Young leaves of dandelion make delicious sandwiches, the tender leaves being laid between slices of bread and butter and sprinkled with salt. (Once the leaves are mature, they are too bitter to be eaten.) The young leaves may also be boiled as a vegetable, spinach fashion, thoroughly drained, sprinkled with pepper and salt, moistened with soup or butter, and served very hot. Some grated garlic or nutmeg, a teaspoonful of chopped onion, or grated lemon peel can be added to the greens when they are cooked. A simple vegetable soup may also be made with dandelions.

Dandelion beer and dandelion wine are common drinks in many parts of the United States and Canada. In England, dandelion stout is a favorite.

The roasted roots are used to make dandelion coffee. The prepared powder is said to be almost indistinguishable from real coffee. It is obtainable at most health-food stores and vegetarian restaurants. Dandelion coffee is a natural beverage without any of the injurious effects that ordinary coffee has on nerves and digestive organs.

It exercises a stimulating influence over the whole system, helping the liver and kidneys do their work and keeping the bowels in a healthy condition, without causing insomnia.

We are told by English medical herbalist T. H. Bartram that dandelion coffee not only prevents formation of gallstones, but "Hepatitis, or inflammation of the liver, and jaundice, when uncomplicated, readily yield to [it]."

Two Forgotten Plants of Noble History

Chicory and endive have fallen on hard times—the one a dusty roadside herb, the other, its only relative, a vagrant. But chicory and endive were among the seven bitter herbs of the Last Supper, invested with miracle healing power. Chicory appears in the oldest complete herbal we have, from the first century A.D., and both chicory and endive were respected by all the great sages of Western medicine. With good reason:

Chicory juice, says one expert, "is a folk remedy for tumors and cancers of the liver, stomach, and uterus. Powdered seed are applied for indurations of the spleen. The leaf, boiled with honey, is used as a gargle for cancer of the mouth. . . . The juice from its macerated leaves is sedative and soothing." It relieves edema (swelling from water retention) and has been used as a remedy for asthma, dysmenorrhea, dyspepsia, and as if that weren't enough, it was always regarded as an aphrodisiac, its seeds used in love potions.

The latex of endive—a milky substance in the plant—has been used for cancer of the uterus, tumors of the liver, spleen, and throat, and indurations [hardening] of the spleen. Endive is used to increase bile flow and with chicory is said to dissolve gall stones.

Woman, 86, Claims Osteoporosis Gone after Drinking Juice of Three Bible Plants

We are told of an 86-year-old woman who found that after drinking 1 cup of the combined juices of chicory, endive, and escarole (another of the bitter herbs eaten by the Jews just before their exodus from Egypt) once a day for 6 months, her osteoporosis had all but disappeared. Because of the bitter taste, she mixed in carrot juice or beet juice to sweeten it. She feels this has significantly strengthened her bones and says she would recommend it to any older person who is worried about falling and breaking brittle bones.[8]

A Bitter Herb Jesus Ate Strengthens Weak Heart, Slows Rapid Heartbeat

Egyptian researchers have discovered that chicory root has two heart benefits. It slows a rapid heartbeat (tachycardia), and it also has a mild heart-stimulating effect, somewhat like digitalis. My friend Carlson Wade recommended trying a cup or two of chicory coffee, which he himself drank as a protective liver tonic.

A Bible Food for Stones, Gravel, and Male Birth Control

Chicory coffee is reportedly excellent for cleansing the liver and spleen, as well as for treating jaundice. It is also protective. In one study, 70 percent of lab animals given chicory extracts survived a dose of acetaminophen high enough to be fatal, that killed 100 percent of untreated animals.

Tea made from chicory root and endive is said to be good for getting rid of gallstones. Add 3 tablespoons of chopped chicory root to a quart of boiling water, reduce heat, simmer for 20 minutes, remove from heat, add 1/2 cup of finely cut raw endive, cover and steep for 45 minutes. Drink 2–3 cups between meals, and again about 2 hours before bedtime.

A decoction of 1 ounce of chicory root to a pint of boiling water, taken freely, has been found effective in jaundice, liver enlargements, and gout and rheumatic complaints, and a decoction of the freshly gathered plant has been recommended for gravel.

---

[8]John Heinerman, *Heinerman's Encyclopedia of Healing Juices,* 1994.

Chicory-root coffee shows promise as a male birth control. Scientists in India gave boiled water extracts of dried powdered chicory to lab animals, while a control group received no chicory, only water. Those that had been drinking the chicory-root water showed high infertile sperm counts. One scientist states that drinking extra-strong chicory-root coffee, up to 6 cups per day, should make an average man's sperm infertile for about a week.

A Bible-Food Remedy for Sexually Transmitted Diseases and for Tuberculosis

Watercress—the fifth bitter herb of the Last Supper—has been used as a remedy for tuberculosis, still a major problem in many Third World countries and recently reemerging in the United States, and for various sexually transmitted diseases.

In one reported case,[9] a person suffering from chlamydia, an infectious sexually transmitted disease, symptoms of which are frequent pain and discomfort in the urinary and genital tracts and painful urination, was advised to drink a combination of watercress-turnip juice twice a day. The high sulfur content in the watercress helped kill the viruses causing the chlamydia, and the turnip juice made it more palatable to drink. In 7 weeks, the person using this remedy was reportedly cured.

In another case, a Vietnam War veteran was suffering from tuberculosis at a Veteran's Administration hospital. None of the usual drugs that doctors were giving him seemed to help much. The watercress-turnip juice combination was then given to him, with liquid Kyolic garlic mixed in, as well: two small glasses every day with meals. To his doctors' astonishment, the man experienced a remarkable improvement. Reportedly, it was the sulfur compounds in the watercress and Kyolic garlic that did the trick in this stubborn case of drug-resistant TB.[10]

---

[9]Heinerman, *op. cit.*
[10]Heinerman, *op. cit.*

In San Francisco, in the late 1800s, many Chinese railroad workers were dying from tuberculosis. Legend has it that they discovered on their own, through experimentation, that watercress helped treat tuberculosis. Some who recovered after eating it took the secret back to China, where they planted it and began using it medicinally.

A Bible-Food Remedy for Gingivitis

One of the ways the Chinese use watercress is to treat gingivitis. This is an inflammation of the gums, with swelling, redness, a watery discharge and bleeding. Left untreated, it progresses to pyorrhea, a degeneration of the gum tissue supporting the teeth. Together, these two conditions are known as periodontal disease. Most people have it, to some extent, as they grow older, because not even brushing and flossing can get rid of the bacteria that cause it, which are hidden in deep pockets between the teeth and gums. In southern China, people simply chew watercress to get rid of these symptoms.

A Bible-Food Remedy for Shingles

One prominent researcher suggests that taking two 500-milligram tablets of the amino acid lysine three or four times a day might help relieve the distressing and unsightly symptoms of shingles.

But watercress is one of several Bible healing foods that contain a high degree of lysine. Many types of beans (see Chapter 14) are also rich in lysine, namely black-bean sprouts, lentils, lentil sprouts, and fava beans; also parsley (see next chapter).

An All-Purpose Miracle Remedy from the Bible

"Watercress," says famed French herbalist Maurice Messegue, "has a purifying action. Take a glass of its juice in the morning, and the poisons will all vanish. . . . Its effectiveness in ridding the system of intestinal parasites is well known. I recommend it for chronic bronchitis . . . for diabetes because it lowers the blood sugar, for neuralgia, for toothache, and for loss of hair. In other words, it is in my opinion an herbal remedy of the utmost value. For external application I use it as I do cabbage, in poultices and in compresses for gout, rheumatism, and muscular pain. The juice of this plant applied to the skin is an excellent cure for dermatitis and acne." In small quantities, watercress is thought to act as an oral contraceptive that can produce temporary sterility.[11]

+ + +

The remaining two herbs of the Last Supper were mint, whose astonishing powers are revealed in Chapter 2, and sheep sorrel, whose secrets are revealed in Chapter 5.

"And They Shall Eat the Flesh . . . Roast with Fire . . ."
Exodus 12:8

In Exodus, God commands the Jews to eat a roasted or burnt shank of lamb. Today we know that meat should never be eaten raw or rare—it must be well done, roasted to rid it of harmful bacteria. Among the many harmful microorganisms to which the Jews were exposed were those that cause venereal disease—a major punishment resulting from the worship of Baal, a widespread practice, particularly among the Moabites and Midianites at the time of Moses (Numbers 22:41), which involved extremely licentious rites.

To Prevent and Heal Herpes

The Jews of antiquity knew nothing of viruses or bacteria, but they followed the Bible and the Mosaic laws which required them to eat certain foods rich in lysine, which halts the growth and spread of the herpes virus in the cells of the body. Lysine seems to wrap a protective coating around each cell, preventing the virus from getting in. Two Biblical foods high in lysine are milk and meat.

---

[11]From *Health Secrets of Plants and Herbs* by Maurice Messegue. Copyright © 1975 by Opera Mundi. Copyright © 1979 by William Collins & Co., Ltd. By permission of William Morrow & Company, Inc.

CHAPTER 4
THE HEALING POWERS OF *CHAROSET*

The rituals of The Lord's Supper were introduced by Jesus at the end of the last Passover ceremony that he attended. But it is important to remember that the first half of that final evening's proceedings were traditional Jewish rituals that pay homage to God.

Passover marks the birth of the Jews as a people over 3,000 years ago, as well as its emergence as a nation under Moses' leadership. God commanded the Jews to remember it each year—"to keep the passover"—at the same time, every April, in the same way (Exodus 12:26–7). It is a ceremony which has remained unchanged for 30 centuries and existed 1,000 years before Jesus was born.

It begins on an evening close to Good Friday—it varies slightly each year because the ancient Hebrew calendar was different. Since God spared every first-born Jewish child, all first-born sons fast on the day before Passover in gratitude.

Placed before Jesus was a ceremonial meal—with appropriate prayers—that included not only bitter herbs, unleavened bread, and a burnt shank of lamb, but also parsley, symbol of renewed faith, and hope for a bright future—and a sweet dessert, known as *Charoset* (or *Haroset*).

The Healing Powers of *Charoset*

Charoset is a combination of finely chopped apples (at least a half apple per person) and chopped walnuts, to which chopped or mashed raisins, dates, cinnamon, wine, and honey may be added. (For more details on raisins, wine, and honey, see pages 210 and 343). These ingredients, mixed together, symbolize the mortar that the ancient Hebrews used to make bricks as slaves in Egypt.

Contained within this sweet dish are curative plant medicines that can relieve heart pain . . . dissolve and eliminate gallstones and kidney stones . . . help an underactive thyroid . . . make skin blemishes, ugly warts, age spots, acne, psoriasis, and herpes disappear, and more.

A famous feature of this ceremony is called *Karpas*—in which either of two Bible healing plants, parsley or celery, symbolizing new life and rebirth, is dipped into salt water to remember the tears shed in bondage. One of these plants can help heal hernias, joint pain, diabetes, and urinary disorders (see page 52). The other is a vegetable medicine that kept a 96-year-old woman free of cataracts, able to read without glasses, for nearly half a century . . . that relieves gout, bursitis, neuritis, and rheumatism . . . that contains calcium blockers and other plant chemicals that help prevent and treat irregular heartbeat, help lower blood pressure and cholesterol, and much more (see page 59).

The Miracle in *Charoset* That Relieves Heart Pain

In Jesus' time, walnut trees grew on the shores of the Sea of Galilee. His seamless coat is said to have been dyed a rich brown using walnut leaves. Josephus, in the first century A.D., states that in his day extremely old trees of this species were abundant in Palestine, especially around the Lake of Gennesaret. In the Moffett translation of the Bible, Song 6:11 reads: "Down I went to the walnut-bower, to see the green plants of the dale." Solomon's "nut garden" was a walnut-bower. Its fine shade, fragrant leaves, and delicious fruit made it a favorite.

Walnuts contain omega-3 fatty acids, which have an anti-inflammatory effect similar to powerful drugs, without the side effects, for ailments such as arthritis, rheumatism, and heart disease.

Reportedly, an infusion made from the woody partitions inside the walnut is excellent in cases where the coronary vessels have become hardened, and for cardiac pains and fever. Remove the dividing walls of four or five walnuts, soak them in water for 1 day, leave them overnight, and then boil them for a few minutes (about 20 minutes) the next morning. Drink this tea in the morning on an empty stomach. A world renowned European herbalist states: "When taken regularly it will alleviate the feeling of constriction and pain in the chest. This infusion is also effective in cases of high temperature accompanied by pains in the heart. Some relief is frequently noticed after the first cup, but if the pains continue, the tea should be sipped frequently until they and the fever have disappeared."

In 1992, researchers at the Loma Linda University Medical School reported that Seventh-Day Adventists who rarely eat nuts suffer heart attacks and coronary deaths at twice the rate of those who routinely ate nuts five times a week. Closer analysis revealed that eating moderate amounts of walnuts, without increasing total dietary fat and calories, "decreased serum-cholesterol levels and favorably modifies the lipoprotein profile in healthy men."

These conclusions were based on two experimental diets, lasting 4 weeks each, in which 30 percent of calories were derived from fat—a level recommended by the American Medical Association.

Hundreds Cured of Kidney and Gallstones in 2 Days

In the early '60s, Chinese doctors reported curing hundreds of patients of all ages of kidney and gallstones, using 2-1/4 cups of raw walnut meat deep fried in pure olive oil (for more details on olive oil see Chapter 13) until crisp. The walnut meat was then ground to a coarse powder and mixed with 2-1/4 teaspoons of dark honey to form a paste. This was then given to each patient for 2 days, at the end of which most stones had partially dissolved, and turned soft and been eliminated.

The Miracle in *Charoset* That Helps an Underactive Thyroid

I recently asked an herbalist friend of mine why his sudden fondness for walnuts. He told me he had been bothered for years with an underactive thyroid (hypothyroidism), with fatigue, mental sluggishness, a tendency to overweight, and, lately, swollen ankles. He cited a study in which fresh walnut juice had caused levels of thyroxine—the thyroid hormone—to increase 100 percent.

Since eating a handful of walnuts daily, the swelling in his ankles had subsided, he said, and judging from the way he felt he expected a definite improvement on his next thyroid blood test.

The Miracle in *Charoset* That Fights Cancer

Studies have shown that black-walnut shells contain a crystalline compound—ellagic acid—which is effective in treating high blood pressure, skin cancer, and muscular paralysis due to electrical shock. Grapes (see page 214), strawberries, black currants, raspberries, and cashews also contain this valuable substance.

Laboratory animals that were fed ellagic acid experienced 45 percent fewer tumors and a delay in onset of the tumors by up to 10 weeks, when exposed to a chemical that induces skin cancer, compared to another group without ellagic acid. Walnut shells—if used for their ellagic-acid content—should be placed in boiling water, and brewed this way for a half-hour or so. This solution may then be strained, sweetened to taste, and taken as tea.

"Administered as a drug," according to one newspaper account, "ellagic acid prevents esophagus, liver, skin and lung cancer in rats and mice. . . ." Scientists are quick to point out that ellagic acid can be used only as a preventive before a cancer starts, and not as a treatment.

A single daily helping of fruits or vegetables that contain ellagic acid could cut the risk of stroke almost in half, according to Dr. Elizabeth Barrett-Connor and Dr. Kay-Tee Khaw in a report in the January 29, 1987, issue of *The New England Journal of Medicine*.

How *Candida* Infections Vanished?

In one study, the fresh husks of black walnuts destroyed candida (*Candida albicans,* which causes yeast infections) better than a commonly prescribed antifungal drug. To extract the antifungal ingredient—Juglone—from the husks, take the shells of a dozen green walnuts and break them into pieces. Add the pieces to a quart of boiling cabbage juice. Cover and simmer on low heat for 15 minutes. Remove from heat and allow to stand for another 20 minutes. Use this solution to douche the vagina two or three times daily, until symptoms disappear.

The Secret in *Charoset* That May Help You Shed Pound after Pound

Walnuts are our richest dietary source of serotonin, which makes you feel full. A study of more than 25,000 Seventh-Day Adventists showed that those who ate the most nuts were the least obese. It is important to remember, however, that Seventh-Day Adventists are vegetarians. You might experiment to see if eating a handful of walnuts helps you control food cravings.

A Powerful Sedative in *Charoset* That Can Give You a Good Night's Sleep

Walnuts contain a powerful sedative (ellagic acid) that can put you in la-la land long enough to get a good night's sleep. It's in the meat of the walnut. American Indians used to use walnuts to stupefy fish. They'd simply sprinkle some shelled crushed walnuts in the water. The fish, who never saw walnut chunks before, would gobble them down and soon be asleep. In suspended animation, the fish would float to the surface, where they were easily scooped up by the Indians.

It is a little-known fact that the sweet aroma of walnut wood—from shavings and sawdust—has a relaxing and soothing effect similar to smoking marijuana. Walnut wood is not on any controlled substance list. It's a natural tranquilizer, given by nature for comfort and pleasure.

"Skin Blemishes . . .
Just Seem to Disappear as If by Magic"

"Certain skin blemishes, ringworm and even warts just seem to disappear as if by magic, whenever green or immature black walnut is used on the skin," says Dr. John Heinerman. "Just make a couple of incisions into its outer shell . . . and rub the juice on whatever you want cleared up." If you experience a slight burning sensation or brown stain, there's no need to worry. These will soon pass, he says, adding, "Practically all kinds of warts, dark ugly age spots and ringworm have been successfully eliminated with this treatment."[1]

He says that 2 tablespoons of walnut leaves, added to boiling water, stirred, covered, and removed from the heat and allowed to steep for 30 minutes is an excellent wash for acne, and that older people who have been troubled with eczema and psoriasis reported considerable relief after washing their afflicted body parts with this same tea several times a day. He says it not only relieves the itching and inflammation, but actually helps to heal the skin, too.

Burdock root (see pages 79 and 86) is sometimes added for greater effect, he says: 1 tablespoonful of coarsely chopped, dried root is simmered for 10 minutes before the walnut leaves are added and the mixture is steeped for 40 minutes. You can also drink this tea, he says.[2]

According to English herbalist Maude Grieve, the bark and leaves of walnut "are of the highest value for curing . . . herpes, eczema, etc., and for healing indolent [painless] ulcers; an infusion [tea] of 1 oz. of dried bark or leaves (slightly more of the fresh leaves) to the pint of boiling water, allowed to stand for six hours, and strained off is taken in wineglassful doses, three times a day, the same infusion being also employed at the same time for outward application. Obstinate ulcers may also be cured with sugar, well saturated with a strong decoction of walnut leaves."

---

[1] John Heinerman, *Heinerman's Encyclopedia of Fruits, Vegetables and Herbs,* West Nyack, NY: Parker Publishing Company, Inc., 1988.

[2] John Heinerman, *Heinerman's Encyclopedia of Nuts, Berries and Seeds,* West Nyack, NY: Parker Publishing Company, Inc., 1995.

Excellent for Constipation

Walnuts are especially good for those suffering from constipation. "When drug-store laxatives do not produce the desired results," says a well-known European herbalist, "walnuts may solve the problem. They are recommended for people with liver disorders, and although most liver patients cannot tolerate fat they will find that moderate quantities of walnuts will agree with them quite well."

The Miracle in *Charoset* Chosen by Jesus as His Symbol of Salvation

The palm tree, with its long tapering stem rising 80 feet or more, and its great terminal cluster of feathery leaves that make it stand out conspicuously, has always been a symbol of spiritual uplift, hope, and survival. David the Psalmist is quoted in the Old Testament as saying:

The righteous shall flourish like the palm tree . . . Those that

be planted in the house of the Lord shall flourish. . . . They

shall bring forth fruit in old age. *Psalms 92:12–14*

Dates—the fruit of the palm—have been called the "food of the desert." So common were they in the Jordan Valley that Jericho was known as the "city of palm trees" (Deuteronomy 34:3). Whatever other foods the multitudes lacked during lean years, they always had dates, since the average palm produces about 100 pounds of fruit every season for 100 years, and palms grew in abundance, always near water. Whenever a weary traveler saw palm trees, it was a sure sign of food and water nearby.

Legend has it that Jesus commanded a palm to bend so that He could pick dates for His mother after Joseph had refused to do so. It did this so willingly that He blessed it and chose it as a symbol of salvation for the dying, promising that when He entered Jerusalem in triumph it should be with a palm in His hand.

St. Christopher is said to have used a palm staff when he carried the small and weak, including the infant Jesus, across the raging river. Jesus told him to thrust his staff into the ground and it sprouted into a date palm, a miracle that resulted in the conversion of Christopher. Angels are said to have carried a palm from heaven to Mary, mother of Jesus, after the crucifixion.

To the ancient and medieval Christian martyrs, angels were said to bring palm "branches" to convey their souls to heaven. On All Souls Day palm leaves are cast into a fire and their rising into the sky as smoke is taken as proof of victory by the souls who are that day released from purgatory.

The use of palm leaves in processions seems to have originated at the time of the restoration of the temple by Judas Maccabeus and has been continued to this day by Jews at the Feast of the Tabernacles and by Christians on Palm Sunday and Easter.

Charoset Ingredient Studied for Anti-cancer Activity

Dates—the fruit of the palm—are being studied for anti-cancer activity. According to medical botanist Dr. James Duke, former head of the Germplasm Resource Laboratory of the United States Department of Agriculture, in his book, *Medicinal Plants of the Bible:*

> "A nut cataplasm [a poultice made from crushed date pits] is said to help testicle tumors. The fruit, prepared in various manners, is said to remedy cancer of the stomach and uterus, abdominal tumors, hardnesses of the liver and spleen, and ulcerated and non-ulcerated cancers."

Dr. Jonathan Hartwell, formerly of the National Cancer Institute in Bethesda, Maryland, carefully screened thousands of plants for anticancer activity, and his reports appeared in "Plants Against Cancer," a survey in the scientific journal *Lloydia* (1967–71). Hartwell cites the medicinal use of dates in connection with cancers, indurations or tumors of the abdomen, gum, liver, mouth, parotids, spleen, stomach, testicle, throat, uterus, and viscera.

Medical anthropologist Dr. John Heinerman says, "A drink made of fresh, pitted dates in any kind of juice (orange, carrot or pineapple) would be the most logical way to take it internally, while a handful of pitted dates made into a puree could be spread on external eruptions with apparently satisfying results."[3]

The immediate services of a doctor should always be sought in matters as serious as these. Self-treatment is not recommended. The use of dates should be regarded as an unproven but apparently harmless supplement to existing cancer therapy, if your doctor approves.

The Miracle in *Charoset* That Helps Prevent Thinning Bones

Dates are rich in boron—a mineral that can prevent the thinning of bones that occurs with age. New research shows that boron dramatically increases blood levels of natural estrogen, a hormone that prevents the thinning of bones known as osteoporosis.

After menopause, bone loss occurs in women at a tremendous rate, particularly in the hips, knees, and spine. It happens to men, too, at an advanced age, but the disease is noticeable far sooner in women.

Dr. Forrest H. Nielson of the U.S. Department of Agriculture's Human Nutrition Research Center, found that when postmenopausal women got 3 milligrams of boron a day, their calcium losses dropped by 40 percent.

Dr. Nielson discovered that boron caused the most active form of estrogen, estradiol 17B, to *double* to levels found in women on estrogen replacement therapy.

Without boron, your body cannot retain calcium, but the average American gets only half the boron needed. This may explain why people who take lots of calcium tablets and eat lots of high-calcium foods still suffer from osteoporosis.

Dates, grapes, raisins, beans, almonds and honey—all Bible foods—are the richest sources of this essential mineral that literally holds your bones together.

---

[3]*Heinerman's Encyclopedia of Healing Juices,* 1994.

The Miracle in *Charoset* That Relieves Celiac Disease, Constipation, and Insomnia

Celiac disease, also called sprue, is a chronic intestinal disorder in which the body cannot tolerate gluten, an elastic protein substance found in bread dough, resulting in diarrhea. Dates contain protein carbohydrate complexes and mineral salts that halt this reaction to gluten, according to one expert. Figs, another popular Bible food, work in a similar way. Dates also have a dynamic laxative effect and can relieve acid in the gut and heartburn. But because dates are intensely sweet, they should not be used by those with blood-sugar problems, such as diabetes and hypoglycemia.

A Bible Food That Causes Bacteria to Shrivel Away Keeps Your Body Tissues Soft and Pliable

A major benefit of apples[4] is that they provide potassium—which kills germs by withdrawing their water: they literally dry up and shrivel away. Potassium also keeps tissues soft and pliable, and fights hardening of the arteries. You can prove this by using apple cider vinegar as a meat tenderizer (see below). Apples also provide pectin, a water-soluble fiber that vastly reduces cholesterol and protects your heart.

---

[4]There has been a great debate as to whether apples existed in the Holy Land in Biblical times. Quinces, grapes, and even bananas have been suggested as possibly being what the Bible means, when it talks about apples. Some experts point to the lush varieties of apple that grow there now, in abundance, as evidence of their presence in Biblical days. Others insist that the common apple is not a native of Palestine, but is a comparatively recent introduction there, and that at best only a few wild apples grew in the mountains—small, wretched, and woody—barely able to survive the heat. But the fact is, there really were lush eating apples in the Holy Land in Biblical times, and we know this because the Talmud—the 39 books of Biblical commentary, dating from the first century A.D.—speak of them as food and medicine. They were considered a particular delicacy, notable for their pleasant aroma. Apples, grapes, and plums were considered healthful and were served to invalids. Apple wine was used both as a beverage and if aged as medicine. See *Biblical and Talmudic Medicine* by Julius Preuss, M.D., published in Germany in 1911, translated and edited by Fred Rosner, M.D., Sanhedrin Press, NY, 1978.

D. C. Jarvis, M.D., author of the best-seller *Folk Medicine,* greatly favored apple cider vinegar—for medicinal purposes—because it carries everything over from the apple except the sugar, which turns acid in fermenting to form vinegar.

The acid in apple cider vinegar is extremely valuable, said Dr. Jarvis, because it can eliminate many ailments by changing your system from alkaline to acid. It also kills bacteria in the lungs and intestines—so much so, in fact, that waste matter in the intestines loses its smell.

Thirdly, the acid in apple cider vinegar dissolves calcium and other thick, clogging mineral deposits in your system, so they can move out—in exactly the same fashion that acid dissolves calcium and mineral deposits off tea kettles and furnace pipes, said Jarvis.

These solid calcium and mineral deposits—which can be the cause of various aches and pains—are alkaline before the apple cider vinegar dissolves them.

You can easily see how this happens, said Dr. Jarvis, by submerging an egg shell in apple cider vinegar. It will soon begin bubbling and softening, and will gradually disappear.

The same effect can be observed by adding soap to milk. This will make the milk alkaline, thick, and even lumpy. Pour in some apple cider vinegar, and the acid in the vinegar immediately dissolves the lumps. (Needless to say, milk with soap and vinegar in it should not be taken into the body as food.)

Many Ailments Relieved with This Wonderful Bible Healing Food

Among the many ailments that yield to apple cider vinegar, according to Dr. Jarvis, are hardening of the arteries, inflammation of the kidneys and bladder, itching scalp, hay-fever and allergy symptoms such as eye tearing and runny nose, sinus seepage, postnasal drip, sinusitis, and facial pain or neuralgia.

The pain of paranasal sinusitis can be relieved, he says, by taking 1 teaspoonful of apple cider vinegar in a glass of water each hour for seven doses. Sip slowly. This will usually relieve the pain of facial neuralgia, he adds.

One teaspoonful of apple cider vinegar in a glass of water four times a day will result in marked relief of arthritic pain in the small joints of the hands and feet, over a 2-week period, says Jarvis.

A Bible Food Remedy for Inflammation of the Kidneys

"Several years ago," said Mrs. B., "I was subject to attacks of pyelitis, an inflammation of the kidneys. I would become quite ill, with chills, headache, nausea, fever, a racing pulse, and a nagging pain in my left kidney that would not go away. I'd get a tremendous urge to urinate, and when I did it burned, and was cloudy with pus. My doctor gave me antibiotics and prescribed bed rest. Nothing really worked to rid me of this trouble, until a friend suggested trying apple cider vinegar, two teaspoonfuls in a glass of water daily. The condition cleared right up. After I'd been free of it for a few months, I discontinued the apple cider vinegar. A couple of weeks later, the pyelitis came back. Again I was able to get rid of it with the apple cider vinegar."

Biblical Food Remedy for Vaginitis

An old but effective folk remedy for vaginitis is to add 3 cups of apple cider vinegar to a hot bath and soak in the tub for 20 minutes. Reportedly, vinegar baths and douches help restore normal acidity to the vagina, which can make candida, trichomonas, and gardnerella disappear.

Bible Healing Food Halts MS

Miss L. A. writes: "I was diagnosed as having MS in April 1975 by [two doctors]. My whole left side was weak and my left leg was so stiff that at times I could not go up and down the stairs. I was taking every kind of vitamin supplement there is but that didn't seem to improve me. Around the first of June I remembered a book I had read . . . written by an M.D. . . . . He said vinegar builds strong muscles. I started drinking about one ounce a day mixed with honey.

"About a week later, I went to see my doctor and my feet did not tremble any more. He said I was definitely better. I was still weak though so I started drinking a half glass a day. The improvement was dramatic. I have most of my strength back now . . . I don't know why, but vinegar has helped me more than anything else."

How This Bible Food Melts Away Fat

Apple cider vinegar contains powerful enzymes that help dissolve clumps of fat, and wash them right out of the system—so powerful, in fact, that meat soaked in apple cider vinegar is tenderized. When you drink it, even in such small quantities as 2 tablespoons in fruit or vegetable juice, moments later it is breaking up accumulated fat in cell tissues, says one expert.

I well remember when *Folk Medicine* by Dr. Jarvis became a big best seller around 1958–60, and his apple cider vinegar remedies were very popular. At that time, a group of women that included my mother used to eat lunch together and have lively discussions. One frequent topic was diets. Dr. Jarvis claimed it was easy to slim down with apple cider vinegar. All you had to do, he said, was sip a couple of teaspoons of it in a glass of water at each meal. No special diet. Just sensible eating. He claimed that a woman could go down three dress sizes in about 5 months this way—that a woman who wore a size 50 dress would be able to take a size 42 in a year (that's over 100 pounds) effortlessly!

My mother, who had never been able to make her weight budge, lost 12 pounds in 3 months, on this "diet," going from 139 to 127. Two other members of the group lost 10 pounds and 16 pounds, respectively, in 3–4 months. The winner, however, was a woman who went down two dress sizes in a year—a loss of about 30 pounds.

How the Holy Oil of the Tabernacle Protects Against Botulism, Staph Infections, Candida, and Tuberculosis

Cinnamon was one of the principal ingredients used in the manufacture of the precious ointments or "holy oil" which Moses was commanded to use in the Tabernacle for anointing the sacred vessels and the persons of the officiating priests (Exodus 30:23). It had to be imported from India and was therefore very costly and precious.

Cinnamon is a powerful antiseptic that kills many decay- and disease-causing bacteria. It kills the microorganisms that cause botulism and staph infections. Its leaf juice has strong activity against the germs that cause tuberculosis.

It suppresses completely the cause of most urinary tract infections (*Escherichia coli* bacteria) and the fungus responsible for vaginal yeast infections (*Candida albicans*). It contains a natural anesthetic oil, eugenol, which makes it useful for treating cuts and bruises. It stimulates the uterus, and therefore should not be used by women during pregnancy.

Recent research has demonstrated that certain spices—namely cinnamon, nutmeg, turmeric, and bay leaf—help the body use insulin more efficiently, thereby lowering elevated blood sugar levels. Cinnamon also helps break down fats in your digestive system, and also helps reduce blood pressure.

Miracle Herb from Last Supper Removes Poisons from the Body

At the Passover table, parsley symbolizes new beginnings because it is one of the first herbs to appear in spring. But parsley is much more than that. Parsley juice is valuable for removing poisons from the body.

Parsley has a marked action upon the tubules of the kidney, neutralizing and promoting excretion of waste products containing uric acid. By virtue of a substance it contains called apiol, it assists in the concentration of urea.

Parsley is an excellent diuretic; it drains excess fluid from the body. It is used medicinally for a variety of illnesses but more particularly for kidney inflammation, inability to urinate, painful urination, prostate pressure, gravel, kidney stones, and other urinary disorders. Culpepper wrote: "The seed is effectual to break the [kidney] stones and ease the pains and torments thereof . . ."

Reported cases:

"Ever since I started to take parsley, I got relief both from bladder irritation and prostate pressure. Now, after over a year, I feel so grateful I want to pass the information on to others that suffer as I did."—Mr. R. B.

Mrs. M.D.R. reports, "I was incapacitated by what was diagnosed as toxic poisoning accompanied by a tough case of pyelitis (inflammation of the kidneys). For two years I helped support a general practitioner and a neurologist. At the end of that time I could not walk across the room without help, I had lost 50 pounds, and my pocketbook was a mere shadow of its former self. . . . An acquaintance asked me if I had tried parsley tea. . . . As I had never done this, he gave me these instructions: 'Take a fresh bunch of parsley . . . wash it in cold water. Place in a dish and cover with scalding hot water. Cover to keep warm. When cold, pour off the liquid and drink during a 24-hour period. Repeat daily until cured.'

"I've recommended this to many people. They never fail to get a cure, regardless of whether it is a kidney or bladder complaint. I've never known it to require more than three weeks for a cure and have known several cases where only three days were necessary. My own case required between two and three weeks for a cure, and there has been a lapse of 35 years without a recurrence.

"A few months ago, I heard that a friend was having kidney trouble. Without further investigation I set her the above instructions. About a month later I received a two-page letter stating that she had been under a doctor's care for six months with two hospital confinements. She received my letter on the day that she returned from the last hospital trip and was ready to try anything once. In three days her urine was perfectly clear and she was ready to resume her household duties in her mobile home. In a week's time, she was covering the park to catch up on her social obligations and tell the world about her wonderful cure."

Hopeless Diabetic Sent Home to Die Still Alive 30 Years Later Thanks to 3 Healing Bible Foods

Ted V., a man with advanced diabetes, was told by doctors his condition was hopeless and was sent home to die at age 60. At age 90, he was still alive, in excellent health! He had started eating a combination of garlic, parsley, and watercress. His blood sugar dropped from over 200 to 110. And he went on happily using this remedy for many, many years.

Mr. C. D. suffered from prostate enlargement, with infection and pus and finally complete stoppage of urine. He was extremely frightened and had fever and chills. He was rushed to a hospital, where a doctor quickly inserted a tube to drain his bladder. He could not urinate without the tube. He was told he needed surgery, but they could not operate since he had diabetes. He was advised to try parsley tea. After drinking this tea, he could urinate freely without a tube, his sugar dropped to normal, and surgery was happily avoided. Many others report similar relief.

Throws Away His Canes

Parsley tea seems to have a beneficial action in some types of rheumatism. We are told of an elderly man who could barely hobble around with the aid of two canes. The man started drinking parsley tea and became well enough to discard the canes.

These Women Claimed Menopausal Joint Pains Gone with a Bible Healing Food

Writing to the editor of a health publication, Miss M. H. asked, "By what natural means would you deal with menopausal rheumatism?" The editor replied: "Parsley, containing apiol, has been found to bring relief in a number of cases of rheumatism in women passing through the 'change of life.' How is it taken? Place a handful of fresh parsley in a two-pint enamel milk saucepan and cover with one-and-a-half pints of cold water. Bring to a boil. Simmer no more than 10 seconds. Remove vessel from the gas; allow to cool; strain when cold. Those who like a strong infusion can add more parsley, as this common culinary herb is quite harmless."

Reported uses of parsley:[5]

"A woman I know drank parsley tea for six weeks to clean out her kidneys. She swears it not only did the job, but also kept her change-of-life rheumatism under control. Now, whenever she feels the slightest twinge of rheumatism she drinks the tea for a while and says that takes care of it."—Miss T. T.

"So many women suffer from rheumatism during the menopause, and at one time I did too. But I found relief by drinking parsley tea. Parsley is a good remedy for so many things, and it is perfectly harmless."—Mrs. C. B.

"During the change of life, I suffered joint pain in my right knee. The doctor prescribed some tablets, which did not bring any relief but upset my stomach. I then asked a friend of mine who believes in old-time remedies what she would use if she were me. She suggested parsley tea, and I found that after I used it over a period of several weeks my knee became normal.

"I mentioned this remedy to one of my relatives who was also going through the menopause and complaining of a painful shoulder. And she, too, got very good results from using the tea, as she has no more pain."—Mrs. E. P.

---

[5]Richard Lucas, *Magic Herbs for Arthritis, Rheumatism and Related Ailments,* West Nyack, NY: Parker Publishing Company, Inc., 1981.

Bible Food Helps Prevent Hernias

The ancients believed that parsley would "fasten loose teeth" and "brighten dim eyes"—which holds up scientifically, since parsley contains 22,500 units of vitamin A per ounce, four times as much vitamin C as does an equal weight of oranges, and has an iron content far surpassing that of spinach (5.73 mg per ounce, versus 1.2 for spinach). Dorothy H. Anderson, M.D., of Columbia University reported tests on animals in which vitamin A increased resistance to hernias—a frequent problem for older people. A deficiency of vitamin A, she found, increased susceptibility to this ailment.

Instant Allergy Relief with This Bible Food

Dr. Heinerman tells how, at a Natural Living convention where he was scheduled to speak, he began sneezing continuously. Although he had no idea as to the cause, during dinner in the building's cafeteria he developed a strong craving for some parsley that was freshly cut, washed, and on display at the salad bar. He piled his plate full of parsley sprigs, covered them with some oil-and-vinegar dressing, and croutons, and devoured the entire plate of parsley. "Something wonderful soon happened," he says. "My frequent sneezing stopped completely! I still don't know what it is in the parsley that made this happen, only that the leafy herb is good for allergies!"[6]

A 1984 study by W. W. Busse, et al., in the *Journal of Allergy and Clinical Immunology* (73:801) shows that parsley inhibits the secretion of histamine, a chemical produced by the body that triggers allergy symptoms.

How to Use This Miracle Healing Food

The ancients used parsley to absorb the inebriating fumes of wine. They also ate it to quickly neutralize the smell of garlic. Parsley is

---

[6]John Heinerman, *Heinerman's Encyclopedia of Healing Juices,* 1994.

famous for neutralizing odors, due to its high level of chlorophyll, the active ingredient in many breath fresheners.

Parsley tea taken after meals is good protection against indigestion. Just steep a few sprigs of it in boiling hot water, sweeten to taste, and drink. Eating fresh parsley leaves is even better.

When making parsley tea, the roots can also be used. Dried parsley roots are available at many health-food stores. They are much more powerful than the leaves. Therefore, the manufacturer's instructions should be followed.

Caution

Parsley juice can stimulate uterine contractions during labor. This is due to a chemical it contains called apiol. During the early 1900s, large doses of apiol were used to induce abortion, despite its unpleasant side effects (intoxication, giddiness, flashes of light, vertigo, ringing in the ears). Normal amounts of parsley, of course, may be eaten by pregnant women. And it is generally considered safe for healthy, nonpregnant, nonnursing adults.

Nursing mothers should be aware that parsley can dry up the milk supply. But after the weaning period, parsley tea can be used to inhibit milk production and relieve the discomfort of overfull breasts. Eating fresh parsley is an old folk remedy for breast tenderness caused by water retention—it flushes excess water out of the body.

A Natural Alternative to Prescription Drugs for Gout

At Passover ceremonies, celery can be substituted for parsley. Celery is a member of the parsley family, and is mentioned in the Talmud, the 39 books of Biblical commentary dating from the first century, as a remedy for infections and tumors. Celery's most famous use, however, is as a remedy for gout.

Celery neutralizes uric acid in the body. The immediate cause of gout is an excessive accumulation of uric acid in the joints—from eating too many sweet and starchy foods. Uric acid forms hard crystals in the joints that cause excruciating pain.

The pain hits suddenly, almost always in the big toe, wrist, ankle, or thumbs. The skin becomes shiny, red or purplish, swollen, and excruciating to touch. Unlike arthritis, where the pain is deep and aching, in gout the pain is sharp and agonizing. There may be fever or chills, with a rapid pulse. Attacks can last 4 days or more, increasing in frequency.

When uric acid crystals collect in the kidneys, serious kidney damage can follow. Excess spillage of uric acid into the urine may produce kidney stones.

Celery seed is hypo-uremic—it lowers uric acid. Plus it contains about 20 different anti-inflammatory agents. Celery seed tea may be prepared by placing 1–2 teaspoons of freshly crushed seeds into a cup of boiling water. Steep for 20 minutes, strain, sweeten to taste. Dose: 1 cupful three times a day. It may also be taken in the form of celery seed extract tablets, four a day.

For some people, this works just as well as standard medicines, such as allopurinol (Zyloprim), sodium bicarbonate, phenylbutazone, or colchicine—without any side effects. Colchicine, for example, was discovered by some unknown Egyptian genius around 500 B.C. and has been in steady use ever since. No one knows why it works but it does bring quick relief. But it is very strong medicine and can cause nausea, vomiting, and other side effects.

Reported cases:

Mr. F. T. says: "Since I started drinking celery seed tea daily and adding fresh celery to my meals, I have no more rheumatism. And thank God I no longer suffer attacks of gout in my right toe which used to send me into terrible spasms of pain. Hope you'll pass the good word along to others."

"I'm so glad I found out about celery tea," says Mrs. W. M. "It is the only thing that took away the awful bursitis pain I had in my shoulder, and brought back the movement. I drank the tea faithfully every day and followed a light diet."

Celery seed also contains a diuretic substance that causes pounds of excess water to drain away, and has been used for weight loss, and to relieve high blood pressure, and congestive heart failure. Celery seed stimulates uterine contractions, and has been used by some women to bring on their periods, or to relieve the bloated feeling caused by premenstrual fluid retention. It has lowered blood sugar levels in diabetes.

Sciatic Pain Relief

Sciatica is a painful inflammation of the sciatic nerve which runs down the back of the thigh and leg. For relief, my mother drinks strong celery seed tea before each meal. For many people, this actually clears up the condition. Celery seed tea can be purchased at your local health-food store. But celery seeds are available right off the spice rack at your local supermarket. You can also get them by allowing garden celery to grow till it flowers.

Facial Neuralgia Pain Vanished

"A friend of mine told me she was completely relieved of her facial neuralgia by drinking fresh celery juice. I asked if I could borrow her juicer as I wanted to see if celery juice would help my painful neuritis attacks which I suffer with almost every winter. I drank two pints of the juice daily, and by the end of the week the pain was gone. I kept drinking the juice for 3 more weeks to make sure the pain would not return. That was 5 years ago. I bought my own juicer, and whenever I feel even the slightest twinges of pain, I immediately start drinking celery juice and the neuritis attack does not happen."—Mrs. L. S.

A Natural Calcium Blocker

Celery contains calcium blockers and other plant chemicals that help prevent and treat arrhythmias, and other compounds that help lower blood pressure and cholesterol. Celery is high in apigenin, a chemical that expands (dilates) the blood vessels and may help prevent high blood pressure.

Researchers at the University of Chicago Medical Center have found that very small amounts of a compound in celery, 3-n-butyl phthalide, can lower blood pressure in animals by 12–14 percent, and cholesterol by about 7 percent. The equivalent dose in humans can be supplied by about four ribs of celery. After eating a quarter pound of celery every day for a week, a 62-year-old man's blood pressure dropped from 158 over 96 to 118 over 82.

Bible Healing Food Keeps Woman, 96, Free of Cataracts

At 96, my great grandmother Celia swore that celery juice, placed in her eyes with a dropper, had cleared up her cataracts 40 years earlier, restored her sight, and kept it that way. Her vision was so sharp she could read in the dark without glasses.

She prepared it by mashing some celery into a pulp with a fork; then she strained out the juice, added some water, and put drops of it in her eyes. The celery had to be garden-fresh and green (and presumably free of pesticides). And she used pure spring water. She applied the celery water two to three times a week.

+   +   +

Celery preparations are considered generally safe by the Food and Drug Administration. Nevertheless, people with specific conditions should talk to their doctors first before using them. This is especially true of people with kidney problems, and pregnant or nursing women. Celery tea, juice, oil, or extracts should never be used to try to induce an abortion.

CHAPTER · 5

A MIRACLE LEAF FROM THE LAST SUPPER: THOUSANDS CLAIMED IT SAVED THEIR LIVES

. . . and the leaf shall be for medicine. *Ezekiel 17:12*

Another miracle plant on the table at the Last Supper was sheep sorrel, one of the bitter herbs. Its pleasant acid taste makes it a good dressing for meat, which is exactly how it was used.

Sheep sorrel—a gift from the Lamb of God—came near to being regarded as a miracle herb by doctors over the centuries, because of its strong infection fighting power, power to relieve blockages of the stomach and intestines, to restore a sick person's appetite, relieve nausea and vomiting, abscesses and ulcers. It has a long history as a folk remedy for cancer in Europe and America.

Sheep sorrel's most famous use is as part of an anti-cancer remedy—a simple four-herb tea called Essiac—revealed by an Ojibway (Chippewa) medicine man in Canada 75 years ago. It is one of the most remarkable stories in all of medicine, because many doctors have said it relieved pain, restored strength, when all else failed. Thousands claimed their lives were saved by it, while most doctors say it's completely worthless.

The Remarkable Story of Essiac

In 1922 a Canadian nurse named Rene Caisse, working at a hospital in northern Ontario, saw an elderly lady being bathed, and noticed that one breast was just a mass of scar tissue. So she asked about it. The lady, who was nearly 80, said that some 20 years earlier, while living in a mining camp with her husband, she developed tumors on her breast. Doctors in Ontario diagnosed it as advanced cancer, and said the breast would have to be removed.

Because they had no money for surgery, they returned to the camp where an Ojibway medicine man—a friend of her husband's—said he could heal it. He prepared an herbal brew, which she drank daily. Her breast began to improve. He showed her how to make the tea, so she could continue drinking it. She did this for over a year, and the tumors disappeared. More than 20 years later, she still seemed fine.

Rene asked the woman how to prepare this tea. "My thought was that if I should ever develop cancer, I would use it," she said. See recipe on page 79.

The ingredients—sheep sorrel, burdock root, slippery-elm bark, Turkish rhubarb—have been around for years (three out of four are Bible plants) and are legal and deemed safe for purchase from health-food stores and herbal distributors in the United States and throughout the world (see A Closer Look at Essiac, on page 84.)

Given 6 Months to Live, Her Aunt Recovers

In 1924, Rene's aunt was operated on, and the doctors found she had cancer of the stomach, with liver involvement—and told her she had 6 months to live. Rene told her aunt's doctor about the Ojibway Indian tea, and asked if her aunt could try it. He gave his consent. After drinking this herbal tea daily for 2 months, Rene's aunt recovered and lived another 21 years.

The doctor, R. O. Fisher, M.D., of Toronto, was so fascinated by this miraculous recovery that together they began experimenting on mice inoculated with human cancer cells. The results were so impressive that Dr. Fisher decided to try this herbal mixture on some of his advanced cancer patients. These patients, too, showed definite improvement.

Rene named the tea Essiac—her name spelled backwards. Other doctors heard about it and began sending her their advanced cancer patients.

Diabetes Vanished, Pancreas Normal Again

In 1925, a doctor persuaded Rene to treat a woman who had cancer of the bowel complicated by diabetes. Since no one knew what effect Essiac would have on a patient taking insulin, her doctor, Dr. J. A. McInnis, said he would discontinue the insulin, and if the diabetic condition got worse she could take it again. "To our surprise," said Rene, "the diabetic condition improved with the Essiac . . . and continued to improve until there wasn't any diabetes at all."

As for the cancer in her bowel, according to Rene: "At first [it] became larger and harder and almost caused an obstruction in the bowel. However, after a few more treatments it softened and reduced in size until it entirely disappeared. . . . Essiac treatments were discontinued after 6 months of weekly injections* and the patient continued in good health"

In 1926, Dr. Frederick Banting, co-discoverer of insulin, reviewed this case and concluded: "Essiac must actuate the pancreatic gland into normal functioning, otherwise the patient would have had to take treatment for the rest of her life, just as she would have had to take insulin."

While no diabetic should stop taking prescribed medication on this basis, still, decades later, we find this comment by Julian Whitaker, M.D. in one of his newsletters, referring to Essiac: "I've

---

*Some Essiac ingredients were given by injection—because it worked faster that way—and the rest were given as a tea to drink. If all the ingredients were injected it caused a violent reaction. Unfortunately, which herbs went into the injectable solution is not known. Essiac is used today only as an herbal drink, containing all four herbs.

seen records of diabetic patients who were taking insulin and were able to stop it completely after the use of this herbal formula."[1]

8 Doctors Claim It Relieves Pain, Can Do No Harm

On the strength of what doctors were seeing with their own eyes, in 1926, eight of them signed a petition to the Department of National Health and Welfare in Ottawa asking that Rene be given facilities to test her remedy on a large scale. In their petition they said: "We believe the treatment for cancer by Rene Caisse *can do no harm, and that it relieves pain, will reduce enlargement and will prolong life in hopeless cases.* To the best of our knowledge, she has not been given a case to treat until everything [else] has been tried without effect, and even then she was able to show remarkably beneficial results."

In response, Ottawa's Department of Health and Welfare sent two doctors with warrants for her arrest. "But when they found that I was working with nine of the most eminent doctors in Toronto," said Rene, "they did not arrest me." In fact one of them, Dr. W. C. Arnold, was so impressed that he arranged for Rene to continue her work at the Christie Street Hospital Laboratories.

Thousands Come to Seek a New Chance

News of these miraculous recoveries spread quickly, with an ever-increasing stream of patients (about 30 a day) coming to Rene's apartment for treatment. Soon neighbors began complaining about the congestion of cars and people. She took cases diagnosed as incurable. To avoid constant threats of arrest, several doctors and patients helped Rene get permission from Dr. J. M. Robb, the Minister of Health, to treat patients. "Dr. Robb told me I wouldn't be interfered with again as long as I didn't make a charge for my treatments, and had a written diagnosis of cancer from a doctor for each patient."

In 1935, Bracebridge, the little town where Rene lived, near Toronto, leased a building to her for $1 per month, to use as a clin-

---

[1]Reprinted with permission of Julian Whitaker, M.D.

ic. This came about when a local doctor, Albert Bastedo, M.D., referred a terminally ill patient with bowel cancer to Rene, and the patient recovered. The doctor was so amazed at this recovery that he convinced the town council to give her an old hotel that had been closed for nonpayment of taxes.

"Here, for almost eight years, I treated thousands of patients, most of them given up as hopeless after everything in medical science had failed," said Rene. She did it free of charge, always under a doctor's supervision. Dominion Street was as crowded as the shrine at Lourdes with people seeking a new lease on life. Some were carried. Many were brought by ambulance—and their first treatment had to be given to them *in* the ambulance. But after a few treatments they were able to walk into the clinic by themselves each week, some traveling hundreds of miles to do so. They came from all over Canada and the United States.

She had to turn people away who came without a written diagnosis from a doctor. (Some doctors refused to give it.) "They would beg me to treat them . . . it was very heartbreaking at times. Sometimes visiting doctors would examine these patients and give a written diagnosis in pity for the patient."

Rene accepted small voluntary contributions, never more than $2, that barely covered her expenses, and kept bill collectors hammering at her door for the next 40 years. She refused to profit from Essiac, although she was offered thousands of dollars to sell exclusive rights to the recipe you'll find on page 79.

Given Days to Live, Her Mother Recovers

Shortly after the clinic opened, Rene's 72-year-old mother was diagnosed with cancer of the liver, inoperable because of a weak heart. One of Ontario's top specialists, Dr. Roscoe Graham, said she had only days to live. He said her liver was "a nodular mass." Rene began giving daily injections of Essiac to her mother, who had not been told she had cancer, telling her only it was a tonic to make her feel better. After 10 days, Rene's mother rallied, regained her strength, and completely recovered, living another 18 years before passing away at age 90, "with no pain, just a tired heart."

"This repaid me for all of my work," said Rene, "giving my mother 18 years of life which she would not have had, and made up for a great deal of the persecution I had endured at the hands of the medical world."

+   +   +

"During this time many, many doctors, surgeons and scientists visited my clinic, read case histories, examined patients and watched me administer Essiac treatments," said Rene. "Doctors from many parts of the United States came [and] brought or sent patients."

"By God, You've Got It"

Dr. Richard Leonardo, surgical specialist and coroner of Rochester, New York, at first scoffed at the idea of there being any merit in Essiac. He said it was entirely psychological—Rene's personality, not Essiac, that was getting results. Rene told him that the only way to prove or disprove it was to remain in the clinic and see the patients, which he decided to do.

Dr. Leonardo stayed for 4 days examining patients, talking to other doctors. Then, just before he left, he sat down, slapped the armrest of his chair, and said, "Well, by God you've got it! But the medical profession isn't going to let you do this to me. I spent seven years in medical school, and I've written books."

"He told me," said Rene, "that if my treatment of a simple hypo-dermic injection was accepted, he'd have to go home and tear up his books and discard his surgical instruments."

"The Rapidity of Repair Was Absolutely Marvelous"

Dr. Emma Carson, a Los Angeles doctor, traveled to Bracebridge in the summer of 1937 to see for herself if there was any truth to news stories of the impressive results Rene Caisse had been getting with Essiac. She was skeptical and intended to stay only a few days. She wound up spending nearly a month, scrutinizing the records of over 400 patients and examining many of them.

The Huntsville Forester, a Canadian publication, quotes her as saying: "I am simply amazed at what I have found . . . The farther I investigate, the stronger becomes my conviction that Miss Caisse has made a cancer treatment discovery of world-wide importance."

In a press release picked up by several newspapers, Dr. Carson wrote: "The vast majority of Miss Caisse's patients are brought to her for treatment after Surgery, Radium, X-Rays, Emplastrums, etc., had failed to be helpful, and the patients were pronounced incurable or hopeless cases. Really the progress obtainable and the actual results from 'Essiac' treatments and the rapidity of repair was absolutely marvelous and must be seen to be believed."

"The Most Humane, Satisfactory, and Frequently Successful Remedy They Had Found"

In a five-page report, Dr. Carson wrote: "I also visited, examined and obtained data at patients' homes where they were pursuing their business vocations as ably as if they had never experienced the afflictions of cancer . . . I could scarcely believe my brain and eyes were not deceiving me, on some of the most seriously afflicted cases. . . .

"Several prominent physicians and surgeons who are quite familiar with the indisputable results obtained in response to 'Essiac' treatments . . . conceded to me that the Rene M. Caisse 'Essiac Treatment' for cancer is the most humane, satisfactory and frequently successful remedy for the annihilation of cancer 'that they had found at that time' . . ."

Relief of Pain in Many Difficult Cases Witnessed by Doctor

Dr. Benjamin Guyatt, a professor of anatomy at the University of Toronto, was another independent investigator. He made dozens of inspections of Rene's clinic during the 1930s, and wrote as follows:

"In most cases, distorted countenances became normal, and pain reduced as treatment proceeded.

"The relief of pain is a noticeable feature, as pain in these cases is very difficult to control. On checking authentic cancer cases, it was found that hemorrhage was readily brought under control in many difficult cases. Open lesions of lip and breast responded to treatment. Cancers of the cervix, rectum and bladder had been caused to disappear. Patients with cancer of the stomach, diagnosed by reputable physicians and surgeons, have returned to normal activity.

"The number of patients treated in this clinic are many hundreds and the number responding wholly or in part, I do not know. But I do know that I have witnessed in this clinic a treatment which brings about restoration, through destroying the tumour tissue, and supplying that something which improves the mental outlook of life and facilitates re-establishment of physiological function.

"It is my privilege to do all in my power to bring the cancer sufferer this remedy 'Essiac' which has brought relief and restored health to many in the past."

According to Rene, Dr. Guyatt visited her clinic almost every month for 3 years. "But," she wrote, "in spite of these good reports and the petitions signed by the doctors, the [Royal Cancer Commission] reported that they had found no benefit in the treatment."

55,000 Sign Petition

In 1938, over 55,000 people, including many doctors, signed a petition supporting a bill that had been presented to the Legislature of Ontario to allow Rene to continue treating patients who had been deemed incurable by doctors, without constant harassment from the Ontario Ministry of Health and the threat of arrest for practicing medicine without a license, using an unapproved method, refusing to reveal the exact herbs used in Essiac, and refusing to confine herself to testing it exclusively on mice.

As for practicing medicine without a license, she said, "I am a nurse, not a doctor, therefore I always made sure that every case was diagnosed by a qualified physician, and as often as possible administered treatment under the observation of doctors."

As for confining herself to testing it exclusively on mice, she said, "I felt it was inhuman for them to ask me to give up treating patients while I showed them whether it would work on mice. . . . I have done a great deal of animal research. . . . I found that on mice . . . after 9 days of Essiac . . . the growth would regress until it was no longer invading the living tissue."

Rightly or wrongly, she never revealed which herbs she used, or how, to anyone except a few close friends sworn to secrecy.

Rene had a compelling reason for not revealing her recipe. She said that every herbal remedy researchers got their hands on disappeared once they got its formula—discredited in favor of far more expensive drugs and treatments.

She said she would have gladly given her formula to the medical community if only they had conceded that Essiac had some merit, and had promised that it would be used to help suffering humanity. But they refused.

So she kept her secret—until a year before she died. At that point, she sold the formula for $1 to a drug company she thought would distribute it widely. But tests dragged on—and were still going on when she died at age 90 (following hip surgery). Rene was fed up. She wanted it used immediately on suffering humanity.

Compelling Testimonies

As a result, hearings were held by the Royal Cancer Commission in March 1939. The six doctors on the panel were all surgeons, radiologists, and diagnosticians. The chairman was an Ontario Supreme Court judge. Out of 387 people who came in support of Rene—all former patients—49 were allowed to testify. They all said she had saved their lives after they had been diagnosed as incurable—with very little time left—by doctors and specialists.

Reported testimony before the Commission:

Tony Bazuik, a railroad watchman, had received radium treatments for lip cancer that left his mouth so swollen and sore he could not eat or breathe through it. The pain forced him to quit work. Friends gave him money for a trip to Bracebridge to see Rene Caisse. "His face was so disfigured it was unbearable to look at," she said. He felt immediate relief after his first dose of Essiac, but could not return for a second visit. Even so, after only one treatment, his lip returned to normal. He went back to work, never had a recurrence, and almost 40 years later, at age 79, he told a Canadian magazine he could: "Eat for one man, work for three, and sleep like a baby."

Annie Bonner had been diagnosed with cancer of the cervix which was inoperable because it had spread to other organs. "I suffered agonies for 10 days with radium needles," she said. Then she had x-ray treatments every day—sometimes twice a day—except when she was too badly burned. So weak she could not stand without help, she was down to 90 pounds (from 120).

After 9 weeks in the hospital, and a year of x-ray treatments, the cancer spread up her right side to her shoulder. Her arm swelled to twice its size and turned black. It was too painful to be touched. Her doctor advised her to have her arm amputated. He said it was dead and would remain useless.

Just before checking into a hospital to have the arm amputated, she decided to try Essiac treatments with Rene Caisse. "I was so weak that I had to lie down in the back of the car," she said. "But after a few treatments I began to feel much better. The swelling gradually went down in the arm and my appetite improved."

After 4 months on Essiac, her arm was back to normal, her weight was up to 150, and x-ray exams showed she was cancer-free. "I am feeling quite well," she wrote, "able to do all my own housework. I thank God for sparing me."

She was outraged to learn that even though she had been faced with the loss of her arm after a year of x-ray treatments, the Commission listed her case as "recovery due to radiation."

Walter Hampson testified that he had been diagnosed as having cancer of the lip. After receiving the pathologist's report, his doctor urged Mr. Hampson to go immediately for radium treatment. The patient refused and came to Rene's clinic instead for Essiac treatments. "I cured Mr. Hampson," said Rene, "and he went before the Commission on July 4, 1939. . . . In spite of the fact that he had never had an operation, other than having a small nodule removed for analysis, this case is listed in the Royal Commission's report as recovery due to surgery." He was still living, with no recurrence, when contacted 23 years later.

May Henderson was told by her doctor that she had tumors in both breasts, and needed a double mastectomy. Then she was told she had a large tumor in her uterus. "My color was muddy yellow, my hair thin and lifeless and my eyes gray and stony. I hemorrhaged so badly I thought I would die, and couldn't stand up for any length of time." Her doctor said she was beyond help. But she gave his written diagnosis to Rene, and was started on Essiac.

"At first," she said, "the lumps seemed to grow harder, but then the turning point came and I discharged great masses of fleshy material." She told her story to the Committee in March 1939. *In 1977—40 years later—at age 82, she said she was healthy and never had a recurrence.*

Nellie McVittie was down to a mere 86 pounds when she was carried—bleeding—into Rene's clinic one day in 1935. Her doctor said she had cancer of the uterus and neck of the womb. The neck of the womb had been cauterized and subjected to radium treatments. At Rene's clinic she was given Essiac treatments for about 2 months. "I got relief almost immediately," she later wrote, "and have had no more recurrence of my old trouble since then."

Herbert Rawson, 48, was diagnosed by two doctors, with carcinoma of the rectum, confirmed by x-rays, in 1935. He had a hard mass with sloughing and bleeding and great pain. When he refused surgery, his doctor gave him a written diagnosis and permission to treat with Essiac. Treatments began in April

1935, and the last of 30 was given in May 1936, at which time he showed a good improvement in weight. Except for 1 month of rest, he was able to work all during treatment. No trace of cancer was found in 1936 when he was examined by three physicians. He died of a stroke at age 73, having survived his ordeal by 25 years.

John Thornbury testified that his wife, Clara, had been diagnosed by x-ray 2 years before as having probable cancer of the stomach, and had been so weak, at 72 pounds, that he'd had to carry her into Rene's clinic. Mrs. Thornbury testified as well, saying that she now weighed 107 pounds, and could do all her own work. *(She lived to be 91—having survived her ordeal by 36 years.)*

John Tynan testified he had cancer of the bowel and rectum, which had been diagnosed by four doctors. The growth had broken through the bladder wall, and he had been operated on twice, and told that nothing could be done. Four years after treatment by Rene, he had gained 39 pounds, and was in good health.

The Royal Commission said that x-ray reports were not acceptable as diagnoses. They demanded pathological reports. When Rene presented patients who'd been diagnosed with cancer by the government pathologist, the head of the College of Physicians and Surgeons said, "even the pathologist could be wrong."

The Commission would not consider any recovery due to Essiac unless there had been no other treatment previously given. But in the majority of cases, patients were sent to Rene only after everything else had failed.

The head of the College of Physicians and Surgeons said if Rene's patients had been cured by Essiac without having been given orthodox treatments, then they had not suffered from cancer. In these cases, the Commission said that the doctors had all been mistaken in their diagnoses. In other words, in the 49 cases they agreed to hear, over 100 doctors had been wrong, because most patients had seen more than one doctor, and some had seen three or four.

Nearly all recoveries were attributed to surgery, radiation, deep x-ray therapy, cobalt, and nitrogen mustard gas—even though most had suffered relapses and been diagnosed as terminal by the time Essiac was begun.

During the course of the hearings, several doctors recanted their diagnoses. Others testified that former patients of theirs had not benefited from Rene's treatments and had since died.

Πot a Cure, But Brings Comfort, Relieves Pain

Rene freely admitted that a great many of the people who came to her could not be helped, and that all she could hope to do was make them comfortable, and perhaps extend their lives a bit. She said this treatment made tumors smaller, after six to eight treatments, and easier to remove surgically, with much less risk of spreading; that it relieved pain, prolonged life, and that in some patients not too far gone, remission was possible.

The Commission rejected Essiac as having any merit as a cancer remedy, saying that they had no choice, since they had no idea what was in it. Rene said she'd gladly reveal what was in it, if they would admit that people had been helped by it. They refused.

In 1942, Rene Caisse, fearing imprisonment, closed her clinic. For the next 30 years, she continued to treat patients in great secrecy in her home. She was constantly under surveillance by officers of the Canadian Health Department, facing a 7-year prison sentence if caught giving anything to help a cancer patient. When people came to her begging for help, she'd give them some free Essiac, pleading with them to hide it until they were safely out of sight.

"Remarkably Beneficial Results"

In 1959, at the age of 70, Rene was invited by Dr. Charles Brusch—President Kennedy's physician—to treat both terminal cancer patients and laboratory animals with Essiac, at the Brusch Medical Centre in Massachusetts. This she did, under the supervision of 18 doctors. After 3 months, Dr. Brusch and his research director, Dr. Charles McClure, issued this statement:

"[Essiac] has been shown to cause a decided recession of the mass and a definite change in cell formation [in mice]. . . . Clinically, on patients suffering from pathologically proven cancer, it reduces pain and causes a recession in the growth; patients have gained weight and shown an improvement in their general health . . .

"Remarkably beneficial results were obtained even on those cases at the 'end of the road' where it proved to prolong life and the quality of that life. . . . This . . . has convinced the doctors at the Brusch Medical Centre that Essiac has merit in the treatment of cancer. The doctors do not say that Essiac is a cure, but they do say it is of benefit. It is non-toxic . . ."

While Rene was at the Brusch Medical Centre in 1959 questionnaires were sent to some of her former patients, to see if they were still alive, and if they ever had a recurrence. And from time to time, Rene herself sent out letters of inquiry. Signed statements came back as follows:

+ Mr. Tony Bozuik, 22 years, no recurrence (40 years by 1977, age 79).
+ Mr. Jack Finley, 20 years, no recurrence (age 60 in 1959).
+ Mrs. E. Forsythe, 24 years, no recurrence.
+ Mr. Wilson Hammell, 22 years, no recurrence (39 years by 1976).
+ Mr. Walter Hampson, 15 years, no recurrence.
+ Mrs. Lillian Heller, 11 years, no recurrence.
+ Miss May Henderson, 20 years, no recurrence.
+ Mrs. D. H. Laundry, 11 years, no recurrence (age 78 in 1959).
+ Mr. John McNee, 30 years, no recurrence (age 91 in 1959).
+ Mrs. Nellie McVittie, 23 years, no recurrence (age 65 in 1959).
+ Mr. Herbert K. Rawson, 28 years, no recurrence.
+ Mrs. Jessie Slater, 11 years, no recurrence.
+ Mrs. J. H. Stewart, 16 years, no recurrence (age 76 in 1959).
+ Mr. Norman Thompson, 20 years, no recurrence.

+ Mrs. Clara Thornbury, 22 years, no recurrence (age 75, lived to age 91).
+ Mrs. G. Tibble, 25 years, no recurrence.
+ Mrs. Eliza Veitch, 18 years, no recurrence (age 76, lived to age 83).
+ Mrs. Lena Wagner, 18 years, no recurrence.
+ Mrs. Lizzie Pearl Ward, 14 years, no recurrence.
+ Mr. Frank Walter, 20 years, no recurrence (37 years by 1976).
+ Mrs. Hattie M. Wurts, 20 years, no recurrence.

"There's Something To It"

In a Winnipeg newspaper, the *Free Press,* for November 5, 1977, Dr. Brusch is quoted as saying, "If it wasn't any good the Sloan-Kettering Cancer Institute would not have continued testing it all these years. They were trying to find out what it was . . . there's something to it."

This article cites two of Brusch's own carefully documented cases:

Patrick McGrail, 60, had been suffering from cancer of the esophagus, in the advanced stage. A former gourmet chef, he could not eat or sleep because of constant pain. "I had an operation and 10 chemotherapy treatments and it was terrible," says McGrail. "I could have done better just drinking this Essiac. It's saved me. The pain is gone. I'm gaining weight. I'm going to live."

(When last heard from, McGrail had gained 20 pounds and was still alive 11 years later, still drinking an ounce of Essiac nightly before bed.)

George Gallagher, 60, vice president of a large company, found he had cancer in July 1976. Six months later, he was operated on and took chemotherapy twice. After seeing people being kept barely alive, losing hair, and in great pain, he went home and began treatments with a naturopath. But he continued losing weight (down to 90 pounds) and suffering. The end seemed near when he started taking Essiac. "The results were amazing in the first 3 days," said Gallagher's son. "His blood count jumped out of the danger zone and back up to where it is considered healthy. For the first time in six months his appetite came back . . . his pain went away and he could get a restful sleep. He's been taking Essiac for a couple of months now, drinking it like cold tea. My dad has gone up six pounds in weight. He's started to have an interest in life again. He's reading again and exercising. He can really feel the Essiac working."

But the article also goes on to quote Dr. Joseph Whiteman, director of the Ontario Cancer Research Foundation, who "like almost everyone in cancer research before him is down on Essiac."

"It has been tested in a preliminary way by a couple of doctors on a group of patients who are terminal cases so to speak and none of them have made any significant responses," says Whiteman. "They have had no results. . . . We have a thick file of documentation on Essiac, and I have been over it carefully. My opinion is that Essiac is not a useful remedy. I think in the past there was always the problem of whether patients really had cancer or were responding to treatment they previously had. When taking Essiac some seemed to have improved but most of them had some kind of spontaneous remission or something—some spontaneous lift just from the fact that they were hopeful.

"I don't believe anyone with cancer should use Essiac," Dr. Whiteman said. "I wouldn't recommend it. I feel the same about Laetrile. I think the substance or value of Laetrile and Essiac is about even. I don't think much of either of them."

About 4 months after that interview, Dr. Whiteman was suddenly stricken with stomach cancer and died on March 8, 1978.

"I Am 100% for Essiac"

This same 1977 article quotes Dr. Charles Brusch, M.D., as saying: "I am 100% for Essiac or I would not have been using it. . . . I never use the word cure because they'll always say there has been a remission. But there will be a control for cancer—like high blood pressure or diabetes. You'll be able to control it."

In another interview in 1977 for *Homemaker's* magazine, a Canadian publication, Dr. Brusch said, "Essiac has tremendous merit to supplement any therapy a cancer patient may be using. . . . I regard it as essential to back up any other therapy."

In 1990, Dr. Brusch was still endorsing Essiac. He claimed to have been using it himself since 1984, when he had several cancer operations. "I have in fact cured my own cancer," he claimed, "the original site of which was the lower bowels, through Essiac alone."

How to Make Essiac

It must be stressed at the outset that in giving this information, no cancer cure is claimed. No one can guarantee pain relief or cures, nor is any food a cure-all for any ailment. You are advised to seek a doctor's advice immediately for any condition you may have. Self-treatment is not recommended, nor should any foods listed here be used as the sole means of treating any ailment, unless your doctor approves.

Today, premixed, commercially prepared Essiac is unapproved for marketing in the United States and Canada as an anti-cancer medicine. But a number of over-the-counter herbal products have sprung up, sold only as herbal tea, that claim to contain the same herbs Rene Caisse used.

I favor the do-it-yourself method of preparing this herbal tea by buying the herbs you need, mixing them together, and steeping them in boiling water, because it's hard to tell whether a premixed product follows Rene Caisse's exact formula. I wouldn't feel safe otherwise.

In January 1995, in a move to guarantee public access to Essiac, Rene's close friend and assistant for over 40 years, Mary McPherson, turned over notarized copies of the original Essiac formula in Rene Caisse's handwriting to the Town of Bracebridge in a simple ceremony at the town hall.

Shortly afterward, the recipe was printed in its entirety in both the *Bracebridge Herald-Gazette* (January 11, 1995) and the *Bracebridge Examiner* (March 29, 1995).

The *Examiner* article—which appears to be reprinted from 1982—quotes Mrs. McPherson as saying, "I want people to know exactly what Rene's Essiac is like." (Referring to all the commercial imitations.) She first met Rene in 1935 when her mother was suffering from cancer, and received treatments at Rene's clinic. Her mother was cured, and lived another 30 years, in good health, passing away in 1965, at the age of 86.

Mary then worked with Rene, helping her brew the Essiac, assisting her in running the clinic and looking after patients.

In 1945, Mary's own husband, Clifford, was stricken with cancer. She says that Rene's Essiac treatment cured him, and he lived another 36 years, passing away "only last year" at the age of 81.

Although she worked with Rene for over 20 years, helping her brew Essiac, she says she never knew the specific ingredients until after Rene's death in 1978.

"Rene always told me there was an envelope with my name on it in a dresser drawer in her house on Hiram Street," Mary recalls, "and I was to have it once she passed away. The envelope contained the recipe for [Essiac]."

Here are some important points to remember about the four ingredients:

1. *Sheep Sorrel:* This bitter herb from the Last Supper is a common plant in Canada, the United States, and in most temperate regions of the world, where it grows in open areas and meadows, and is gathered in early summer. It can be started from seeds, and if the leaves alone are gathered, a planting can last 3–4 years. It is a perennial miniature of garden sorrel. It must be green in color and have an aroma of sweet grass. If you gather it in the wild, make sure you bring someone along who can teach you to recognize it, because its arrow-shaped leaves are similar to other plants, some of which are dangerous. There appear to be several store-bought types of sorrel on the market today of an inferior quality, which may or may not be related to the sorrel family. Sheila Snow, who spent 2-1/2 years inter-

viewing Rene Caisse for a book on this subject called *The Essence of Essiac* (1994) says that since this is the primary herb in Essiac, one must become thoroughly acquainted with its appearance, aroma, and taste, which is bitter.

2. *Burdock:* Burdock is a Bible plant referred to in Isaiah and Hosea (see page 00). The roots look like carrots and can be cut into slices to dry. When dried, it has a sweet taste. The root must be harvested in October from the first-year plant. Rene's long-time friend and assistant, Mary McPherson, said she was worried about false imitations. "I have seen a fine powder called Essiac," she says. "In fact, true Essiac is full of burdock root chunks." (It is the only plant in the formula that is cut, not powdered.)

3. *Slippery Elm Bark:* Slippery elm bark is a Bible plant referred to in Genesis (see page 89). It's available at any reputable health-food store and it must be a light brown powder. It tastes much like flour. One expert points out that sometimes the commercial product is adulterated with flour or other starchy substances which create a gravy-like decoction, so beware. Ask for pure powdered slippery elm bark—made from the inner bark. It should be light beige.

4. *Turkish Rhubarb Root:* This product may be purchased in health-food stores, as a powder, or in root form. The plants are native to China and Tibet. Rene preferred this variety because its medicinal properties were stronger and the taste less bitter than garden rhubarb. It is yellowish-brown in color. Common rhubarb may be substituted, but the plant must be at least 3 years old.

Below is Rene Caisse's original recipe as transmitted to her friend and colleague, Mary McPherson. *(Use a measuring cup, not a scale.)*

Essiac

1 pound (16 oz.) of sheep sorrel herb *(powdered)*

6-1/2 cups (52 oz.) of burdock root *(cut)*

1/4 pound (4 oz.) of slippery elm [inner] bark *(powdered)*

1 ounce Turkish rhubarb root *(powdered)*

"Mix these ingredients thoroughly and store in glass jar in dark dry cupboard.

"Take a measuring cup. Use 1 ounce of herb mixture to 32 ounces [1 quart] of water depending on the amount you want to make. [Most herbalists recommend using pure spring water or distilled water.]

"I use 1 cup of mixture [8 oz.] to 256 ounces [2 gallons] of water. Boil hard for 20 minutes (covered) then turn off heat but leave sitting on warm plate [or heating element of stove] overnight, covered.

"In the morning [after it has been sitting 10–12 hours] heat steaming hot and let settle for a few minutes, then strain through fine strainer into hot sterilized bottles. [Cap while hot.] Let sit to cool. Store in dark cool cupboard. Must be refrigerated when opened. When near the last when it's thick, pour in a large jar and sit in fridge overnight, then pour off all you can without sediment [and use].

"This recipe *must* be followed *exactly* as written. I use a granite preserving kettle (10–12 quarts), 8 oz. measuring cup, small funnel and fine strainer to fill bottles."

+   +   +

This simple recipe—which at present would cost about $40 a year—is what all the fuss was about. In an article called "Rene Caisse's formula: It's one of the worst-kept secrets in Muskoka" (*Herald Gazette,* December 22, 1993), staff writer Doug Specht says: "For $40, you can buy enough herbs to make a year's worth of tonic. All you add is two gallons of pure spring water, brew in a stainless steel container, strain, then bottle and store in a cool, dry place." (Just make sure the herbs are organically grown, free of pesticides.)

Pre-mixed versions of this tea cost considerably more. But you can buy the dried herbs and mix them yourself, for pennies a serving. (See Where to Buy Herbs, page 89.)

This recipe produces a large amount of Essiac (6 quarts or 192 1-ounce doses), presumably because it's the recipe Rene used in the 1930s when she prepared it for hundreds of people at a time. That's a 6-month supply, at the rate of an ounce a day. You can try making larger or smaller amounts using the basic proportion of 1 ounce of herb mixture to 32 ounces of water.

Rene always used a measuring cup, never a scale. Most herbalists recommend granite or stainless steel pots, amber glass bottles with airtight caps, a small fine-mesh stainless steel strainer, a large stainless steel spoon, a stainless steel funnel, pure spring water or sodium-free distilled water. When finally ready, they recommend pouring the brew into hot sterilized bottles, one at a time, using the funnel, capping the bottles firmly and allowing them to cool. When cool, tighten the caps again, and store bottles in a cool dark cupboard until needed. Once opened, it must be stored in a refrigerator but never frozen.

Dosage

Reportedly, these are Rene's instructions for taking Essiac:

1. Take 1 ounce of Essiac with 2 ounces of warm water every second day at bedtime, on an empty stomach, at least 2–3 hours after supper.

2. Do not eat or drink anything for at least 1 hour after taking Essiac.

3. Do not take any medications at the same time as Essiac. Allow at least 3 hours between them. Or ask your doctor if they can be taken sooner.

4. Continue the treatment every other day for 32 days, then take the treatment every 3 days.

5. Once you start using a bottle of Essiac, keep it refrigerated but never in the freezer.

Rene believed that small amounts of Essiac taken over an extended period of time were safer than frequent stronger doses.

Non-toxic

Rene always claimed that Essiac is made from non-toxic herbs, and the doctors in their statements about Essiac seemed to agree:

> "We believe the treatment for cancer by Rene Caisse *can do no harm, and that it relieves pain, will reduce enlargement and prolong life in hopeless cases.*"—statement of eight doctors, to the Department of National Health and Welfare at Ottawa, October 27, 1926.

> "Essiac has merit in the treatment of cancer. The doctors do not say that Essiac is a cure, but they do say it is of benefit. *It is non-toxic. . . .*"—statement issued by Charles Brusch, M.D., and Charles McClure, M.D., of the Brusch Medical Centre, Cambridge, Massachusetts, Fall 1959.

"Since no evidence has ever been presented at any time by any person, scientists or otherwise, that there is the slightest toxicity, or undesirable reaction, to the use of Essiac, and evidence has been presented that is overwhelming that it has proved of great benefit, it is difficult for me to understand the reluctance of the medical profession to its use," said Rene (*I Was "Canada's Cancer Nurse," The Story of Essiac,* by Rene Caisse, R.N., 1980).

The Turning Point

Rene noticed there was usually a crisis at some point, after which the patients seemed to feel better. Often they'd report an enlarging and hardening of a tumor; then it would begin to soften and the patient would report discharging large amounts of pus and fleshy material. After this, the tumor would seem to be gone, and they suddenly felt completely normal.

For example, the *Vancouver Sun* for June 3, 1992 reports the case of a 70-year-old woman with an ovarian tumor. Told she had 2 months to a year to live, she quit chemotherapy after 5 months and told her doctors she preferred to die in peace. "I was not even human," she said. "I was sick to my stomach. I had headaches, fevers. I was not eating. I was going downhill very fast." Then she heard about Essiac, tried it, and is certain is saved her life. After 6 weeks on Essiac, she awoke one night, thinking she had wet the bed. She looked and saw thick, grayish matter pouring from her. Over the next 2 weeks she excreted "awful stuff." But she says, "I started to feel so good, I couldn't believe anybody could feel so good. I felt better than I had in 10–15 years." When she returned to the clinic for a scheduled examination, the doctor just said, "I'm giving you a clean bill of health." Then he walked out. He didn't ask what she had taken, what she had done. He didn't seem to care.

Other Conditions Helped

That's not all. The woman in this case history had developed diabetes and was taking insulin before she started taking Essiac. After her ovarian tumor disappeared, she noticed she was having a reaction to insulin and slowly tapered off her insulin injections. Did Essiac cure her diabetes? "All I know is that I take nothing for diabetes now," she said.

Her husband, 71, had a prostate problem for years. At night, every half hour he'd have to get up to urinate. It was painful and exhausting. Doctors told him his condition wasn't serious enough yet to warrant surgery. He started taking Essiac, and instead of urinating he got up one night and excreted a large amount of pus. He had a wonderful night's sleep and hasn't been bothered with any prostate symptoms since then.

In a publication called *Fifty Plus,* for April 1994, we are told of a 28-year-old woman who was suffering from a thyroid condition. She was taking a prescription drug, which she had been told could clear up the condition. It didn't. The cyst on her thyroid gland got bigger, and she began to suffer from weight gain, irritability, fatigue, irregular menstruation. Her doctor recommended that her thyroid be removed before it turned cancerous. She decided against it. Then a friend told her about Essiac, and showed her how to make it. Since starting on Essiac, she has been told that the cyst on her thyroid is draining away. The hard lump in her throat has softened to the point where it's almost invisible to the naked eye.

At 90, Rene Caisse had outlived most of her opponents in her battle to get Essiac recognized as a powerful remedy against disease. Alert and very active, right to the end, she died following hip surgery, a few months before Christmas 1978. Her longevity and freedom from disease have been attributed to the Essiac she took twice a week for nearly 50 years.

"Essiac supplies the body with the resistance required to prolong life, to relieve pain and to cure if taken before the malignant cells have invaded and destroyed the vital organs," she wrote.

"Ulcers are very often a forerunner of cancer and can and are being cured by Essiac. It acts on all the glands in the human body, restoring them to health and activity. It gives the patient a new mental outlook—a happy healthy outlook, which the disease had taken away."

Some AIDS patients report that drastically low T-cell counts have risen to normal since they started using Essiac. Although the focus on Essiac has been as a cancer treatment, it has reportedly alleviated and sometimes cured many chronic and degenerative conditions because it cleanses the body as well as the liver and strengthens the immune system.

A Closer Look at Essiac

Three of the herbs in Essiac have been mentioned individually, at one time or another, by various experts, as having anti-cancer properties. And three out of four of these herbs are from the Bible.

"A Miracle Herb"

Writing about sheep sorrel—a bitter herb from the Last Supper—famed French herbalist Maurice Messegue says: "Certain doctors in the sixteenth and seventeenth century came near to regarding it as a miracle herb for cases of infection, fevers, scurvy and poisoning.

"I once knew a farmer who treated himself with nothing but sorrel, and personally I have found it very useful. . . . I recommend it for all urinary or digestive malfunctions, for blockages of the stomach and intestines, for hemorrhoids, for mouth and throat ulcers . . . and for fighting fevers in general.

"Used externally it is an excellent treatment for skin troubles such as herpes and acne, as well as for abscesses and ulcers. Its roots and its seeds are particularly useful for diarrhea, stomach ache, colic and dysentery."[2]

Sheep sorrel contains oxalic acid, which can interfere with calcium metabolism—if you consume immense quantities every day for weeks, says herbalist Steve Brill.[3] "Still, I've never heard of anyone getting sick from eating normal quantities of sheep sorrel. A European woman I know raves about enjoying sorrel soup with fruit and bread for dinner every day, attributing her good health to this vegetable. However, you should avoid anything with oxalic acid if you have kidney disease or rheumatoid arthritis."

Dr. Jonathan Hartwell, formerly of the National Cancer Institute, in Bethesda, Maryland, carefully screened thousands of plants for anti-cancer activity, and his reports appeared in "Plants Against Cancer," a survey in the scientific journal *Lloydia* (1967–71). Dr. Hartwell cites sheep sorrel's use in cancer of the face, hand, and throat. John Heinerman lists it among specific herbs used for breast and internal cancers, in *The Treatment of Cancer with Herbs* (1980). James Duke, Ph.D., formerly head of the Germplasm Resources Laboratory of the U.S. Department of Agriculture, mentions sheep sorrel's use for cancer and skin tumors, in *Medicinal Plants of the Bible* (1983). Aloe emodin, isolated from sorrel, shows "significant anti-leukemic activity" (*Lloydia,* 1976; *39*:223–4).

---

[2]From *Health Secrets of Plants and Herbs* by Maurice Messegue. Copyright © 1975 by Opera Mundi. Copyright © 1979 by William Collins & Co., Ltd. By permission of William Morrow & Company, Inc.

[3]From *Identifying and Harvesting Edible and Medicinal Plants* by Steve Brill and Evelyn Dean. Text: Copyright © 1994 by Steve Brill. Text and illustrations: Copyright © 1994 by Evelyn Dean. By permission of William Morrow & Company, Inc.

Burdock

Burdock is one of the many burr-producing plants of Palestine, referred to in Isaiah 34:13 and Hosea 9:6, according to experts cited in *Plants of the Bible* by Harold N. Moldenke, Ph.D., and Alma Moldenke.

Two Hungarian scientists in 1966 found "considerable antitumor activity" in a purified fraction of burdock. A chemical in burbock called arctigenin was identified as a growth "inhibitor" in 1970 (*Chemotherapy, 15*:250). Japanese researchers at Nagoya University in 1984 found in burdock a new type of substance which they named the B-factor, for "burdock factor," that reduces cell mutations (*Mutation Research, 129*:1:25, 1984). Burbock is active in the test tube against HIV (*Bulletin of World Health Organization,* 1989, 67:613–18).

"Burdock is one of the best and safest herbal medicines," say Steve Brill and Evelyn Dean.[4] "Many people swear by this herb, relating miracles that would put many doctors to shame. Burdock is used for liver dysfunction, urinary tract disorders, and weight loss. . . . As a general detoxifier and immune-system stimulant, it helps people without clear-cut pathologies who don't feel well. . . .

"People with sugar metabolism problems or chronic weakness often have stomach, kidney, liver and/or lymphatic problems. Burdock root, with its high mineral levels, will build, stabilize, and detoxify these organs. . . . It's helpful for colds, with antimicrobial action. . . . Its demulcent action soothes the upper respiratory tract's mucous membranes. . . . The combination of diuretic and antibiotic effects make this an excellent herb for cystitis."

Burdock root-catnip tea is a great remedy for breaking up, dissolving, and eliminating some stubborn kidney stones and gallstones, according to medical anthropologist Dr. John Heinerman.[5]

Burdock can eliminate many acute and chronic skin problems. The result? Clear, vibrant skin. Dr. Heinerman says that bur-

---

[4]*Identifying and Harvesting Edible and Medicinal Plants, op. cit.*

[5]Heinerman, *Heinerman's Encyclopedia of Fruits, Vegetables and Herbs,* West Nyack, NY: Parker Publishing Company, Inc., 1988.

dock is *the* most important herb for treating chronic skin problems. He says it's one of the few that can effectively treat eczema, acne, psoriasis, boils, herpes and syphilitic sores, sties, carbuncles, cankers, and the like. He recommends drinking burdock tea or using it to wash the skin.[6] To make the tea, bring 1 quart of water to a boil, reduce heat to simmer, add 4 teaspoons cut, dried burdock root, cover, and let simmer for 7 minutes, remove from heat, allow to steep 2 hours longer. Drink 2 cups per day on an empty stomach. Or capsules, four per day, may be taken instead (available at health-food stores).

French herbalist Maurice Messegue writes: "My father was once visited by a farmer who was covered with boils and was in very great pain and distress. The treatment prescribed was entirely that of burdock infusions to be taken internally, and baths and tinctures externally. In eight days all the boils had disappeared."[7]

Burdock root is considered relatively safe, but it is a uterine stimulant that should not be used by pregnant women.

Turkish Rhubarb

Rhubarb, too, is relatively safe but is a strong laxative that should not be used by pregnant or nursing women, or those with chronic intestinal problems, such as colitis. Heinerman says: "Rhubarb has demonstrated some excellent tumor-blocking abilities." He cites the first supplement of volume 20 of *Pharmacology,* which revealed that two of the laxative compounds in rhubarb—rhein and emodin—at a relatively high dose, also blocked Ehrlich and mammary tumors in mice by 75 percent.

Heinerman also cites a 1984 issue of *Journal of Ethnopharmacology,* which reported that rhein and emodin inhibited the growth of malignant melanoma at a daily dosage of 50 mg. per kilogram of body weight. The percentages of inhibition were 76 percent for rhein and 73 percent for emodin.[8]

---

[6]Heinerman, *ibid.*
[7]*Health Secrets of Plants and Herbs, op. cit.*
[8]Heinerman, *op. cit.*

Turkish rhubarb (named after a trade route through Turkey) comes from China. It is much larger than the garden variety of rhubarb used in pies, the root being the part used medicinally. John Heinerman, who visited the People's Republic of China in 1980 with a group of medical students, says "in certain parts of mainland China, rhubarb juice and rhubarb tea are used in the treatment of some forms of cancer with good success. About 1/2 cup of the juice twice daily, obtained by putting fresh stalks through a mechanical juicer, are administered to patients. More often, though, tea is made by simmering 2 cups of finely chopped stalks in 1 quart of boiling water, covered, for up to an hour. Afterwards, the liquid is strained off and given to cancer victims in 1-cup amounts two to three times a day."[9]

He says that in clinical studies at the Central Hospital of Luwan District in Shanghai in the early 1980s, nearly 900 cases of upper digestive-tract bleeding, 57 percent from duodenal ulcers, were treated with rhubarb powder, tablets, or syrup, given in 1 teaspoonful equivalents three times a day until the bleeding stopped, usually in 2 days or less. The success rate was 97 percent. This effect from rhubarb, he says, may be due to its tannic acid, which constricts blood vessels.

In 100 cases of acute inflammation of the pancreas (pancreatitis) and 10 cases of acute inflammation of the gall bladder (cholecystitis), full recovery was achieved with 4 tablespoonsful of a decoction of rhubarb between five and ten times a day. Related symptoms such as abdominal pain, high fever and jaundice usually cleared up in 5 days or less.

To make a decoction for any of these problems, says Heinerman, simmer 2-1/2 tablespoons of cut, dried Chinese rhubarb root in 1-1/2 quarts or 6 cups of boiling water, covered, for 40 minutes, or until about half (3 cups) of the liquid remains. Strain this and take as indicated for the aforementioned digestive problems.[10]

In China, rhubarb root is also used for toothache. They fry the root, then steep it in alcohol to create a tincture. Then, using a cotton ball, they apply the tincture directly to the painful tooth for 5 minutes. Rhubarb contains at least six pain-relieving chemical compounds.

---

[9]Heinerman, *op. cit.*
[10]Heinerman, *op. cit.*

Slippery Elm

The elm is thought by some scholars to be the terebinth tree under which Abraham entertained the three angels (Genesis 37:25). Slippery elm has no reported ill effects. Its unusually soothing quality is due to an abundance of mucilage-containing cells in the bark. When the bark, in strips or powdered form, comes into contact with water, the mucilage cells swell enormously, thus producing a smooth, lubricating effect. It has been used to cover wounds and to soothe a sore throat, inflamed nipples (mastitis), ulcers, colitis, and other gastrointestinal ailments. It has even been used to treat syphilis, gonorrhea, hemorrhoids, and burns, and bring boils to a head.

Slippery elm's reputation for speeding the healing of broken bones is legendary, dating back to the first century. The story is told of a Mormon settlement in Caldwell, Missouri, that was attacked by bandits in 1838. Many settlers were shot and wounded. One young boy had his entire hip joint completely blasted away by gunfire. His mother prayed to God for help. A Voice told her to carefully wash out all the dirt from his open wound, then to get some roots and bark from a nearby slippery-elm tree, pound them into a soft, mushy pulp with a rock, and pack this directly into the wound until it was full, and dress it with clean linen. This soft pulpy material was replaced every few days. The boy completely healed in about 5 weeks. A pliable cartilage had grown over the missing joint and socket, enabling the boy to walk normally and to lead a normal life.

Slippery elm shows promise in treating heart attacks and a wide range of inflammatory diseases. That is because slippery elm contains a protein called CR1 (complement receptor one) that limits damage from heart attacks in lab animals. In those treated with CR1, the area of damage was more than 30 percent less than in animals that were not treated with it. Only two plants—slippery elm and yarrow—have CR1.

Where to Buy Herbs

Unless you're an expert at identifying, harvesting, and preparing medicinal plants yourself—capable of going into the woods and wildcrafting them (which involves getting on your hands and knees and clipping off or digging out the right parts)—or unless you know and trust someone who can do this for you, you have to either buy a pre-mixed version of this tea (which may or may not follow Rene's exact formula), or purchase the herbs and mix them yourself.

If local natural-food stores are not available, you may try ordering by phone from the following list of experienced herb dealers (who are in no way connected with the author or publisher of this book). Ask for organically-grown brands:

Gilbert Blondin
P.O. Box 20111
Ottawa, Ontario K1N9N5
819-777-8070
(Pre-mixed herbs brewed as tea.)

Indiana Botanic Gardens
P.O.B. 5
Hammond, IN 46325
Orders: 1-800-644-8327
Customer Service: 1-800-514-1068
Local: 219-947-4040
Fax: 219-947-4148
(Recommended for purchase of individual herbs.)

Muskoka Natural Food Market
Box 2228
Bracebridge, Ontario P1L1W1
705-645-5471
(Recommended for purchase of pre-mixed dry herbs.)

Nature's Herb Company
Box 118, Dept. 34, Q
Norway, IA 52318
1-800-365-4372
(Recommended for purchase of individual herbs.)

Nature's Way Products, Inc.
10 Mountain Springs
Springville, UT 84663
801-489-3635
(Recommended for purchase of individual herbs.)

Still Deemed Unproven

No one has ever been able to explain why this herbal tea got results in thousands of cases when Rene Caisse prepared it, or when certain people she trusted with the formula—such as President Kennedy's physician—made it and used it, but never when various health authorities tested it.

For example, in 1977, Gilbert Blondin of Hull, Ontario, watched his wife, mother of three young children, recover from a lymphosarcoma 3 months after she began taking Essiac directly from Rene Caisse. Fourteen years later, when her story was told in *The Canadian Journal of Herbalism* for July 1991 ("Old Ontario Remedies 1922: Rene Caisse, Essiac" by Sheila Snow), she was still free of cancer. When Rene refused any offer of financial remuneration, her husband returned to paint her living quarters and do some needed repairs on her house which had been neglected because of her preoccupation with patients. She was so touched by his generosity that they became friends. It is believed she taught him how to prepare the recipe for his wife in order to avoid the long trip to Bracebridge every 2 weeks.

As word spread of his wife's recovery, people came to Blondin for help, and when demand for the brew increased, he quit his trade to work full time producing it. After some controversy in the court system as to whether it was a food or a drug, the final court ruling was that his product was considered to be a food, and is still sold on that basis in Canada. (For information, call 819-777-8070.) I recently spoke to Mrs. Blondin by phone, and was able to verify that she is still alive and well 22 years after Rene Caisse's treatment.

During the entire 50 years that Rene Caisse spent helping—and in many cases saving—the thousands of patients who came to her, she was threatened with arrest and imprisonment for doing so, and the herbal remedy she gave them was declared worthless.

A report issued by the Health Protection Branch of the Canadian Health and Welfare Department finds that "no clinical evidence exists to support claims that Essiac is an effective treatment for cancer." In 1982, says the report, 74 doctors who had been supplied with Essiac reported on 87 cancer patients, of whom 78 showed no benefit. Of the remaining nine cases, four still had worsening cancer, two died, and in three cases the disease had stabilized. Of this last group, all three had received other forms of treatment which could have stabilized the disease.

The report says that these findings were verified in 1983 when the National Cancer Institute in Bethesda, Maryland, tested Essiac and found that the drug showed no anti-tumor activity.

They do not say how the herbal mixture was prepared. In animal tests at Sloan-Kettering, years before, a single ingredient had been tested, and when the full formula was used it had been prepared incorrectly, leading to such disappointing results over a 3-year period that Rene refused to cooperate and ceased sending them herbs. "They froze it," she said. "They might as well have been using water."

They do not say if any of the patients were given intramuscular injections of some of the ingredients, as Rene always gave in advanced cases, along with a solution of Essiac to drink.

They do not say if any of the patients experienced relief of pain, improved appetite, weight gain, or a sense of well-being.

The report concludes: "At the same time, it is acknowledged that Essiac is not harmful to a person's health providing it is not substituted for proven forms of cancer therapy. In fact, there may be positive psychological effects for some cancer patients. In recognition of this, Health and Welfare Canada has historically authorized emergency releases of Essiac on compassionate grounds." [A process so laden with red tape that in 1988 in all of Canada only 100 people were able to get it from a company now out of business.]

Today, Essiac is regarded as a wacko folk remedy by most doctors in the United States, where few people have ever heard of it. But in Canada, primarily in Ontario and British Columbia, it is taken very seriously by thousands who swear it saved their lives, or the lives of loved ones.

Because it has never been proven officially—even though its supporters have included a Premier of Canada, a Health Minister, numerous prominent doctors, and President Kennedy's personal physician—it can't be called a cure for anything.

Clearly, in the absence of strong scientific evidence, Essiac cannot—and should not—be relied on as the sole means of treating any serious or life-threatening condition. It should be discussed with your doctor, reviewing all the evidence, and used only with his or her approval.

Postscript

As this manuscript was being prepared, I came across the following items of interest from Julian Whitaker, M.D.

"I strongly recommend those with diabetes and cancer at any stage to begin a program including Essiac tea. It is easy to take, and it does not taste bad. Brew the tea by following the instructions on the package, and store it in bottles in your fridge. Drink it at least one hour before meals.

1. "If you have cancer, drink two fluid ounces three times a day. To give it a chance to work, take it for at least 12 consecutive weeks, without interruption.

2. "If you have diabetes, drink two ounces twice a day. For general health maintenance take two two-ounce cups twice a day for two weeks, then one cup a day."

A year later, in the May 1996 issue, Dr. Whitaker wrote:

"[Here's] what I would . . . do if I had any type of cancer. I'd take 10 grams of vitamin C a day, 200 to 300 mg of coenzyme Q10, two ounces of Essiac tea three times a day, and shark cartilage.[11] For prostate cancer I'd add another natural agent called modified citrus pectin."

Modified citrus pectin, says Dr. Whitaker, is made from the pulpy part of grapefruit, oranges, and other citrus fruits, "modified" into particles small enough to be absorbed into the bloodstream. "It's been called 'cellular teflon' because it prevents cancer cells from adhering to anything," says Dr. Whitaker. "It's non-toxic, has no side effects, and early research is very promising. The recommended dose of modified citrus pectin is one to two heaping teaspoons of powder (13 g) in water per day. . . . If your prostate cancer has metastasized to the bones or other organs, I recommend you get started on Dr. Burzynski's antineoplasm therapy (the clinic number is 713-597-0111)." Dr. Whitaker describes meeting a patient who did this, whose PSA dropped from 960 to 2.4, and who, 15 months after diagnosis was apparently well on his way to recovery.

+   +   +

Readers are cautioned that Dr. Whitaker's comments, quoted above, are not shared by most orthodox medical practitioners. Dr. Whitaker believes that conventional cancer therapies have done more harm than good for the past 50 years, and that various watchdog agencies and national societies work mainly to eliminate other choices. He believes all persons with this disease should thoroughly investigate alternative therapies. Most doctors would violently disagree.

What should you do if you have any of the symptoms in these pages? You should seek qualified medical help immediately for any condition that has been bothering you. All recognized authorities state that self-treatment is inadvisable without a licensed and qualified doctor's approval. No cancer cure is claimed here. These quoted items are presented solely as an aid to informed discussion.

---

[11] Shark cartilage is covered in this book in Chapter 9.

CHAPTER · 6

A MIRACLE BERRY FROM THE CROWN OF THORNS

Then the soldiers . . . stripped him and dressed him in a scarlet cloak; and plaiting a crown of thorns they placed it on his head and a stick in his right hand . . . They spat on him, and used the stick to beat him about the head . . . Then they led him away to be crucified. *Matthew 27:27–30*

The soldiers took him . . . and dressed him in purple and, plaiting a crown of thorns, placed it on his head. . . . They beat him about the head with a stick and spat at him. . . . Then they led him out to crucify him. *Mark 15:16–21*

Now there was a man called Joseph . . . of Arimathea . . . This man now approached Pilate and asked for the body of Jesus. Taking it down from the cross, he wrapped it in a linen sheet, and laid it in a tomb cut out of the rock . . . *Luke 23:50–54*

According to Christian legend, the Crown of Thorns is believed to have been made of hawthorn—as was the staff of Joseph of Arimathea, the man who took Jesus down from the cross. For thousands of years, this herb has been said to possess miraculous healing powers—the leaves and berries for digestive and urinary problems, the berries and seeds for kidney stones and dropsy (water retention). As a tea it was said to cure nerve problems. Hawthorn's most famous use, however, is as a remedy for heart and circulatory problems.

Miraculous Healing Power

"The hawthorn berry," says Dr. Eric Powell, "is probably the finest general heart tonic ever discovered. It is absolutely harmless and can only do good. Will never be contra-indicated in any type of heart affected, although in some instances other remedies may be called for."

"It is without equal as a remedy for most heart cases," says Dr. Powell, and he speaks with some authority as he himself was cured with hawthorn when given up to die of heart disease as a child. He says he has been prescribing hawthorn berry extract for his patients "for some 35 years with the most pleasing results."

In modern medicine, hawthorn berry extract is used to treat both high and low blood pressure, rapid or feeble heartbeat, fluid build-up, inflammation of the heart muscle, arteriosclerosis, valvular heart disease, and angina. It improves circulation, opens clogged arteries, helps clear artery walls, and strengthens the heart muscle, promoting longevity. It is particularly good for the heart problems of old age, and the insomnia of heart sufferers.

A Priest's Accidental Discovery

The healing power of the hawthorn berry was discovered quite accidentally. John Wesley, an eighteenth-century English clergyman, noticed that when his horses became winded and exhausted they'd nibble on hawthorn berries, and recover quickly. Wesley began using hawthorn berries with excellent results as an energy tonic for members of his church. Then, in the late 1800s, a Dr. Green of County Clare, Ireland, acquired a great reputation—and became quite wealthy—by means of a medicine he kept secret. On his death in 1894, his daughter stated that the remedy was a tincture of the ripe berries of English hawthorn.

An Explosion of Interest

This ignited an explosion of interest in the medical world, and innumerable articles by doctors appeared, citing their amazing experiences with hawthorn. Typical is this one by Crawford R. Green, M.D., of Troy, New York, which appeared in the *Homeopathic Recorder* in May 1908: "The action of [hawthorn] is so broad that there are few heart conditions it does not include, and none that contra-indicate it. In fact, it may be regarded as approaching a specific for cardiac conditions in general.

"It acts both as a powerful heart tonic and as a stimulant. It profoundly affects the circulation, strengthening the weak pulse and regulating its rhythm, correcting alike tachycardia, brachycardia [low pulse], or simple arrhythmia [irregular pulse], apparently regardless of cause.

"Its action in valvular heart conditions is truly remarkable, whether the mitral or aortic area be affected. It seems to have positive power to dissolve valvular growths of calcareous or vegetative origin. It is of value, too, in heart conditions caused by, or associated with anemia.

"[Hawthorn] has saved many lives in cases of organic disease with failing compensation [circulation]. In the pronounced edema of such conditions, it manifests a diuretic action in every respect rivaling that of Digitalis . . .

"In heart pains of various kinds . . . [Hawthorn] often gives relief when other remedies fail. In angina pectoris it is of indubitable value. Jennings has reported its use in a series of 40 cases of true angina with remarkably good results.

"As a heart stimulant and sustainer in infectious fevers [hawthorn] is of the greatest service. In diphtheria, typhoid, pneumonia and all other toxemic conditions, it may be confidently prescribed as a routine measure upon the least sign of a flagging heart. In such conditions, it gives results far safer and far more effective than alcohol, Digitalis or Strychnia. When employed in this manner, I have frequently seen lives saved with it when I am confident that any other form of stimulation would have failed. In two cases of typhoid fever I have seen heart murmurs disappear within 24 hours after its administration, reappear within a few hours when the remedy was experimentally discontinued, and again disappear upon its readministration."

"Absolutely Safe"

"In fatty degeneration of the heart, where, above all, we must guard against the danger of over-stimulation, [hawthorn] is an absolutely safe remedy," wrote Dr. Green. "In the tubercular wards, it has been shown that [hawthorn] will often tide a patient over critical periods when adrenaline is of too transient action, and Strychnia . . . would expand the heart and as surely kill the patient. In shock, in collapse, in syncope [fainting spells] of cardiac origin, [hawthorn] gives excellent result when administered alone or in conjunction with any other stimulant that seems immediately indicated.

"A summary of the symptoms for which [hawthorn] has been administered would be . . . feeble and irregular pulse; valvular murmurs; edema; dyspnea [labored breathing]; pallor; cutaneous chilliness; blueness of fingers and toes; circulatory disturbances; heart inflammations; heart pain—all these symptoms and many more . . ."

Seemingly hopeless cases were being cured with this spectacular healing plant. Without modern drugs or surgery, heart victims— some barely able to walk a few feet without terrible pain—were transformed from living skeletons to hearty, robust men and women able to run, kick, jump, and keep stride with anybody.

Recovers from Near-Death in 2 Days

Dr. X, 55, was suffering from painful heart spasms (angina), with labored breathing, upon the slightest exertion. He had to climb several flights of stairs daily, which caused severe attacks of pain radiating to his left shoulder and arm. If he tried to move, these pains would shoot up the side of his neck and into his face.

He grew so weak he could barely shuffle from one chair to another in his room without having an angina attack. His sleep was interrupted by nightly angina attacks. He could not sleep lying down, as this caused an attack. He got what little rest he could in a Morris chair. Nitroglycerine gave him only a few minutes of relief.

His doctor—a Fordham University professor—decided to try hawthorn berries: 20 drops of a tincture three times daily in water, gradually increased to 50-drop doses.[1]

In 2 days, dramatic improvement could be seen. Intervals between attacks grew longer. Dr. X could eat more and get some sleep. In 4 weeks, he could go up and down a flight of stairs, and he resumed work. In 6 months, Dr. X was performing operations, without suffering from angina attacks.

A New Lease on Life

"I cannot resist the temptation," wrote A. H. Gordon, M.D., "of recording another brilliant success in the use of [hawthorn]. . . . December 3, 1899, I was called upon to visit Mr. H., of this city, who had been afflicted with heart disease for many years; occupation, traveling salesman; age about 38 years. . . .

"I found the patient confined to bed, cyanotic, his limbs enormously swollen, almost complete suppression of urine, a very rapid, intermittent, irregular, and at times, almost imperceptible pulse. He was not able to raise himself in bed without immediate symptoms of collapse appearing; he spoke with great difficulty . . . it was only a question of a few days when the final end must come.

"An examination of the chest showed an enormously enlarged and dilated heart with leakage [and] regurgitation of the aortic and mitral valves. . . . It is in just such cases as these that I have seen [hawthorn] exert its wonderful powers, and I administered it to this dying man, having assured [his friends and family] that although the case seemed hopeless, I had known it to have restored [healthy circulation] in many similar cases.

"He received [hawthorn] in the usual dose every 3 hours day and night for 4 days, and no other medicine of any kind. At [the end of that time] he was sitting up in bed, dropsy [swelling from water

---

[1]In certain cases, a plant will give up its active ingredients more easily when prepared with pure or diluted alcohol (not rubbing alcohol), or brandy, vodka, or gin. This is called a tincture. Tinctures are available from most health-food stores.

retention] having entirely disappeared, urinary secretion restored, pulse fairly good, respiration unimpeded, appetite very good, skin normal in appearance, a complete restoration of [circulation] . . . a new lease of life for Mr. H.

"I received a letter from him . . . April 7 of this year to the effect that he was as well as he had been for years and able to attend to his business as usual."

Medical Journals Were Bulging with Exciting Reports

Nor are these isolated cases. Turn-of-the-century medical journals were literally bulging with exciting reports of miraculous healings from tea, extract, and tincture preparations from the humble hawthorn berry:

J. P., an 82-year-old judge, was suffering from heart pains, edema, and asthma. He could walk only a few steps at a time. He sat anxiously propped up in a chair, with a suffocating feeling in his chest, his breathing labored, his limbs greatly swollen, fearing he would die any minute. The swelling extended from his toes up into his abdomen. His heartbeat was weak and irregular. A physician gave him six drops of tincture of hawthorn in water, every 3 hours, soon increasing the dose to 12 drops every 3 hours daily for several days. The judge's heart pains gradually subsided. Two years later, he was taking daily strolls, and hearing law cases on a part-time basis.

Patient was an old soldier. Pulse was only 26. He had attacks of heart failure when no pulse could be found, but the wife would keep rubbing him and giving him stimulants, and finally the heart would start beating slowly. He seemed practically dead during attacks. Digitalis was tried, but it produced such a rapid trembling, distressed feeling in his heart with cerebral confusion that he disliked taking it. Hawthorn was given and the old man had no more attacks! Before that, he had them frequently, especially after any unusual exertion.

A girl, 14, was suffering from valvular leakage of the heart, following rheumatic fever. She was not expected to live. Her lower limbs were swollen from dropsy (water retention), her circulation weak. Nothing seemed to help her. Then she was given hawthorn tincture in five-drop doses three to four times daily. The dropsy disappeared soon afterwards and she was up attending school in a short time. Three years later, she told her doctor she was as well as she had ever been, could run, climb stairs, and attend to her usual duties without any return of trouble. Her doctor, seeing these results, used this remedy in three other similar cases with the same results.

Too Good To Be Forgotten

Modern research seems to confirm these findings. "[Hawthorn] is too good an herb to be forgotten," says one medical doctor. "Hawthorn is considered by experienced physicians in Germany—and I agree with them from my own experience—as an herb beneficial to the heart and as a kind of 'Elixir of Life'."
According to this doctor:

1. Hawthorn improves coronary artery circulation
2. It improves the metabolism of the heart muscle cells with better oxygenation
3. Improved circulation and oxygenation make it possible for a heart damaged by degeneration to remain efficient for a longer time
4. Hawthorn relieves cerebral circulatory disturbances in pre-sclerosis of the brain; like vaso-motor headaches; vertigo and uncomfortable sounds; loss of mental alertness and forgetfulness.

"Hawthorn is a so-called Basic Therapy without any habit-forming action or any side effects," says this doctor. "It can be taken for years to *prevent* acute decompensation of the heart in old age. It is tolerated very well, and, what is important, can be combined at any time with other cardiac glycosides, if needed. Hawthorn is an excellent remedy for the 'degenerative' condition of the heart, i.e., interstitial myocardial fibrosis as a result of gradual narrowing of the arteries. The main indication for its use is the 'senile heart,' a functional condition due to old age with a tendency to decompensation [lack of circulation] after an increased burden such as exertion, infection and toxic conditions. . . ."

Recent Scientific Findings

In 1969, W. Starfinger, M.D., reported on 125 patients who were treated with a hawthorn extract (50 mg), 15 drops, three times a day, decreased to twice a day after 3–5 days, then once before bedtime as a permanent medication, for the following conditions:

+ 18 cerebral and cardiac circulatory disorders due to senility

+ 26 hypertension and hypotension cases with myocardial damage

+ 16 liver damage cases with myocardial damage

+ 20 cases of coronary spasms caused by climacteric (menopause) with circulatory disorders of the cardiac muscle

+ eight cases of cardiac arrhythmias

+ 19 focal infection intoxications with insufficient coronary circulation

+ various cases of coronary insufficiency and myocardial damage related to diabetes (three), multiple sclerosis (two), nephrectomy (one), spastic asthmatic bronchitis (four), a spinal deformity with heart displacement (one), aorta/mitral valve disorder (one), head wound (one), bladder calcium (one)

In every case, the hawthorn extract was well-tolerated, with no side effects. In the case of the circulatory disorders, dizziness, forgetfulness, sleep disorders, and so forth improved, along with a general feeling of improved health. The myocardial damage resulting from liver damage reacted well. In cases of focal infections, the hawthorn extract was a valuable aid for eliminating coronary spasms. In eight patients, the hawthorn extract was administered to promote cerebral and cardiac circulation as geriatric therapy. A surprising effect was observed: premature fatigue states were eliminated; there was harmonious sleep; gaps in memory disappeared; and memory and retention ability were dramatically increased.

Other findings:

+ In 1951, a yellow substance was found in English hawthorn that produced dilation of the coronary vessels.

+ That same year, 100 heart patients requiring continuous therapy were given the liquid extract with fine results. Marked subjective improvement was noted in patients with mitral stenosis, and with heart diseases of old age. In other patients, digitalis could be either temporarily discontinued or considerably reduced when hawthorn extract was given.

+ In one reported case (1968) a patient whose heart action was so strident and turbulent that it could be heard 5 or 6 feet away, was given fluid extract of hawthorn. In 2 weeks, his heart had so quieted down that a stethoscope had to be used to hear it. The tremendous pulsing of his collar, tie, and shirt front had completely subsided.

+ In 1981, a double-blind test was conducted with 120 patients suffering from loss of cardiac output. The researchers found that in comparison to the placebo group, the hawthorn group exhibited significant improvement in heart function and reported considerably less shortness of breath or palpitations.

+ A 1990 experiment found that a mixture of hawthorn and motherwort might prove an effective preventive and/or treatment for atherosclerosis. Also, dried hawthorn flowers were tested pharmacologically and found to have a positive inotropic (muscle stimulating) effect.

In Every Case Blood Pressure Was Reduced, Often Dramatically

In another study, men and women with high blood pressure were given a tincture made from hawthorn berries. Some of these patients had arteriosclerosis of unknown origin. Some had chronic nephritis. All had old-standing hemiplegic lesions (paralysis on one side of the body), and several suffered from mild dementia.

No ill effects were complained of by any of the patients. In every case the systolic and diastolic pressure was reduced, often sharply.

No other treatment was given, except tincture of Crataegus (hawthorn berry), 1 drachm (1 teaspoonful) three times daily in water, taken by mouth. The blood pressures returned to their former levels about 14 days after stopping the hawthorn doses. The patients were at rest in bed on a light diet during the entire treatment.

Frightening Heart Palpitations Relieved, Acts Like a Calcium Blocker

We are told of a 65-year-old woman who suffered for years from frightening heart palpitations. Her doctor said it was nothing to worry about. But still the palpitations would come on suddenly for no apparent reason. Then a friend told her to try an over-the-counter health-store remedy containing hawthorn berry extract.

In 20 minutes, she felt relief. Now whenever the palpitations start, she takes a hawthorn capsule and it seems to calm her heart and make her feel normal again.

Various flavonoids in hawthorn have been shown to keep blood vessels open in a manner similar to calcium channel blockers. Hawthorn extracts also increase heart energy resulting in improved heart function and revitalized circulation.

Leg Pain Relieved

Intermittent claudication is the narrowing of leg arteries, due to cholesterol build-up, causing pain on walking short distances. In studies, people with intermittent claudication showed better blood flow and walking ability after being injected with hawthorn extract. The dosage for hawthorn extract—available in health-food stores—standardized to contain 1.8 percent vitexin-4'-rhamnoside or 10 percent procyanidins is 200 to 250 milligrams three times daily. It should never be used as a substitute for prescribed medication, and should only be used if your doctor approves.

Uses, Limitations, Safety

"Much more is now known about the potential of hawthorn, and it has been established that it really is a specific plant for cardiovascular diseases," says Rudolf Fritz Weiss, M.D. It is most helpful, he says, for:

1. "Senile hearts, that is patients with degeneration of cardiac muscle, or with coronary artery disease and concomitant problems. [Hawthorn] has rightly been called the drug to care for the aging heart. The anginal symptoms of coronary disease in particular tend to disappear with [hawthorn] therapy.

2. "Hypertensive hearts, in failure or not, mainly to maintain heart muscle in good condition, that is prevent or treat complications, primarily coronary disease.

3. "Weakness of myocardium [the middle layer of the heart wall] after infectious diseases such as pneumonia, influenza, diphtheria, scarlet fever, etc. Also for muscular insufficiency requiring digitalis, as follow-up therapy [in addition to digitalis, to enhance its effect].

4. "Cardiac arrhythmias, mainly extrasystoles and tachycardiac attacks, in the latter case by [intravenous injection]."

It is now definitely known that hawthorn does not contain any digitalis-type glycosides, according to Dr. Weiss. In Europe, where hawthorn is more widely used, it is often given in addition to digitalis or when the side effects of digitalis need to be avoided.

It is not the drug for cutting short an anginal attack, Weiss stresses—nitroglycerine continues to be the drug of choice for that. It has a long-term sustained effect on degenerative, age-related conditions, and is completely safe for long-term use, he says, adding that no toxic effects have been noted.

Using the Berries, Flowers, and Leaves of This Plant

Hawthorn tea can be made from the flowers or the leaves. Two teaspoons of the mixture are infused for 20 minutes, using a cup of boiling water, and taken morning and night, initially also at midday, according to Dr. Weiss. Since hawthorn tea does not have much flavor, it is advisable to add 1 or 2 teaspoons of honey. Sugar, he notes, is of benefit in heart disease.

A tea of hawthorn berries has a brown-red color of fruity odor and a pleasant taste. According to one medical doctor, "As [the tea] is not poisonous, the dosage need not be so accurate. An average dose of the tea for an adult would be a teaspoonful in water, 3 or 4 times a day."

A tincture is made by pouring boiling water over hawthorn berries, and steeping them like tea or soaking them in gin or vodka. Tinctures are best left to professionals to make, and are available from many health-food stores.

Hawthorn tincture may be taken in doses of 10–20 drops three times daily, or the fluid extract may be taken in doses of 10 drops three times daily, says Dr. Weiss.

"To get the best results with elderly patients," says Weiss, "hawthorn needs to be given not just for weeks, but for many months at least, preferably 20 drops of the tincture, the fluid extract or a good [commercial] preparation, morning and night, diluted with a little water. This method has the advantage that patients find it easy to remember to take the drops. . . .

"In more acute cases or if symptoms become more severe at times, a teaspoonful of the extract can safely be taken at once, two or three times daily, though only for a limited period, up to some weeks if necessary. [Hawthorn] is unusually well tolerated. Overdosage is highly unlikely. On the other hand, it appears that increasing the dose beyond the level mentioned will not increase the effect. Cardiac side effects are virtually unknown. Gastric symptoms will sometimes occur, though it has not yet been established if these [actually] are connected with [hawthorn]."

However, author Michael Castleman notes that large amounts of hawthorn may cause sedation and/or a significant drop in blood pressure, possibly resulting in faintness, and that it should not be used by pregnant and nursing women.

Author Richard Lucas says that doses of hawthorn extract should be taken before meals, with a little warm or cold water, and that for young children five drops are sufficient according to medical herbalists. Hawthorn is also sold as a non-prescription homeopathic remedy in pill form. These tiny pills may be taken in the third or thirtieth potency, he says.

However, Dr. Eric Powell of England says of these pills: "Experience leads us to prefer the 30th potency, although excellent results follow the 3×. For the 30th potency take 5 pills on rising and 5 on retiring daily."

CHAPTER · 7
"THE HAND OF GOD" A HOUSEHOLD PLANT THAT SAVES LIVES

Joseph of Arimathea . . . came and removed the body [of

Jesus]. He was joined by Nicodemus . . . who brought with him

a mixture of myrrh and *aloes,* more than half a hundredweight.

They took the body of Jesus and . . . wrapped it, with the

spices, in strips of linen cloth. *John 19:38–40*

Images of the aloe vera plant—a gift to baby Jesus, later used to anoint His body at burial—have been found carved on Egyptian walls from 4,000 B.C. The Egyptians believed that aloes had magic healing power and assigned them royal status second only to the pharaoh. Arab traders introduced the use of aloe to other parts of the world. Jesuit missionaries planted it around settlements in the New World, starting probably in Barbados around 1590.

Legend has it that the Indians of both Central America and Mexico were so amazed at this plant's ability to relieve so many ailments—cough, abscess, arthritis, bursitis, cataracts, burning urine, diabetes, genital herpes, gangrene, cramps, stomach pain, intestinal problems, leg ulcers, varicose veins, yeast infections—to name just a few, that they called the plant, with its long leaves reaching toward heaven, "The Hand of God."

The word *aloe* is derived from the Arabic *alloeh,* meaning "bitter, shiny substance." Only aloes with *aloin*—the aloe drug—have actual healing power. There are over 300 kinds of aloe, but only three are readily available that produce the miracle healing juice called aloin. They are:

1. *Aloe vera,* also known as *Aloe barbadensis* (referring to the island of Barbados where it once grew in abundance). This is most widely sold in the United States.

2. Closely related to it is *aloe succotrina,* named after the island of Socotra near Yemen. This is the aloe of the New Testament used to embalm Jesus' body. Because of its disagreeable smell, it was mixed with fragrant myrrh when wrapped among the burial clothes. A lot of it was used, as shown by the immense quantity of this mixture brought by Nicodemus. In Jewish burial, unlike Egyptian burial, bodies were not eviscerated. Therefore, the body of Jesus was left intact.

3. The third major aloe is *aloe ferox,* which originated in South Africa and is also known as *Cape aloe.* (There's also a *false* aloe, erroneously named, which is not even a member of the aloe family. It appears throughout the Old Testament, but is actually only a type of wood, eaglewood, used for incense and perfumery.)

All true aloes have similar characteristics so that aloe succotrina of the New Testament, used to embalm Jesus, has much the same qualities as aloe vera which is grown today throughout Europe and the United States.

But number one on the list, *aloe vera,* actually has more aloin in it, 18 to 25 percent; number two, *aloe succotrina,* has 7-1/2 to 10 percent aloin; number three, *aloe ferox,* has 4.9 percent aloin.

All have long, tapering, spiny-edged, fleshy green leaves that exude a mucilaginous sap when broken. All are perennial, in bloom most of the year in warmer climates, less frequently where it's cold.

Most plants will shrivel up after a few days without water, but aloe vera continues to put out new shoots for up to 7 years without water. Alexander the Great is said to have conquered the island of

Socotra for its large aloe vera crop. His troops reportedly took the plants into battle to heal their wounds. The plant would survive long periods of time without being in the ground.

Astonishing Facts about This Bible Plant

Most people are familiar with aloe's reputation as a healer for the skin. But what is not commonly known is that aloe vera can be ingested (in juice or capsules). Users claim its all-natural elements regenerate internal tissues and organs in the same way it regenerates the skin tissue.

Taken internally, it is said to have a healing effect on arthritis, ulcers, diabetes, and more. Testimonials on the medical benefits of using aloe juice internally tend to come mostly from arthritis sufferers who claim greater mobility and relief from pain and swelling. Others report remarkable relief from stomach ulcers and gastrointestinal problems. Some diabetics claim their need for insulin was reduced or eliminated.

An aloe vera leaf produces two substances: (1) a yellow or reddish sap, called latex, that is bitter and irritating to the lips. This sap is the juice of the plant and is responsible for most of its healing power. The active principle that makes it work is called *aloin*. (2) The leaf also produces a clear, semi-solid, unpleasant-smelling gel, which enables it to avoid water loss and survive for extremely long periods of time without water. If the leaf is cut, the gel simply heals over. The gel has been used for centuries to soothe and heal burns, cuts, and skin irritations and to soften skin. Studies show that it is the gel that is responsible for aloe's ability to penetrate the skin, allowing the juice to work.

How This Bible Plant Saved a Life

In one of his popular newsletters, Dr. Julian Whitaker, M.D., tells the story of a 10-year-old boy who was diagnosed with a rare brain tumor—meningioma. Surgeons were unable to remove the entire tumor, and it continued to grow, exerting so much pressure that his eyes bulged out. The prognosis was dismal. A friend suggested that the boy drink aloe vera concentrate. Out of desperation, the parents gave him 8 ounces daily to drink.

"Ninety days later," says Dr. Whitaker, "to the surprise of his doctors and the elation of his family, Steve's tumor was in total remission." Today he is quite normal but continues to drink aloe vera juice every day.

Although aloe is available in many forms—juice, gel, concentrate, and capsules—concentrates (the stronger the better) of the whole leaf are your best value, says Dr. Whitaker. "One or two ounces a day of a good product can be used as a maintenance dose, but I would recommend up to eight ounces a day for acute illness," he says. Among the illnesses he cites are ulcers of long duration and AIDS.[1]

Aloe juice, also called the aloe drug, exhibits these properties:

1. It has the ability to kill certain bacteria, fungi, and viruses.
2. It has the ability to dilate capillaries, increasing blood supply to the area treated.
3. When applied to injured tissue, the sap or juice penetrates and anesthetizes tissue, relieving pain. It numbs while it heals.
4. It has an anti-inflammatory effect; it reduces swelling of skin and muscles.
5. It speeds up the healing process and growth of new cells.

One researcher claims that aloe vera works because it contains at least six antiseptic agents—lupeol, salicylic acid, urea nitrogen, cinnomonic acid, phenol, and sulfur—that eliminate many internal and external infections. He says the first two of these, plus magnesium, are highly effective analgesics, which makes aloe a good pain-killer. Three anti-inflammatory fatty acids—cholesterol, campesterol, and B-sitosterol—make aloe soothing to the stomach, small intestine, colon, liver, kidney, and pancreas and help heal rheumatoid arthritis, rheumatic fever, ulcers, and allergies. It explains why for thou-

---

[1]Reprinted with permission of Julian Whitaker, M.D.

sands of years aloes have helped heal and cure a monumental list of human ailments and deserve to be called the "Medicine Plant."

"The Hand of God" A Bible Plant for Arthritis Relief

Recently, I received a booklet in the mail from a distributor of aloe products, full of detailed letters and photos of arthritis sufferers who claim miraculous relief since using what folk healers have called "The Hand of God"—a reference to the finger-like shape of aloe leaves and the fact that they point toward heaven:

> In a signed letter, one woman says she had constant, unrelenting pain throughout her body from arthritis—stiff joints, swelling in her legs and knees. She could hardly walk or get out of a chair. She went to several doctors, and to a local clinic, and was given a lot of medications that didn't help. After 7 or 8 years she was in so much pain she thought she had bone cancer. Her husband finally convinced her to go to the Mayo Clinic, where she was diagnosed with rheumatoid arthritis and give 18 gold shots, which gave her swollen cracked lips, and blisters all over her body, including her mouth. Told to quit work, she could not even hold a cup of coffee. She was taking codeine, Aleve, Naprosyn, ibuprofen—and more. Nothing worked. Then she got a booklet explaining the wonders of aloe vera. She started taking aloe-vera capsules. Gradually, the swelling went away in her fingers, toes, wrists, and ankles. In 6 months, she was completely free of pain—able to go dancing on Saturday nights with her husband again.

> She shared her "secret" with a friend who was barely able to walk, with a cane. In 3 months, she was walking on her own, without any help. At one point, she stopped taking the aloe-vera capsules and was unable to walk again without a cane. She started taking it again and got better.

A cerebral-palsy victim writes that she ordered some aloe-vera capsules. "I've been taking them for a month," she says, "and I can really feel the difference in my body. . . . they help my muscles and my pain. I will take them the rest of my life."

A 70-year-old man with excruciating pain down his legs due to two collapsed discs was told by doctors that it was permanent, irreversible, and would get only worse. At 82, he started taking aloe-vera capsules. In 2 months, the swelling was down, and he has no more pain in his back or legs!

An 85-year-old farmer writes that his hands pained him so much he couldn't grip anything. After a very active life, he needed help just putting on a shirt. His leg would swell up at the end of a day. He'd have to get up two or three times a night to urinate. A horrible pain struck him between his left knee and hip, forcing him to use crutches. It hurt so much to lie down, he had to sleep sitting up. Then he started taking aloe-vera capsules. Within a week he could see a difference, and gradually he got the use of his hands back. The frequent need to urinate at night stopped. His leg suddenly stopped hurting. He felt so good he went out and did some work on the farm. He is now able to work 12 to 14 hours and says he feels like a new man.

. . . the cases go on and on.

One man says that the arthritis in his hands was so bad that his fingers began to curl: "I couldn't close my hand or make a fist. There were knots in both elbows the size of golf balls, and I was unable to raise my arms above my shoulders." His condition began to improve when he began drinking 2 ounces of aloe-vera juice a day. Today, 5 years later, he says he has no more pain in his hands and that the knots on his elbows have disappeared.[2]

---

[2]From *Aloe Vera: Nature's Soothing Healer* by Diane Gage © 1988, 1996. Published by Healing Arts Press, Rochester, VT. Reprinted with permission.

Aloe vera also works on arthritis when it is applied externally. Some aloe users say they feel relief when they rub the gel directly onto the skin over an aching joint or muscle.

Controlling Blood Pressure, Diabetes, and Other Problems[3]

We are told of a man who used to be on medication to treat high blood pressure, but the drug made him drowsy. A friend told him that aloe vera works to treat high blood pressure, so he started drinking 6 ounces a day of aloe-vera juice. Within a short time, his blood pressure dropped from 150/100 to 120/80, which is normal. Without aloe vera, it shoots back up.

A diabetic patient claims that aloe-vera juice helped make his life insulin free. "It took about nine months," he says, "but I haven't had to take insulin for years." He points out that one of his customers also stopped taking insulin after drinking aloe-vera juice for a year.

Another diabetic says he'd suffered two heart attacks, had acute bronchitis, gout, uremic poisoning, and kidney stones and was receiving cortisone shots for bursitis and arthritis. He was given some aloe vera for his fifty-eighth birthday. In 3 months he was off insulin, and the gout, kidney stones, and arthritis all disappeared.

A woman suffering from phlebitis in her legs, with a tendency to develop blood clots, says that after taking aloe-vera juice she never had the problem again.

A victim of multiple sclerosis, who could walk only with crutches, purchased some aloe-vera gel and drink. Six days later, she was walking around without crutches. She claimed the aloe drink took away the soreness and inflammation in her joints, which had made it so painful for her to walk.

---

[3]Gage, *op. cit.*

Another woman says doctors wanted to amputate her leg. She wouldn't let them. Instead, she changed to a vegetarian diet and started drinking aloe-vera juice daily. After being crippled for a year, she says she no longer uses crutches, that her body is free of tumors, and that she saved her leg.

Healing Stomach Ulcers

In April 1963, in the *Journal of the American Osteopathic Association,* Vol. 62, in a report entitled, "Aloe Vera Gel in Peptic Ulcer Therapy: Preliminary Report," Drs. Blitz, Smith, and Gerard say that they used aloe-vera gel as the sole medication, in most cases, for the treatment of peptic ulcers in 18 patients. They state that all patients but one completely recovered, the exception being a girl who didn't stay with the program.

The researchers stated, "Clinically, aloe vera gel emulsion has dissipated all symptoms in patients considered to have incipient peptic ulcer. Duodenitis . . . treated with aloe vera gel, resulted in uniformly excellent recovery, except in one patient. In case of peptic ulcer about which there could be little doubt . . . aloe vera gel emulsion provided complete recovery."

In double-blind studies evaluating aloe vera's effectiveness in treating ulcers, Carrington Laboratories tested a drug it extracted from aloe vera against Cimetidine, one of the major ulcer drugs. "Aloe vera definitely had a healing effect on ulcers," said Clinton Howard, director of the facility. "Most of the current ulcer drugs on the market work by reducing the production of hydrochloric acid in the stomach. Ours may have a surface action effect, and coat the stomach in much the same way as the drugs Mylanta and Maalox." It is not known yet whether this aloe-based ulcer drug, called Carrysin, makes the natural coating in the stomach work better or if it serves as a partial coating itself.[4]

The research also indicated that this aloe-derived drug worked as an immune stimulant. "The active ingredient in aloe vera stimulates our body's macrophage, one of the white blood cells that con-

---

[4]*Aloe Vera: Nature's Soothing Healer* by Diane Gage, *op. cit.*

trols the immune system," says Howard. "We also discovered that Carrysin causes macrophage to put out increased amounts of prostaglandin, an anti-inflammatory product."[5]

Reported cases:

One businessman says he had stomach ulcers for years and had been told by doctors to quit working and avoid stress. While he was on vacation, a fellow tourist told him about aloe vera. He began drinking aloe vera daily and started feeling much better. He hasn't had any problems in 5 years.

Another man tells of having had two operations for stomach problems before he began drinking aloe vera. As long as he drinks the aloe-vera juice, he doesn't have any problems.

A woman was scheduled for surgery for bleeding ulcers, but the night before the operation, she was detained by family problems and had to go to her sister's house to help out. The sister had aloe juice, which this woman drank for 2 weeks without realizing its healing power. Later, when she returned home, she went to her doctor for an X-ray and no ulcer showed up. The doctor didn't believe it and took another set of X-rays. He wanted to know what she used.

Another man says he used to have an ulcerated stomach and a hiatal hernia, until he began drinking 4–8 ounces of aloe-vera juice daily. Now he says he can eat spicy foods or anything else he wants, without any side effects, not even heartburn.

A 59-year-old woman says she had ulcers nine times and was ready to have part of her stomach surgically removed when she read about aloe-vera juice. "I didn't realize you could drink it," she says, "so I tried some. It had a strange taste, but it cured my ulcer."

[5]Gage, *op. cit.*

A woman says that whenever she experiences heartburn and indigestion, she drinks aloe-vera juice. "It knocks it out in five minutes," she says.

Hair Growth Stimulated, Acne Healed

In a 1973 study, Egyptian doctors from the University of Cairo investigated the effects of aloe in cases of alopecia (hair loss), acne, and seborrhea.

They said that in one group all patients showed rapid hair regrowth. One of them, a boy aged 12 years, had hair growing in the bald area in 1 week.

In another group, aloe vera decreased the loss of hair and completely stopped it from falling by the end of the first month. Two of the patients showed regrowth of hair in the bald areas within 3 months.

Also treated were three women, ages 23–25, with acne vulgarus. In 1 month, two of the women were completely free of acne, the third showing marked improvement with little signs of it.

Max B. Skousen, Director of the Aloe Vera Research Institute in West Valley City, Utah, and author of *The Ancient Egyptian Medicine Plant: Aloe Vera Handbook,* finds that aloe vera helps fight skin breakouts. To treat acne, he says to cleanse the face morning and night. Then apply aloe-vera juice or gel and let it dry. This acts as an astringent to reduce oily skin and also stimulates the tissue to heal without scarring. He suggests using aloe-vera ointment directly on pimples and other sores to enhance healing and reduce scarring.

Speeds Healing of Sore Gums

Tooth pain can disappear completely with continual applications of aloe-vera gel directly onto the tooth. Aloe vera was found to be just as effective as two anti-inflammatory drugs (indomethacin and prednisolone)—with the added benefit of being nontoxic—in studies by Eugene R. Zimmerman, D.D.S., professor of pathology at Baylor College of Dentistry.

Another doctor reports applying an aloe-vera gel directly to dentures to help the gums heal. "The average period of time to wait to remove stitches after extracting teeth," he says, "is three days. When we use aloe vera, we can remove the stitches the following day. . . . when aloe vera is used many patients don't need to take any pain medication after surgery."

He uses this gel for denture patients with sore mouths, and also to reduce irritation and inflammation around exposed roots and sore gums caused by temporary crowns. Yet another dentist states: "After an extraction I place some aloe vera on a piece of gauze and have the patient bite down. This helps ease the pain and aids in healing. My uncle . . . after his wisdom tooth was removed . . . placed the inside of an aloe vera leaf on his gum and the pain immediately subsided."

In emergency cases, this doctor rubs aloe vera in and under the gum to cleanse and soothe the area until the patient can see a periodontist.

Shingles Completely Healed

One expert—Bill Coates, R.Ph., of Coates Aloe International—states that aloe vera used topically (on the skin) kills bacteria and viruses, such as the herpes simplex virus, which causes fever blisters, and the herpes zoster virus, which causes shingles. In her book, *Aloe Vera: Nature's Soothing Healer,* Diane Gage says:

> A woman from Carson City, Nevada, can attest to aloe vera's role in healing shingles. She says that her uncle developed shingles after having his leg amputated. Antibiotics and other prescription drugs failed to cure the condition. So she began bathing the affected areas with an aloe-based bath and shower gel, applying jojoba oil and then applying aloe vera gel. In addition, her uncle drank three ounces of aloe vera juice before each meal. By the second day, the shingles began to improve. By the seventh day, all but a couple of sores had disappeared, and within a month he was completely healed.[6]

---

[6]Gage, *op. cit.*

"Within a Week the Bedsores Were Gone"[7]

As an anti-inflammatory agent, aloe vera dissolves dead, devitalized cells like those found in decubitus ulcers and bedsores. One woman became interested in aloe-vera products when they healed her mother's painful and persistent bedsores. "My mother began using a bottle of aloe vera lotion and within a week the bedsores were gone," she says.

Reportedly, today many nursing homes are using aloe-vera gel, because it does a better job on early stage bedsores than anything else they've tried.

Leg Ulcers Healed

In 1973, a medical paper titled "Use of Aloe in Treating Leg Ulcers and Dermatoses" appeared in *Dermatology,* January–February, Vol. 21, No. 1, in which the authors report on three cases of chronic leg ulcerations:

> The first was a 50-year-old merchant who "stood during his work, had chronic varicose ulcers on the left leg of 15 years' duration, surrounded by eczema. . . . The ulcers were deep, foul-smelling and their bases were dirty and fixed." The report states that with applications of aloe gel, healing began within a week, and after 6 weeks one ulcer was completely healed, and after 10 weeks the other was. The last ulcer took 11 weeks to heal.

> The second patient, a 51-year-old man, had edema with enormous swelling of the left leg and foot with roughness and corrugation of the skin. He had chronic and foul-smelling ulcers of 7 years' duration, a huge one on the back of the left leg, and two smaller ones on the other side. He complained of throbbing pain during the first 2 weeks of

[7]Gage, *op. cit.*

treatment with aloe gel, but this soon disappeared. The small ulcers healed within 6 weeks; the larger showed vast improvement in 9 weeks.

The third patient, a 22-year-old man, had suffered a burn on the middle of his left leg 8 years earlier, and an ulcer developed there. It was now increasingly painful to stand on. He had varicose veins in the leg, with redness of the skin around the ulcer. It was dirty with running pus and dead flesh on the lower part. "After five weeks of aloe treatment there was good progress of healing of the ulcer [which] progressively decreased," says the report.

Healing Burns

Over the years aloe vera has been widely used in treating radiation burns. Modern research on this began in 1935, when C. E. Collins, M.D., used it to treat x-ray burns and found that the wounds healed more quickly and left less scar tissue when treated with fresh aloe-vera gel.

"We have noted . . . that the application of the leaf is extremely soothing, and allays the discomfort considerably. This was noted especially in breast [cancer] cases, in which the axilla received a large amount of radiation and became quite painful. . . ."

. . . said Drs. Fine and Brown, in their medical paper, "Cultivation and Clinical Application of Aloe Vera Leaf," on the treatment of radiology burns in 1938. In a study funded by the U.S. Government in 1959 to test the effectiveness of aloe-vera ointment on radiation burns, it speeded up the healing time and reduced scar tissue.

Reported cases:

A man with skin cancers covering both arms underwent a radical procedure in which doctors burned them off, leaving him in extreme pain. His wife began treating him with aloe ointment and spray. His arms healed almost completely in 11 days, and now look healthy and normal.

Another man accidentally dumped a pot of scalding hot water on his right foot. He was immediately taken to an emergency room, where a doctor treated him for third degree burns, and showed him how to repeat the procedure at home. He complied, but 4 days later his foot was so horribly swollen and painful he went to a second doctor. Same treatment. Now running a high fever, he decided to follow his sister's advice and try an aloe-vera "jelly." Within 3 hours, the swelling disappeared and his fever subsided.

"Some people apply the sliced-open aloe leaf directly on the burn," says one expert. "Others allow the aloe vera gel to drain from the leaf into a container to try to keep the gel as free as possible of the yellow sap, which can irritate a burn. They then soak a bandage in the gel and wrap the bandage around the burn. Still others combine these two techniques by placing the cut piece of leaf on the wound and covering it with a bandage; the bandage then remains moist and does not cling to the wound."[8]

Healing Allergies, Dermatitis, and a Kidney Infection

A researcher tells how he was born with a wide range of severe allergies, resulting in itchy, watery eyes, sinus congestion, infections, and large patches of severe dermatitis all over his body. Tests revealed he was allergic to nearly 200 separate substances. Allergy shots did not help. Ointments and ultraviolet light didn't help much either.

Then he began drinking 100 percent pure aloe-vera juice. To his amazement, all his allergies completely disappeared. His dermatitis cleared up, along with a persistent kidney infection. Even his hemorrhoids healed with his extra use of an aloe-vera ointment.

He says that for 10 years he has not had a cold, flu, or any other type of major infection. All his symptoms return if he quits drinking the aloe. As long as he drinks it he remains symptom-free.

_____

[8]Gage, *op. cit.*

A Powerful Bible Healing Plant
Fights AIDS

Since 1987, AIDS patients have known that aloe juice, or a drug derived from it—polymannoacetate—will provide relief for symptoms of AIDS. And it keeps those who have the virus but no AIDS symptoms from developing the disease. It's not a cure, but in the majority of cases tested, excellent results have been achieved in stopping the progress of the disease.

"A substance in the aloe plant shows preliminary signs of boosting AIDS patients' immune systems and blocking the human immune-deficiency virus's spread without toxic side effects,"

. . . says Dr. H. Reg McDaniel, as quoted in an article, "Aloe Drug May Mimic AZT Without Toxicity," in *Medical World News,* December 1987.

Patients Improved an Average of 71 Percent

In this study, the symptoms of 16 AIDS patients were significantly reduced when given 1,000 mg a day of this aloe-based drug (polymannoacetate) for 3 months. At this point, less seriously ill patients improved by an average of 71 percent, advanced cases 20 percent.

"Fever and symptoms of night sweats, diarrhea and opportunistic infections were either eliminated or significantly improved in all patients, with corresponding drops in HIV antibody positive cell cultures and HIV core antigen levels," says McDaniel.

No toxic effects were noted in a total of 29 patients who received the aloe-vera drug. And there is good reason to believe that pure aloe-vera juice itself can relieve the symptoms of AIDS, since the drug is present in the plant.

"Symptoms Disappear Almost Completely"

An article in the *Dallas Times Herald,* July 12, 1988, quotes Dr. Terry Pulse as saying that 20 ounces of aloe-vera juice (stabilized so as not to lose its strength on exposure to air) were administered orally to

69 AIDS patients who had been classified as those who would "never improve or get better." Afterward they were able to "return to work." Pulse says these patients "go back to their standard energy level, their symptoms disappear almost completely—and that's in 81% of the patients that I put on this drug."

"The sooner you can get a patient on this drug, the better off they are," says Pulse. His patients take 20 ounces of the liquid daily, "and I keep them on it indefinitely," he says, some for over 2 years.

"We have had deaths," he says, "but in those patients, most can be attributed to having gone and gotten chemotherapy for skin cancers, or whatever, or have taken other drugs in combination that knocked out their immune system, such as AZT."

What does all this mean? "It means," says Pulse, "that until there is a magic bullet, this is a stopgap measure and it buys them time at a fraction of the cost of AZT."

How to Grow This Bible Healing Plant at Home

Aloe vera can't be grown outdoors in most areas of the United States, because of harsh winter temperatures. But it can be grown indoors easily.

Aloe vera can be grown from cuttings or seeds, but it takes much longer from seeds. Start with cuttings from someone else's plant, or from a garden shop. The width of the pot must be at least half the length of the aloe leaves. A plant with 12-inch leaves needs a container at least 6 inches wide.

This plant likes bright but not direct sunlight, and fresh air at least during the summer. It grows best in a large window where the temperature is between 75 and 85 degrees Fahrenheit.

Aloe vera does not need constant watering. It stores a lot of water in its thick leaves. To determine when to water it, poke your finger into the soil up to the first knuckle. If it's dry to that point, water.

The soil should dry out between waterings. Use a sandy soil with good drainage. If the water is slow to drain, add pumice to the soil—half soil, half pumice.

Feed your aloe plant once a month, except in winter when it rests. Use a low-nitrogen fertilizer. Follow package instructions.

It will grow rapidly. You can either plant new shoots separately or place the entire plant into a larger pot. New shoots send out their own roots and detach easily from the mother plant.

Most growers claim the leaves should be about 3 feet long to be effective for healing. But the leaves of a house plant can be used at 1 foot. Only mature plants have full medicinal potency. An outdoor aloe reaches maturity in 1-1/2 to 5 years.

Most aloes growing on windowsills will never flower. The plant will remain small, but will reproduce frequently, sending up new shoots, called pups. It's fun to grow and can be a pleasant addition to your home or office—your own first-aid kit in a pot.

CHAPTER · 8
THE AMAZING HEALING POWER OF A GRAIN BLESSED BY JESUS

One of his disciples, Andrew . . . said to him, "There is a boy here who has five *barley* loaves and two fish; but what is that among so many?" Jesus said, "Make the people sit down." . . . so the men sat down, about five thousand of them. Then Jesus took the loaves, gave thanks, and distributed them to the people as they sat there. . . . When everyone had had enough, he said to his disciples, "Gather the pieces left over . . ." They gathered them up, and filled twelve baskets with the pieces of the five *barley* loaves that were left uneaten. *John 6:1–13*

Barley and wheat were the most important grains grown throughout the Holy Land ("a land of wheat and barley," Deuteronomy 8:8). Barley was more popular because it could grow in poorer soil and survive heat and drought better. Wheat was for the rich. Barley, the tougher, chewier, and less durable of the two, was for the poor—a universal symbol of poverty and humility. To make it taste better, working class people would often mix fava beans, lentils, honey, and several other ingredients with the barley, and the bread so made was called barley cakes. A poor or lowly person was scornfully referred to as "a cake of barley bread."

Bread was closely associated with Christ, not only because of his miracle of the feeding the masses with five barley loaves, but because He was born in Bethlehem, which means "house of bread." Christ often breaks bread with His disciples. He says we should always bless the bread.

Hot and tasty loaves of bread—which during religious ceremonies was always unleavened to symbolize that it was pure and not "corrupted" by starter leaven from previous breads—were served in light wicker baskets. These pieces of bread, whether leavened or unleavened, were broken by hand, and handed by the head of the household to each member of the family and to guests. The Last Supper began just this way:

> And as they were eating, Jesus took bread, and blessed it, and
>
> brake it, and gave it to the disciples, and said, Take, eat; this is
>
> my body . . . *Mark 14:22*

Medicinally, barley water was used as a soothing remedy for stomach disorders, and to relieve nausea. To prepare it, put 2 ounces of barley in a pot with 6 cups of water. Boil it down to half the amount of water. Strain, sweeten to taste, and drink. Two thousand years later, this remedy still works.

> Sylvia M. had frequent heartburn and indigestion that forced her to take antacids. She moaned that her life was ruined, that she *didn't have* a life anymore—just constant indigestion. The attacks would last for a week and sometimes awaken her in the middle of the night. X-rays showed she had a peptic (stomach) ulcer. Various medicines her doctor prescribed—Zantac, Tagamet, Pepcid, and more—had no effect and were a waste of money, she said. Then she read about barley water, and how easy it was to make. She drank it three times a day. In a week, all her symptoms were gone. X-rays showed her ulcer had vanished. Her doctor was so impressed with this fast healing, he now recommends barley water to all his ulcer patients.

I believe the hidden message in the story of five barley loaves being used to feed 5,000 is that barley is an unusual and important health-giving plant available to everyone.

"Spear Water"

The Jews of antiquity had a remedy for gallstones they called *medekarim,* literally, *spear water,* because "it spears or pricks the gall." This was, in reality, barley water. Here is modern evidence of the ability of barley water to break up bile from the liver—excess amounts of which can back up into the bloodstream, giving the skin a yellowish or jaundiced look.

> A doctor reports the case of a woman who contracted a severe jaundice, who cured herself by boiling a cup of barley grains in 6 to 8 pints of water until they were soft, and drinking the water during the day, from time to time. Her urine became quite clear and the jaundice disappeared. "This sounds almost too simple to be true," says the doctor, "but if it really helps, why should we not try it?" Similar results are being achieved in the tropics in cases of liver trouble and jaundice, he says, using the same simple Bible medicine—barley water.

According to the *Gemara,* a book of Biblical commentaries, "spear water" also referred to barley beer in Biblical days. The two most popular types of barley beer at that time were Egyptian *zythos* and Medean beer, which were regarded as universal remedies.

Anti-cancer Power in a Grain Blessed by Jesus

In *Double the Power of Your Immune System* (1991) John Heinerman tells how green barley juice worked for a woman with melanocarcinoma:

Linda Y., a 33-year-old Chinese American from Los Angeles, shared a recent experience with me that she hoped would benefit some of my readers . . . She [said] that about 8 months earlier, a pigmented mole on her right thigh started giving her some problems, so she consulted several skin specialists. They referred her to a prominent oncologist at UCLA Medical Center. He pronounced it a rare form of melanocarcinoma, which he thought was treatable with combined chemotherapy and radiation. Upon learning of the drastic side effects of both, however, she decided to take her chances with more natural things instead. Someone told her about bakuryokuso from Japan, which she started taking faithfully. She reported that her melanocarcinoma began subsiding within seven weeks of taking the bakuryokuso.

Bakuryokuso is plain green barley juice powder. She took 1 teaspoonful in a glass of juice or plain water with every meal.

Heinerman goes on to say that green barley juice and wheatgrass (see pages 190) are very popular in the East. He says that one product very popular throughout Japan and now available in the United States and Canada is Kyo-Green, which consists of organically grown young barley and wheatgrass, with kelp, unpolished (brown) rice, and Bulgarian chlorella (a mineral-rich algae). He lists the company that produces it as:

Wakunaga of America Co., Ltd.
23501 Madero
Mission Viejo, CA 92691
California phone number: 1-800-544-5800
Nationwide: 1-800-421-2998

Heinerman attributes the power of barley juice and wheatgrass to chlorophyll. Drs. Charles Elson and Walter Troll say that so-called protease inhibitors in barley and other seeds suppress cancer-causing agents in the intestinal tract.

Japanese researchers have discovered a protein—P4-D1—in barley grass juice that seems to protect cells from ultraviolet radiation and a specific carcinogen. This was said to be a result of the stimulation of DNA repair by this protein.

Both that protein and another in barley grass juice—D1-G1— have been shown to have anti-inflammatory activity when injected into lab animals. In addition, both these barley compounds are remarkably free from side effects.

The Miracle in a Humble Grain

Many scientists attribute the healing power of barley juice to chlorophyll. In his book *Nature's Healing Grasses* (1960), H. E. Kirschner, M.D., says: "Chlorophyll, the healer, is at once powerful and bland— devastating to germs, yet gentle to wounded body tissues. Exactly how it works is still Nature's secret [but] to the layman, at least, the phenomenon seems like green magic."

In 1980, Dr. Chiu Nan Lai at the University of Texas Medical Center reported that the more chlorophyll in a vegetable, the greater the protection from cancer-causing substances. Barley is loaded with it.

Ames testing shows that chlorophyll neutralizes the cancer-causing action of mixtures of coal dust, tobacco, fried beef, and other compounds. In this capacity, it is more effective than vitamin A, vitamin C, or vitamin E against mutations from the same mixtures.

Completely Non-toxic
It Has Healed So Many Ailments
It's Hard to Believe (but true)

"The number of surface conditions in which chlorophyll has been successfully used would be unbelievable were they not so well documented," says Ron Siebold, in *Cereal Grass: Nature's Greatest Health Gift*. "Chlorophyll heals wounds . . . stimulates repair of damaged tissues and inhibits growth of bacteria.

"Medical literature is replete with reports demonstrating these effects. Surface wounds and sores due to surgery, compound fractures, osteomyelitis (bone inflammation), decubitus (bed sores), and routine cuts and scrapes all show fast and dramatic improvement with the topical use of chlorophyll. Chlorophyll therapy has saved limbs from amputation . . .

"In hundreds of experiments and trials on humans and animals," says Siebold, "chlorophyll therapy has always been shown to have *no toxic side effects*. Not just low toxicity. *NO toxicity*—whether ingested, injected or rubbed onto a surface. This fact alone makes chlorophyll one of the most unique therapeutic substances known to medical science."[1]

Speeds Healing

D. H. Collings demonstrated that the healing time of wounds is shorter with chlorophyll therapy than with penicillin, vitamin D, sulfanilamide, or no treatment.

Chlorophyll speeds wound healing by increasing the amount of blood nutrients available for tissue repair. It decreases swelling due to its mild blood-thinning, or heparin-like property.

"Burns caused by heat, chemicals, and radiation heal faster with chlorophyll therapy, whether or not they are infected," says Siebold. "Chlorophyll was used to prolong the survival of skin grafts before the development of immune-suppressing drugs which are now used."[2]

Used Successfully for Sinusitis & Heart Infections

There are several reported cases of the successful use of chlorophyll for bacterial endocarditis, an infection of the tissue surrounding the heart. Chlorophyll has also been used successfully to treat chronic and acute sinusitis, vaginal infections, and chronic rectal lesions.

---

[1]Reprinted from *Cereal Grass: Nature's Greatest Health Gift* by Ronald L. Siebold, M.S., © 1991. Used with permission of NTC/Contemporary Publishing.

[2]*Cereal Grass: Nature's Greatest Health Gift* by Ronald L. Siebold, M.S., *op. cit.*

Reduces Pain, Inflammation in Gum Diseases

Dentists and physicians have successfully used chlorophyll to control mouth infections such as pyorrhea and Vincent's angina (trench mouth). "Chlorophyll solutions provide significant relief of pain, reduction of inflammation, and the control of odor for patients with serious mouth diseases," says Siebold.[3]

Peptic Ulcers Healed Faster

"Chlorophyll has also been shown to be extremely effective in speeding the healing of peptic ulcers, wounds which develop internally in the gastrointestinal tract," says Siebold. "Several studies document the use of chlorophyll in the treatment of ulcers resistant to more conventional therapies. The results are quite impressive. In the Offenkrantz study, 20 of the 27 patients with chronic ulcers were relieved of pain and other symptoms in 24 to 72 hours. Complete healing of damaged tissues, as demonstrated by X-ray examination, occurred in 20 of 24 cases within two to seven weeks. These reports included case descriptions of dramatic recoveries from severe, long-standing problems."[4]

Extra Benefit

"Researchers observed a side benefit when chlorophyll was used to treat peptic ulcers," says Siebold. "Chlorophyll tended to 'promote regularity' in the patients studied. According to several investigators, chlorophyll did not act simply to stimulate bowel activity, as does a laxative. Rather, it promoted bowel regularity, stimulating bowel action only when the action was sluggish."[5]

---

[3]Siebold, *op. cit.*
[4]Siebold, *op. cit.*
[5]Siebold, *op. cit.*

Pancreatitis

European investigations report favorable preliminary results in the use of chlorophyll in the treatment of pancreatitis. The chlorophyll is thought to influence several enzymatic reactions which complicate the disease.

Prevents Liver from Making "Bad" Cholesterol

For years, scientists have been trying to find out why vegetarians tend to escape heart attacks, strokes, diabetes, high blood pressure, high cholesterol, "bad" LDL cholesterol, and certain cancers. Dr. Asaf Qureshi, a food consultant formerly with the U.S. Department of Agriculture, thinks the answer can be found in barley.

Dr. Qureshi's father, a doctor, always insisted that his patients from the villages of Punjab (Pakistan) rarely had heart disease because they ate a lot of barley.

In an exciting study that began in 1977, Dr. Qureshi isolated an active compound in barley that suppressed the liver's ability to make cholesterol. It is called tocotrienol—or "Inhibitor 1." Two other inhibitors were also found. All were present throughout the kernels of barley, rye, and oats, particularly in the outer layers.

This is the idea behind a popular cholesterol pill called Mevacor (lovastatin). It blocks an enzyme in the liver that stimulates LDL (the bad cholesterol) output.

In testing the cholesterol of chickens raised on oats, corn, wheat, rye, and barley, Dr. Qureshi found nothing unusual in the blood of corn-fed chickens. Wheat and rye suppressed cholesterol slightly. Oats a bit more.

But barley caused cholesterol to plummet to 76 mg. per 100 liters!

At first, he and his colleagues thought it was just barley fiber doing it. Fiber reduces cholesterol by moving food through the system quickly—reducing absorption time. But when all the fiber was removed from the barley, the chickens' cholesterol still dropped sharply.

They discovered that the three inhibitors in barley deactivate an enzyme in the liver needed to make cholesterol. Not only that, they suppressed the liver's ability to make LDL, the "bad" cholesterol that clogs arteries. Levels of HDL, the "good" cholesterol, remained intact.

These 3 inhibitors in barley are also present in lesser amounts in other grains and vegetables, where they *act as powerful drugs to suppress the liver's ability to produce cholesterol.* This is a major reason vegetarians have much less heart disease, says this expert. They are constantly eating these cholesterol-lowering compounds.

Relieves Chronic Constipation

Israeli scientists tried substituting barley flour for wheat flour in biscuits and scones and gave them to 19 patients suffering from chronic constipation. Each patient was asked to eat three or four barley biscuits a day. Result: Fifteen of them (79 percent) became completely free of constipation, had less gas and abdominal pain, and quit taking laxatives. When they were deprived of these barley foods, virtually all the group became constipated and went back to laxatives within a month.

The less processed the barley, the more healing power it seems to have. Scientists recommend whole-grain barley products: barley flour, barley grits, and barley flakes (a cereal similar to rolled oats). Even the less-powerful Scotch barley and pearled barley found in supermarkets have cholesterol-lowering effects. (Pearl barley is the grain without its skin. Scotch barley is the grain with husks only partly removed.)

With the exception of barley beer (*zythos*), beer is not a good barley source, because almost all the cholesterol-lowering chemicals in the barley used to make it are cast off in the residue. Some of this residue ("spent grain") is made into barley flour for health-food stores and bakeries.

Safe for Those with Gluten Allergies

Barley grass contains no gluten and can be used safely by people with gluten intolerance, better-known as celiac disease: The chlorophyll in barley grass dilutes and enhances the elimination of gluten from the digestive system, according to one expert.

According to John Heinerman,[6] certain allergy specialists in southern California have been recommending green barley-juice powder, mixed with distilled water, to many of their gluten-sensitive patients. The product, called Kyo-Green contains the concentrated juices of young barley and wheat grasses, brown-rice shoots, an algae called chlorella, and giant seaweed kelp. These doctors recommend that their gluten-sensitive patients take 1 rounded teaspoonful of this powder and add it to 6 or 8 ounces of distilled water. This is stirred and taken on an empty stomach for maximum efficiency.

Boosts Energy Dramatically

Heinerman tells of a high-school coach who says he has routinely given glasses of barley-grass-juice powder—Kyo-Green—1 teaspoon mixed with 7 ounces of tomato or V-8 juice, to his athletes before a major game to "boost their energy levels dramatically," and every one of them has done well.[7] Barley-grass-juice powder can be purchased at most health-food stores.

---

[6]*Heinerman's Encyclopedia of Healing Herbs & Spices* (1996).
[7]Heinerman, *ibid.*

CHAPTER ✦ 9
MIRACLE CURES FROM AN OMEGA-3 FOOD BLESSED BY JESUS

I am the Alpha and the Omega, the beginning and the end. I will give unto him that is a thirst of the fountain *of the water of life* freely. *Revelations 21:6*

One of his disciples, Andrew . . . said to him, "There is a boy here who has five barley loaves and two *fish;* but what is that among so many?" Jesus said, "Make the people sit down." . . . so the men sat down, about five thousand of them. Then Jesus took the loaves, gave thanks, and distributed them to the people as they sat there. He did the same with the *fish,* and they had as much as they wanted. *John 6:1–13*

The sea may well be "the water of life" to which God refers in the Book of Revelations. Apparently, to be healthy, we need all the things that sea water contains, the most valuable of which is fish. In the Apocryphal book of Tobit (2:10), for example, we are told how Tobit was blinded by white patches that covered his eyes. In answer to his prayers, the angel Raphael appeared and told Tobit's son, Tobias, to apply the gall of a fish to his father's eyes. Tobias applied the remedy carefully, and the white patches shrank and peeled off. Tobit's sight was restored, and he praised God. (Tobit: 11:11–14).

Fish appear again and again in the miracles and words of Christ. It was on the shores of Galilee that Jesus launched his ministry. Christ's first four disciples were fishermen, and fish for food is described more frequently in the New Testament than anywhere else in the Bible, especially in the wonderful miracle of the Loaves and Fishes (Mark 6:41–2), which says to me: here is an unusual food available to all.

Even more fascinating is the fact that a fish was chosen to be one of the first symbols of Christianity because the first five letters of the word "fish" in Greek stood for the initial letters of the five words: "Jesus Christ, God's Son, Savior." A fish was the secret emblem Christians in hiding used to recognize each other.

The Universal Miracle Cure?

Only in the last decade have scientists begun to understand how right the Bible is, as an astonishing array of ailments cured or relieved by fish comes to light. For example (to name just a few):

AIDS	Clogged arteries	High blood pressure	Osteoarthritis
Arthritis	Colon cancer	High cholesterol	Psoriasis
Asthma	Diabetes	Lupus	Rheumatoid arthritis
Blindness	Enteritis	Macular degeneration	Stroke
Blood clots	Glaucoma	Migraines	Ulcerative colitis
Breast cancer	Heart attacks	Multiple sclerosis	

Fish is an exceedingly remarkable therapeutic and preventive food with enormous lifesaving power—a curative food, full of surprises.

How This Omega-3 Food Works

The "bad guys" in many painful inflammatory conditions are a group of chemicals called prostaglandins, thromboxanes, and leukotrienes.

These chemicals are made from food fat, specifically, cooking oils, margarine, corn oil, safflower oil, sunflower oil, salad oils, and meat and dairy products.

The "bad guys"—known collectively as omega-6 fatty acids—are responsible for a wide range of allergic and inflammatory conditions, such as asthma, rheumatoid arthritis, multiple sclerosis, lupus, Crohn's disease, ulcerative colitis, psoriasis, and eczema, and more.

The "good guys" are drugs that suppress and neutralize these disease-producing chemicals, such as aspirin, corticosteroids, and nonsteroidal anti-inflammatory drugs. The trouble with these drugs is their cost and their side effects, which include weight gain, water retention, susceptibility to infection, depression, high blood pressure, diabetes, peptic ulcers, stomach and intestinal bleeding, acne, excess facial hair, insomnia, muscle cramps, weakness, osteoporosis, and susceptibility to blood clots.

That's where fish oils come in. They have an anti-inflammatory effect similar to powerful drugs, without the side effects—and at very little cost, in capsule form.

The element in fish oils that cools down or neutralizes inflammatory, disease-producing prostaglandins and leukotrienes is called Omega-3 fatty acids.

Omega-3 fatty acids are found in deep-sea fish, such as sardines, tuna, halibut, mackerel, salmon, and herring. Technically, there are two types of fish oil—EPA,* crucial in preventing heart disease; and DHA,* important in brain functions. Most research has been done on EPA.

Even if you don't like fish or sea products, God has provided some vegetable substitutes that have omega-3 fatty acids, namely, flaxseed oil, canola oil, evening-primrose oil, and walnuts. Flaxseed oil, for example, contains linolenic acid, an omega-3 oil that the body can convert to EPA. Linolenic acid exerts many of the same effects as EPA, as well as several of its own. But plant omega-3 oils are generally less than half as potent as those from fish. Both fish oil and flaxseed oil are also available in capsule form.

---

*EPA stands for eicosapentaenic acid. DHA stands for docosahexanoic acid.

How Omega-3 Can Ward off Cancer

"Numerous studies show that fish oil consistently decreases the size of animal tumors, the number of tumors and their tendency to spread," says Artemis Simopoulos, M.D., president of the Center for Genetics, Nutrition and Health in Washington, D.C.

+ COLON POLYPS—In humans, fish oil seems to suppress precancerous colon polyps. In a study at the Catholic University of Rome, patients with polyps who ate fish oil showed suppression of signs of colon cancer in just 2 weeks. In the study, men with colon polyps ate either daily doses of fish oil or a fake capsule for 3 months. Abnormal cell growth—a sign of developing colon cancer—dropped an average of 62 percent in nearly all (90 percent) of the fish-oil group and came to a complete halt in one patient. The doses were equal to eating about 8 ounces of mackerel a day. Dr. George Blackburn, of Harvard, says that high doses of fish oil are necessary at first to correct a deficiency, after which lower amounts are acceptable.

+ BREAST CANCER—Dr. Blackburn finds that fish oil given to breast-cancer patients before and after surgery slows down cancer activity. Rashida Karmali, associate professor of nutrition at Rutgers University, has found that signs of breast cancer in women in the highest risk group were suppressed when they took fish-oil supplements in amounts equal to what Japanese women get from eating fish.

Fish is packed with vitamin D, which seems to ward off postmenopausal breast cancer in women over 50, according to Frank Garland, M.D., of the Department of Community and Family Medicine at the University of California. The recommended dietary allowance (RDA) of vitamin D in the United States is 200 IU (international units) daily. Japanese women eat about six times as much: 1,200 IU daily. When they move to the United States, their vitamin D intake drops and their breast cancer rate rises sharply.

And a study of 6,000 middle-aged men by Therese A. Dolececk, Ph.D., at the MRFIT Coordinating Center in Minneapolis showed that deaths from cancer were lower in men who ate fish regularly.

Omega-3 for HIV

Omega-3 fish oils have actually doubled the life expectancies of HIV patients. According to studies in Tanzania, when people who were HIV-positive were given omega-3 fish oil, along with gamma-linolenic acid (GLA), their life expectancies were *more than doubled.*

The body uses GLA to produce a substance called prostaglandin E-1, or PGE-1 for short. PGE-1 sends protector cells, called lymphocytes, to kill harmful viruses and bacteria. Among these protectors are T-cells, which are like foremen of the crew. These T-cells have the ability to detect foreign invaders, surround and attack them chemically, and to summon other lymphocytes to help destroy them. T-cells also make sure the body doesn't destroy itself.

Omega-3 fatty acids are found in fish and fish-oil capsules, flaxseed oil, canola oil, walnuts, and evening primrose oil. GLA is found in evening primrose oil, borage, and black currants.

Rheumatoid Arthritis

As an anti-inflammatory agent, fish oil can bring relief from the pain, swelling, and stiffness of rheumatoid arthritis, according to Joel M. Kremer, M.D., associate professor of medicine, Albany Medical College, New York.

It significantly reduces leukotriene B4—an inflammatory substance mainly responsible for arthritis symptoms, according to Dr. Kremer. It takes about a month to click in. After that, relief is rapid and lasts as long as you continue to consume fish oil.

The daily doses needed to attain relief range from 3,000 to 5,000 mg of fish-oil capsules with omega-3 fatty acids, according to Dr. Kramer. Since most fish-oil capsules contain 300 mg., that means at least ten capsules a day. But in a Belgian study, 2.6 grams [eight capsules] of omega-3 fish oil daily reduced pain and strengthened hand grip. And several studies have shown this same effect by supplementing the diet with as little as 1.8 grams of EPA fish oil daily (six capsules).

Fish oil also suppresses 40 to 55 percent of the chemicals called cytokines that destroy joints, according to Dr. Alfred D. Steinberg, an arthritis expert at the National Institutes of Health.

Research shows that the irritating chemicals that cause arthritic pain tend to build up again within a month of discontinuing fish oil.

Reported results:

"Several of my patients with rheumatoid arthritis have told me they have less morning stiffness and joint pain when their diet is rich in fish with a high omega-3 fatty acid content," says Isadore Rosenfeld, M.D. "These include sardines, tuna, halibut, mackerel, and salmon. You may possibly improve the symptoms of rheumatoid arthritis if you regularly eat these fatty, cold-water fish. If you cannot afford them or don't like their taste, you may take 6 grams of [fish oil] capsules every day."[*][1]

"After years of taking various medications for arthritis pain, I have been able to control the flare-ups for the past 10 years by eating two to three cans of sardines a week," says one woman.

"I find fish oil very helpful for morning stiffness and joint pain," says a 63-year-old neighbor of mine with a history of rheumatoid arthritis in her knees, shoulders, and hands. She says a capsule a day keeps the pain away. She finds that even if it flares up a bit, she can control it by taking a couple of extra capsules a day for a few days.

In one study by Dr. Kremer, 33 patients complaining of swollen, painful joints with morning stiffness that lasted more than a half-hour were given fish-oil capsules for about three

---

*Dr. Rosenfeld cautions against using fish-oil capsules if you have untreated high blood pressure or diabetes. A diabetic should take no more than 2 grams a day, he says.

[1]From *Doctor, What Should I Eat?* by Isadore Rosenfeld, M.D. Copyright © 1995 by Dr. Isadore Rosenfeld. Published by Random House, Inc., New York, NY. Reprinted by permission of the author.

and a half months. Not only did their symptoms subside, but they were free of fatigue and had energy for longer periods.

A vegetarian diet is also very beneficial for many rheumatoid arthritis sufferers.

Migraines

There's no question that certain foods and beverages can bring on migraine headaches in a person prone to them; foods such as cheeses, chocolate, hot dogs, bacon, processed meats that contain nitrites, foods containing MSG, fermented foods such as beer, yogurt, sauerkraut, yeast, and brewer's yeast, aspartame (Nutrasweet), or lack of caffeine, which occurs in coffee drinkers when they are deprived of coffee. Headaches from these foods may be due to an allergy to them or to a substance they contain called tyramine, which can bring on headaches even in the absence of allergy.

But migraines may also be *relieved* by what you eat. Simple hunger, by lowering blood sugar, can bring on a headache. Headaches that come halfway between meals may be due to too much insulin in your bloodstream (hypoglycemia), due to an overactive pancreas. This can be determined by asking your doctor for a glucose-tolerance test. The solution to that may be to follow a high-protein, low-carbohydrate diet, eating several smaller meals throughout the day, rather than three big ones. A prescription drug, called sumatriptan, available only by injection in the United States but on sale in pill form in Canada and Europe, has relieved even the worst migraines within 2 hours, but should not be used by pregnant women or anyone with angina or coronary artery disease.

Migraine headaches were prevented for about 60 percent of severe migraine sufferers—and greatly relieved in others—simply by taking fish-oil capsules, in a study by Dr. Timothy McCarren at the University of Cincinnati College of Medicine that lasted 6 weeks. Avoiding saturated animal fat can also prevent migraines, according to Dr. McCarren. The study concluded that regularly eating fish, especially salmon, tuna, mackerel, and sardines, can help lessen migraine attacks permanently.

Asthma, Bronchitis, Emphysema

Studies have shown that fish eaters are less likely to suffer from asthma or other respiratory ailments. Eskimos, for example, who eat lots of sea food, rarely suffer from asthma.

English researchers say that regularly eating fish high in anti-inflammatory omega-3 fatty acids, such as salmon, mackerel, sardines, and tuna, may prevent asthma in those who don't have it and help heal those who do.

They had asthma sufferers take high doses of fish oil, equivalent to eating about 8 ounces of mackerel daily, for 10 weeks, which reduced asthma-causing agents in the body by about 50 percent.

At Guy's Hospital in London, asthma patients who took fish oil had fewer breathing difficulties in the so-called late asthma reaction, which usually occurs from 2–7 hours after initial breathing problems.

But fish oil seems to constrict airway passages in asthmatics who are sensitive to aspirin. Others may simply be allergic to fish itself and should avoid it.

Diabetes

Fish eaters are only about half as likely to develop Type II diabetes as are nonfish eaters, according to Dutch researchers at the National Institute of Public Health and Environmental Protection. In a long-term study involving 175 healthy elderly men and women who were free of both diabetes and impaired glucose intolerance, they found—after 4 years—that 45 percent of the nonfish eaters had developed glucose intolerance (a precursor of diabetes), while 75 percent of the fish eaters remained completely free of this symptom. The amount of fish involved? Only an ounce per day. Omega-3 fish oil seems to preserve the pancreas's ability to handle glucose, thereby avoiding diabetes.

Glaucoma

When normal rabbits ate food soaked in cod-liver oil, their eye pressure dropped 56 percent, according to Prasad S. Kulkarni,

Ph.D., of the University of Louisville in Kentucky. "If it works as well in humans as it does in healthy animals, this could be a good prophylactic against glaucoma," says Dr. Kulkarni, who got the idea for this experiment from surveys indicating that Eskimos have very low rates of open-angle glaucoma, on a diet high in fish oil.

Lupus

In England, 27 lupus patients taking fish-oil capsules showed significant improvement, over a 34-week period, while those taking placebo pills got worse or stayed the same. In the United States one prominent medical doctor advises lupus patients to eat sardines packed in sardine oil three times a week.

Eczema

Food allergy is a major cause of eczema, especially in children. In a recent study at Middlesex Hospital in London, researchers estimated that simply eliminating cow's milk, eggs, tomatoes, artificial colors, and food preservatives would help up to three-quarters of children with moderate to severe eczema.

"In addition to food allergies, *dietary oils* are important in the presence of eczema," says Dr. Michael T. Murray. "Specifically, patients with eczema appear to have an essential fatty acid deficiency."

Treatment with essential fatty acids has both normalized the deficiency and relieved the symptoms of eczema in many patients. "It may be particularly important to increase the dietary intake of omega-3 oils, either by eating more coldwater fish (mackerel, herring, sardines, and salmon) or through consumption of nuts, seeds, flaxseed oil, or fish oil supplements," says Dr. Murray.[2]

---

[2]From *Natural Alternatives to Over-the-Counter and Prescription Drugs* by Michael T. Murray. Copyright © 1994 by Michael T. Murray. By permission of William Morrow & Company, Inc.

Psoriasis

Symptoms of psoriasis, especially itching, were "significantly" relieved by eating 5 ounces a day of an oily fish such as mackerel, in a study at the Royal Hallamshire Hospital in Sheffield, England, over an 8-week period. Similar results were achieved in 60 percent of patients taking fish-oil capsules for 8 weeks, in a study by Dr. Vincent A. Ziboh at the University of California at Davis.

Patients with psoriasis must not drink alcohol, which causes increased absorption of toxins from the gut, along with impaired liver function. A weakened liver cannot filter out these toxins. As a result, the psoriasis gets much worse. Herbs famous for improving liver function, such as those mentioned in Chapter 1 in connection with the Last Supper, would be especially helpful.

Wiping out Inflammatory Compounds May Heal Psoriasis

Inflammatory compounds in meat and animal fats can stimulate the skin cells to divide too rapidly, resulting in the skin plaques of psoriasis, according to one expert. Some of these inflammatory compounds—the result of incomplete protein digestion—are called polyamines. Lowered skin and urinary levels of polyamines are associated with improvement in psoriasis.

"The best way to prevent excessive formation of polyamines is to eliminate consumption of meat—with the exception of fish—and other sources of saturated fats while increasing the consumption of polyunsaturated oils, especially omega-3 fish and flaxseed oils," says Dr. Michael T. Murray.

"Several double-blind clinical studies have demonstrated that supplementing the diet with 10 to 12 grams of EPA oils results in significant improvement," he says. "This would be equivalent to the amount of EPA in about a five-ounce serving of mackerel, salmon, sardines, or herring."[3]

---

[3]*Natural Alternatives to Over-the-Counter and Prescription Drugs* by Michael T. Murray, N.D., *op. cit.*

Multiple Sclerosis

People in the fishing industry seem strangely immune to multiple sclerosis, a fact that has not escaped the notice of scientists.

Roy Swank, M.D., a neurologist at the Oregon Health Sciences University in Portland, has been treating multiple sclerosis very successfully with a diet low in omega-6 animal and dairy fats and cooking oils (the "bad guys"), and high in omega-3 foods such as fish (three or more times a week) and a daily teaspoon of cod-liver oil. For 34 years, Dr. Swank kept track of 144 MS patients.

The results of this study are astounding. Minimally disabled patients who followed his dietary recommendations experienced little or no disease progression, and only 5 percent failed to survive the 34-year study. But 80 percent of those who failed to follow the dietary program did not survive the study period.

Writing in the British medical journal *The Lancet* in 1990, Dr. Swank said: "If we got them on the diet before disability set in, 95 percent lived for 30 years without disability. All who did not go on the diet went downhill and most died within 20 years."

Dr. Swank's diet recommends:

1. Elimination of butter, hydrogenated oils (margarine and shortening), and an animal-fat intake of no more than 15 grams per day

2. A daily intake of 40 to 50 grams or approximately 3–4 tablespoons of polyunsaturated vegetable oils

3. At least 1 teaspoon of cod-liver oil daily

4. A normal allowance of protein, mostly from vegetables, nuts, fish, white meat of turkey and chicken (skin removed), and lean meat

5. The consumption of fish three or more times a week

Moderately and severely disabled patients who followed the dietary recommendations also did far better than the group that didn't. The diet prevented worsening of the disease and greatly reduced fatigue.

MS patients are severely lacking in omega-3 fatty acids, according to Ralph T. Holman, Ph.D, of the University of Minnesota and Emre Kokmen, M.D., of the Mayo Clinic. This lack can be partly remedied by eating oils rich in omega-3 fatty acids, he says. Namely, fish oils, which are more potent, and plant oils such as canola and flaxseed oil. It doesn't take much, just a few teaspoons a day.

Dr. Swank's findings deserve serious consideration by anyone with multiple sclerosis, says Dr. Rosenfeld. "The omega-6 fatty acids in animal and vegetable fats stimulate the production of prostaglandins and leukotrienes, body chemicals that promote tissue inflammation and contribute to the development of autoimmune disorders. Omega-3 fatty acids, on the other hand, derived from a variety of deep-sea saltwater fish, have the opposite effect; they neutralize the omega-6 group and enhance the efficiency of the immune system," he says.[4]

A Doctor's Recommendations

"I advise my MS patients to avoid omega-6 fats and to eat fatty fish," says Dr. Rosenfeld. "In fact, that's what I tell most of my patients to do anyway because such a diet may also protect against heart disease.

"From a practical standpoint, that means eating 5 ounces every day of tuna or any other fish that's *very* rich in omega-3. Moderate amounts of skinned poultry or pasta are okay—but forget red meat and whole milk products. Your diet should also be rich in legumes, fruits, and vegetables to make up for the calories you're not getting from fat and animal protein, and to provide fiber. . . . Avoid the forbidden fats in cooking, and instead bake, broil, grill, microwave, or poach your fish. Marinating foods in lemon juice or herbs, diluted fruits juices, or wine will introduce you to exciting new fat-free tastes. You can also braise your fish and vegetables in defatted chicken or vegetable stock.

"If you don't like fish or can't afford to eat it regularly, you can take 2-1/2 grams a day of omega-3 supplements in capsule form, the equivalent of 4 ounces of pink salmon. Since omega-3 oils have a prostaglandin effect similar to aspirin and interfere with blood clot-

---

[4]*Doctor, What Should I Eat?* by Isadore Rosenfeld, M.D., *op. cit.*

ting (a good thing for those prone to coronary disease), do not take them if you have a blood disorder. For the same reason, if you have poorly controlled or untreated high blood pressure it's best not to use them. . . ."[5]

How You May Cheat Death with an Ounce a Day of Omega-3

Eating just an ounce of fish a day cuts the chances of a fatal heart attack in half, according to a Dutch study. And if you've already suffered a heart attack, it can help you escape another one, according to Michael Burr, M.D., of the Medical Research Council in Cardiff, Wales. Burr studied 2,033 men who had all had at least one heart attack. He divided them into four groups:

1. One group was asked to eat 5 ounces salmon, mackerel, or sardines, at least twice a week, or take fish-oil capsules.
2. The second group was asked to cut down on saturated fats, such as butter, cheese, and cream.
3. A third group was asked to increase their fiber intake by eating bran cereal and whole-wheat bread.
4. The fourth group received no instructions and were free to eat as they pleased.

The results after 2 years?

There was no life-saving effect from a low-fat or high-fiber diet. But among fish eaters, the mortality rate dropped 30 percent.

In a study of 84 patients who had had balloon angioplasty to open clogged arteries, at the Washington, D.C., Hospital Center, out of 42 patients who ate both a low-fat diet *and* took fish-oil capsules for 6 months, only eight (19 percent) needed another angioplasty. In an equal number of patients on a low-fat diet *without* fish oil, the rate of recurring blockage was 38 percent—twice as many—according to Mark R. Milner, M.D., the surgeon who made the study.

---

[5]Rosenfeld, *ibid.*

Consistently eating fish both before and after heart surgery keeps arteries open just as well as taking fish-oil capsules, according to Isabelle Bairati, M.D., professor of medicine at Laval University in Quebec City, Canada.

How to Quickly Normalize a Subnormal HDL Count

If your HDL cholesterol—the "good" cholesterol—is subnormal, you can give it a tremendous boost by eating fish rich in omega-3 fatty acids, such as salmon, mackerel, herring, sardines, or tuna, according to Gary J. Nelson, Ph.D., of the U.S. Department of Agriculture's Western Human Nutrition Research Center in San Francisco. In a test, men with normal cholesterol ate salmon for lunch and dinner for about 40 days. The beneficial HDL cholesterol in their blood went way up—within 20 days. Results were surprisingly rapid, says Dr. Nelson. People with subnormal HDL can expect even higher rises from eating fish, he says.

"Omega-3 fatty acids," says Dr. Michael Murray, "have been shown in hundreds of studies to lower cholesterol and triglyceride levels [and] are being recommended to treat or prevent not only high cholesterol levels but also high blood pressure, other cardio-vascular diseases, cancer, auto-immune diseases like multiple sclerosis and rheumatoid arthritis, allergies . . . asthma, lupus, and ulcerative colitis . . . eczema, psoriasis, and many other illnesses. . . .

"If cold-water fish are not readily available, I recommend supplementing the diet with either fish oils or flaxseed oil. The dosages found to be effective when using fish-oil supplements range from 5 to 15 grams of omega-3 fatty acids per day. . . ."[6]

"Much Less Expensive . . . Much Safer"

"Although this can be expensive," says Dr. Murray, "it is still much less expensive than some cholesterol-lowering drugs, and is cer-

---

[6]Murray, *op. cit.*

tainly much safer. Flaxseed oil [another Biblical food] may indeed be the most advantageous oil for medicinal use, especially when cost effectiveness is considered. One tablespoon per day is all that is required. . . . Flaxseed oil can be used as a salad dressing or food supplement, but loses its beneficial quality when cooked."

Dr. Jorn Dyerberg, a leading Danish researcher, says that 4 grams of fish oil taken daily can lower abnormally high levels of Lp(a), a little-known type of cholesterol that some experts think is responsible for 25 percent of all heart attacks in people under 60. After 9 months, the level of Lp(a) in the men tested was reduced 15 percent. Similar results were obtained in Germany in 35 patients with coronary artery disease.

Preventing Blood Clots and Stroke

Omega-3 fish oil prevents blood platelets from sticking together, so that clots cannot form to plug up your arteries. It causes blood platelets to release much less of a clotting substance called thromboxane, according to Norberta Schoene, Ph.D., of the U.S. Department of Agriculture.

Harvard researchers say that eating 6-1/2 ounces of canned tuna can "thin the blood" as much as taking an aspirin. One researcher claims you can get a favorable anticlotting effect from eating 3-1/2 ounces of fatty fish such as mackerel, herring, salmon, or sardines.

Fish also lowers fibrinogen in the blood, another factor that causes clots to form, according to Paul Nestel, chief of Human Nutrition at the Commonwealth Scientific & Industrial Research Organization in Australia.

Dutch researchers have found that men between 60 and 69 who ate fish at least once a week were only half as likely to have a stroke during the next 15 years as were those who ate no fish.

Blood Pressure

"My own blood pressure dropped from 140/90 to 100/70 after I started eating a small can of mackerel fillets every day," says Peter Singer, Ph.D., of Berlin, Germany. For most people, eating fish three times a week supplies enough omega-3 oil to lower blood pressure—and may even eliminate the need for medication in some people.

Dr. Singer found small doses of fish oil as effective in reducing blood pressure as the beta-blocker Inderal, a widely prescribed blood pressure medicine.

Fish-oil capsules do lower blood pressure in those who don't like fish. In tests at the University of Cincinnati, blood pressure fell 4.4 points diastolic and 6.5 points systolic in subjects with mild high blood pressure who took 2,000 mg of omega-3 fatty acids daily for 3 months.

Ulcerative Colitis

Fish oil is being used to treat ulcerative colitis by William Stenson, M.D., at Washington University Medical Center in St. Louis. In one study of 18 patients, Dr. Stenson found that fish-oil supplements reduced an inflammatory agent in the colon—leukotriene B4—by 60 percent. Not surprisingly, patients felt much better and gained weight. Examinations by sigmoidoscopy revealed less inflammation or damage. Nearly half the patients (eight) were able to cut their dosage of prednisone—a drug needed to keep the disease under control—in half.

Crohn's Disease Sufferers Saved from Relapse

Italian doctors have used fish oil to save Crohn's patients from relapse. Out of 78 patients at high risk for a relapse, half were given nine fish-oil capsules daily, specially designed to melt in the colon. The others were given blank pills. After a year, 59 percent of the patients using fish oil capsules were in remission, compared with 26 percent on the placebo.

Fish oil "seems to be one of the truly non-toxic medications to give patients on a long-term basis *to prevent relapse,"* according to Albert B. Knapp, M.D., assistant professor of medicine at New York University's School of Medicine.

Premature Babies Helped

Labor begins when certain body chemicals called prostaglandins stimulate the uterus to contract. If this happens too early, the infant is born prematurely. Omega-3 fatty acids present in fish neutralize these prostaglandins and can delay labor by an average of 4 days, adding up to 4 ounces to a baby's weight, which is helpful to a baby weighing less than 5-1/2 pounds. Women at risk of having a premature baby should start eating fish—particularly salmon, tuna, and halibut—at about the thirtieth week according to one medical doctor. Fish-oil capsules should be avoided by anyone with a bleeding or clotting disorder. *Always check with your doctor before taking them.*

Raynaud's Disease Helped

Raynaud's disease is characterized by fingers that grow pale and hurt in cold weather, or when exposed to cold water or ice. Then, as they warm up, they turn red, become painful and swollen, and tingle or throb. This condition is due to a spasm of the small arteries in exposed areas of the body—fingers, nose tip, ears—when exposed to a drop in temperature. It usually occurs in people with some disorder of the immune system, notably lupus, rheumatoid arthritis, and scleroderma. But it can occur in people who are otherwise completely healthy, except that their fingers get frostbitten quickly on exposure to cold.

Aside from the obvious solutions—stay out of the cold, and if you can't avoid it wear gloves—and as an alternative to drugs, you might try fish oil. In one study of persons with Raynaud's disease who took 12 capsules of omega-3 fish oil daily for twelve weeks, their fingers remained pink and warm after exposure to cold. A 4-ounce serving of pink salmon contains the same amount of omega-3 fish oil as seven capsules. Other rich sources are herring, mackerel, bluefish, sardines, trout, tuna, and whitefish. Omega-3 fish oils cause the inner lining of blood vessels to release prostaglandins, which help prevent the small arteries (arterioles) in exposed areas of the body from going into spasm. Do not take fish-oil capsules if you have high blood pressure or a bleeding or clotting disorder without first checking with your doctor. Limit your dose to 2-1/2 grams a day if you have diabetes.

À Cure for Aging?

At age 68, Otto von Bismarck, the "Iron Chancellor" of Germany, was in feeble health. A lifetime of hard work and overindulgence in food, drink, and tobacco had taken its toll, and he appeared bloated and mentally vague. Then he was introduced to a young Jewish physician named Dr. Schweninger, who promptly put him on a diet consisting almost exclusively of herring.

The effect was miraculous. According to Bismarck's biographer, A.J.P. Taylor, "However curious this seems by contemporary standards, it did the trick. Bismarck's weight went down . . . he slept long and peacefully; his eyes became clear, his skin fresh and almost youthful." According to Taylor, "Every observer noted the change in Bismarck; and it can be seen in his photographs. In 1877 he is bloated, choleric, bursting at the seams." In 1883, just before he met Schweninger, the photos showed "A bearded old man, bewildered at life and hardly able to control his twitchings long enough to face the camera. In 1885 he is fresh, clean-shaven, chin upright, face finely drawn, master of himself, seventy years old no doubt, but a man with a long life before him."

Of course, von Bismarck did not stay on a diet of herring. His diet expanded to include meats and vegetables. But fish remained a major source of rejuvenation for him. He lived to a hale and hearty 83 years of age.

Herring, as we have seen, is a rich source of omega-3 oil, which protects against a wide range of allergic and inflammatory conditions, such as asthma, arthritis, blood clots, clogged arteries, colon cancer, diabetes, heart attacks, high blood pressure, high cholesterol, macular degeneration, ulcerative colitis, and much more.

Herring, like most seafood, is also a rich source of selenium.

The Miracle of Selenium

"It's time to stop ignoring the facts!" says Richard A. Passwater, Ph.D., in his book, *Selenium as Food & Medicine.* "If you want to maintain your good health, increase your resistance to disease, and assure a long and energetic life, it is vitally important that you increase your intake of selenium."

Selenium, he says, plays a vital role in the prevention of heart disease and many forms of cancer. Proper use of selenium can also slow the aging process, strengthen the immune system and improve energy levels. There is increasing evidence that selenium can help prevent and relieve arthritis, forestall the onset of cataracts, and improve resistance to infectious diseases.

"There are even strong suggestions," Dr. Passwater says, "that selenium can improve sexual health and possibly sexual function as well."

Selenium protects the membranes of each of our body's 60 trillion cells. "In so doing," says Passwater, "it prevents the decay of cellular function. . . . [The average reader] may not appreciate the role selenium plays in protecting the body against a whole host of diseases. . . . I have demonstrated selenium's effectiveness repeatedly in my own laboratory . . . I know that selenium is protective against cancer, heart disease, and premature aging."[7] Dr. Passwater continues:

Cancer—"Current evidence suggests that improved selenium nutrition can reduce cancer risk. . . . In other words, the more selenium consumed the lower the incidence of cancer. . . . Recently [circa 1980] several physicians have found that when sufficient selenium is ingested by cancer patients to raise their blood levels of selenium to the desired range, their tumors began to shrink. . . ."

Dr. Gerhard Schrauzer of the University of California says: "If every woman in America started taking selenium today," or had a

------

[7]Reprinted from *Selenium As Food & Medicine* by Richard A. Passwater, Ph.D. © 1980. Used with permission of NTC/Contemporary Publishing.

high-selenium diet, within a few years the breast cancer rate in this country would drastically decline. . . . Selenium is a giant step toward preventing cancer—it is a major breakthrough. . . . If selenium were used properly as a preventive measure against cancer, I think it's possible that it would enable us to cut the mortality rate from almost all cancers by 80 to 90 percent in this country."

Based on epidemiological studies, Dr. Raymond Shamberger of the Cleveland Clinic Foundation advises people to increase their intake of selenium to 200 micrograms a day, because "it can reduce the cancer rate dramatically for some types of cancer, particularly cancer of the colon, breast, esophagus, tongue, stomach, intestine, rectum, and bladder."

The rate of breast cancer among Asian women is one-seventh of the U.S. rate. Dr. Christine S. Wilson, a nutritionist at the University of California, San Francisco, compared the average Asian and American diet and found that Western diets contained about 25 percent of the selenium of Asian diets. She also noted that selenium helps block the formation of peroxides and free radicals, which are believed to trigger various forms of cancer.[8]

Heart Disease—"[Studies suggest that] selenium is an important protective factor in high blood pressure, stroke, heart attack and hypertensive kidney damage," says Dr. Passwater. "Selenium is necessary for the health of the heart muscle itself [and] selenium supplementation is effective in the treatment of chest pains associated with heart disease (angina pectoris)." He continues:

"Chinese physicians recently reported that a congestive heart disease—one that affected children especially—was prevalent throughout vast areas of China. Since this land is known to be low in selenium, the physicians set up a carefully controlled study. In one commune, the people were given 1,000 micrograms of selenium each week. Before long, the incidence of this heart problem—called Keshan disease in China—dropped to zero, and children who were already suffering from heart trouble became well.

---

[8]*Selenium As Food & Medicine* by Richard A. Passwater, Ph.D., *op. cit.*

"Animal nutritionists have noted that animals living in selenium-deficient areas developed such calcification of their hearts, the disease was named white-muscle disease. My early involvement with selenium and heart disease centered on selenium's role in muscle health. Animal nutritionists had determined that selenium deficiencies caused nutritional muscular dystrophy and a degeneration of skeletal muscle called Zenker's disease. A similar degeneration of the Purkinje fibers which cause the heartbeat had been observed in selenium deficiency. In fact, the hearts of most selenium-deficient animals will collapse when surgically removed, while hearts from adequately nourished animals will hold their shape."

Studies have shown that Americans living in selenium-deficient areas are three times more likely to die from heart disease as those living in selenium-rich areas . . . that the heart disease rate in the 55–64-year-old age group was lowest in the selenium-rich states: Texas, Oklahoma, Arizona, Colorado, Louisiana, Utah, Alabama, Nebraska, and Kansas.

Colorado Springs, Colorado, was 67 percent below the national average for heart-disease deaths and Austin, Texas, was 53 percent below.

"Adequate selenium is required to produce the necessary Coenzyme Q required for a healthy heart," says Dr. Passwater.[9]

Cystic Fibrosis—In the late 1970s, Dr. Joel Wallach collected considerable data suggesting that cystic fibrosis in children is due to a selenium deficiency in their mothers during pregnancy. He first noticed that the internal organs of primates with cystic fibrosis looked exactly like organs from selenium- and zinc-deficient animals. He then checked for possible selenium or zinc deficiencies in 120 mothers with children with cystic fibrosis. He found that in 151 cases, the mothers when pregnant, or their newborn babies, had been placed on diets low in selenium.

As a result, 50 cystic fibrosis patients, age 3 months to 37 years, were placed on a balanced diet free of vegetable oils, with selenium

---

[9]Passwater, *op. cit.*

supplementation ranging from 25 to 300 mcg per day. All displayed markedly improved clinical status (normal bowels, reduced lung mucus, increased energy and strength, improved skin and hair, reduced finger and toe clubbing, weight gain, and increased resistance to infections."

Dr. Passwater says, "Wallach's observations imply that there is more hope for cystic fibrosis patients who have not yet had severe pancreatic fibrosis. This is reversible in animals treated with selenium."[10]

Muscular Dystrophy—"It is fairly common knowledge among nutritional researchers that selenium prevents *nutritional* muscular dystrophy in animals," says Dr. Passwater. "Most of these same scientists will quickly point out that this is vastly different from human muscular dystrophy. There is evidence, however, that both nutritional muscular dystrophy and human muscular dystrophy are helped by selenium and vitamin E."

Selenium and vitamin E are required to produce unbiquinone (coenzyme Q) in the body, according to Dr. Passwater, who tells of the case of Mr. S, who went to a clinic where blood tests and a biopsy showed he had late-stage muscular dystrophy. It was incurable. He was told to go home. Nothing could be done. At the suggestion of a friend of his, a medical researcher, who felt that muscular dystrophy was due to a lack of coenzyme Q, he increased the vitamin E he'd been taking from 400 i.u. to 2,000 i.u. and his vitamin C from 500 mg to 3,000 mg daily. He went on a diet rich in cottage cheese and tuna fish to supply selenium.

His triglycerides dropped from 130 to 68. His cholesterol dropped from 240 to 186. And his CPK (creatine phosphokinase—an important indicator of muscular dystrophy) dropped from 610 to 140, which is considered borderline with respect to muscular dystrophy.

Dr. Passwater concludes by saying: "Perhaps the nutritional muscular dystrophy in animals is different from the dystrophy in humans—but maybe it's not. At least some patients are responding to selenium plus vitamin E or Coenzyme Q therapy."[11]

---

[10]Passwater, *op. cit.*
[11]Passwater, *op. cit.*

A leading researcher on the role of selenium in preventing killer diseases, Dr. Gerhard Schrauzer, is quoted in Dr. Passwater's book as saying that the preferred dietary sources of selenium are: whole wheat breads and cereals, organ meats (liver, kidney), and seafoods.

As a supplement, in pill form, he says 150 to 200 micrograms of selenium per day is a good maintenance dose for all ages. Dr. Schrauzer says he, personally, takes 200 micrograms per day, occasionally 300–400 micrograms. He says, "There are no toxicity problems at a regular dosage of up to 800 micrograms per day even over extended periods. Even 2,000 micrograms can be taken for some time without harm, but this is about the limit."

Wrinkles Erased, Skin Smoother, Heart and Memory Improved

Sardines are the mainstay of Dr. Benjamin Frank's "no-aging diet," which he claims can actually make people younger as well as cure many ailments. It was tested on people ranging in age from 40 to 70.

The most striking effect was on the skin of the face. Within a week their skin became smooth, soft, and young looking, with a rosy glow. Within a month or so wrinkles, lines, and age spots began to fade away. Other areas began to show improvement—roughened elbows became smoother, hands became younger looking.

Other organs besides the skin were affected. In older patients with coronary heart disease and congestive heart failure, the heart function was clearly improved. Significant effects were noted with regard to the brain, which responded with an increase in mental alertness and improved memory.

Youth Restorative X: The Secret That May Actually Make You Young Again!

Youth Restorative X—the secret that may actually make you young again—is a nucleic acid called RNA. Sardines are loaded with it.

Essentially there are two kinds of nucleic acids, called RNA and DNA. There is reason to believe that nourishing our cells with RNA nucleic acid by ingesting foods that contain substantial amounts of it can help us live longer, cancer-free lives.

Dr. Frank's diet calls for the consumption of sardines four times a week. The smaller the sardine the better it is, he says. For this reason, Norwegian sardines are favored over American ones. He favors other seafood as well, such as salmon, lobster, shrimp, and oysters. He recommends liver, beans (see page 258) such as lentils and pinto beans, and certain vegetables, including beets, asparagus, and celery (see page 57), all of which contain nucleic acid or substances that create nucleic acid.

Other reported results:

The beauty editor of a national health magazine tried the "No-Aging Diet," found that it worked, and gave it an enthusiastic endorsement.

A college professor tried the "No-Aging Diet." For about 10 days he consumed a can of sardines every day plus 40 tablets of brewer's tablets, which is also high in nucleic acid. At the end of this brief period his skin seemed to have taken on a fresher and more youthful appearance.

Professor Sheldon S. Hendler, Ph.D., a respected biochemist who devoted most of his life to nucleic acid research, called Dr. Frank's No-Aging Diet, "A significant landmark in the history of nutrition."

✦   ✦   ✦

Although fish without scales, such as eels, crabs, shellfish, and even snails and turtles were banned in the Old Testament as unclean because they inhabit stagnant waters that don't flow, they existed in abundance in the clear waters of the Sea of Galilee. According to the Jewish historian Josephus, writing in the first century A.D., "The Sea has fresh water that is very pleasant to drink; the water flows freely and is not muddy." Therefore, there is no such ban on fish without "fins and scales"—including catfish, lampreys, and sharks—in the New Testament.

A Healing Oil That May Make You Immune to Disease

Virtually all species of sharks are known to have an extraordinary resistance to disease. They almost never get cancer. They are impervious to infections. They live for upwards of 100 years. Sharks are virtually indestructible.

The secret? Shark-liver oil, which contains a substance called alkylglycerols—AKGs, for short—a family of compounds that makes sharks virtually immune to disease.

AKGs are found in fish and in the breast milk of mammals, where they provide babies with natural protection and immunity against infection. But nowhere are AKGs more abundant than in the liver of sharks. What this means to you is this:

AKGs stimulate the production of white blood cells—the disease fighters of the body that consume viruses and strengthen the immune system.

AKGs destroy free radicals—highly reactive oxygen molecules in the body that are involved in over 60 painful and chronic illnesses and are a major factor in aging.

Unlike most antioxidants, such as vitamins A, C, E, beta-carotene, selenium, and zinc, which are all effective in scavenging free radicals outside of cells, AKGs are able to penetrate the cell membrane, where free radicals hide, and attack them from within.

Free radicals that have penetrated cell membranes can cause structural damage to the DNA—the circuit or switchboard or blueprint of the cell—and when DNA is damaged, cancer can result. AKGs are uniquely effective in preventing this from happening.

So say Drs. Neil Solomon, Richard Passwater, Ingemar Joelsson, and Leonard Haimes in their book *Shark Liver Oil: Nature's Amazing Healer* (Kensington Books, New York, 1997).

Relief for Cancer, and HIV/AIDS

"I've been using shark liver oil capsules with cancer patients, with patients with chronic diseases—with all kinds of patients," says Antonio Calzada, a medical doctor who operates a clinic in Tijuana. "The result has been remarkable because the patients' quality of life improved immediately, just one or two weeks after beginning shark liver oil treatment."

"We ask them how they are feeling with these new capsules, and they say, 'Oh, Doctor, since you gave me the capsules I am feeling much stronger . . . I have less pain . . .'"

"Shark liver oil has been one powerful way for me to improve my patients' quality of life," says Dr. Calzada, who takes one shark-liver-oil capsule himself every day, just for prevention. He says his energy and ability to concentrate have improved.[12]

Cases reported by doctors:[13]

GG, a 69-year-old woman, had been suffering from chronic lymphatic leukemia for 15 years. Her white blood-cell count had been controlled with oral chemotherapy and steroids, but every 2 months it would skyrocket from 25,000 to over 150,000. After GG's last episode her doctor recommended that she take eight 500 mg capsules of shark-liver oil a day. After 6 months of this treatment, she has had no sudden increases in white blood-cell count that had so long plagued her. In fact, her white blood-cell count is now down to 9,000, which is normal.

One doctor has been recommending shark-liver oil to his patients since 1995. One of the most remarkable cases he's seen is his own grown daughter. She had a persistent cough.

---

[12]Reprinted by permission from *Shark Liver Oil,* by Neil Solomon, M.D., Ph.D., Richard A. Passwater, Ph.D., Ingemar Joelsson, M.D., Ph.D., and Leonard Haimes, M.D. Copyright © 1997 by Neil Solomon, M.D., Ph.D., Richard Passwater, Ph.D., Ingemar Joelsson, M.D., Ph.D., and Leonard Haimes, M.D. Published by Kensington Books, an imprint of Kensington Publishing Corp.

[13]*Shark Liver Oil, op. cit.*

X-rays revealed a mass atop her heart the size of a small grape-fruit. The diagnosis: Hodgkins lymphoma. After trying standard medical treatment and homeopathy, she was almost at Level 4, the last stage, with a 60 percent chance of survival. Her father immediately started her on shark-liver oil with 30–40 percent AKGs, but with vitamins A and D removed to prevent overdos-ing on those vitamins. She started to improve. Her specialist told her to "keep doing whatever you're doing." Her chemo was over, and he gave her steroid injections to keep her blood count up. She developed a lung infection from the steroids, but was able to fight it off, thanks to the shark oil, according to her father. During her radiation treatment, she was able to care for her family, take care of two senior citizens, and deal with the problems of building a new home, to everyone's amazement. In 7 months, she was completely free of the Hodgkins lym-phoma. She continues to take shark-liver oil.

"Dear Doctor: Thank you for getting me to take the shark liver oil you suggested over four months ago. My recent blood work just back this week shows that my T-cell count has risen from 370 to 502. . . . Also, my insulin needs seem to be staying between 5 and 7 units less per day since I started the shark liver oil. I'm also not having as much pain in my legs as before. . . . Again, thanks for all the help."—signed J.S.S., dated July 18, 1996

"To whom it may concern: My name is James. . . . I've been HIV+ for over 10 years now. This last year, my T-cell count came down to 214 from 535. Four months ago [my doctor] put me on daily doses of shark liver oil. My most recent lab work, done last week, shows that my T-cell count has gone up again to 353. The only new factor is the shark liver oil. Also, I'm more full of energy than I have been in a long time. . . ."—signed James, dated July 13, 1996.

The authors note that according to the February 20, 1996, issue of the *Washington Post,* a pharmaceutical company has developed "a vaginal foam that could protect against pregnancy and sexually transmitted diseases." The natural substances in this vaginal foam, tentatively called Maganins, were isolated from animals, including sharks, and have "shown some effect in keeping the human immunodeficiency virus (HIV) that causes AIDS from replicating."

More Miracles from This Healing Oil[14]

The true stories and testimonials of average Americans who have recently been introduced to shark-liver oil in capsule form "hold enormous promise for every person, child or adult, whether suffering from a life-threatening disease or simply trying to stay in the best possible health," say these experts.

Asthma—Swedish scientists have discovered the beneficial effects of shark-liver oil on asthma patients. In every case, the discomforts of asthma began to disappear in just a few weeks with oral doses three times a day containing 50 mg of AKGs derived from shark-liver oil (equivalent to 750 mg shark-liver oil). In some cases, scientists witnessed complete recoveries from asthma after just 6 months of treatment.

Diabetes and Multiple Sclerosis—A woman, 50, with both diabetes and multiple sclerosis complained, "The MS really makes you tired." Since taking shark-liver oil she feels energetic. She says, "I am up and about doing things I haven't done in years. I don't feel like sleeping. I feel good!" (And her blood sugar count is down.)

High Blood Pressure—An older man with high blood pressure began taking shark-liver oil capsules. He then had a blood-pressure test. Even though he skipped taking his blood-pressure medicine for 2–3 days before the test, he tested well within the normal range for the first time in 10 years.

Arthritis—Another man had been suffering from arthritis so badly, he could not even make a fist. Then he began taking shark-liver oil. He noticed the difference in 3 days and is now able even to tie fishhooks for the first time in 20 years.

---

[14]*Shark Liver Oil, op. cit.*

In Sweden, patients undergoing radiation who were given AKGs "showed a much higher survival rate than those . . . who received no treatment other than radiation. . . . The highest survival rate occurred in those patients who received AKGs before, during, and after radiation treatment," says Dr. Joelsson.

No Significant Side Effects

Research on shark-liver oil and its primary ingredient, AKG, is not yet complete, say these experts. "Another 20 years might pass before the complete medical efficacy of shark liver oil is provided. However, because the use of shark liver oil produces no significant negative side effects, we are reluctant to wait 20 years. . . . The reality is that shark liver oil . . . just might be a medical breakthrough, one which could bring with it widespread healing experiences."

(The only side effects that have been noted in shark-liver oil rich in AKGs are, in some cases: belching; a rash if allergic to shark-liver protein; and diarrhea if too much is taken.)

"Remember," say Drs. Solomon, Passwater, and Joelsson, "our claim is not that shark liver oil is a magic potion that will cure all of your ills. However, we do want to stress that studies . . . show that AKGs are effective in enhancing basic immune response."[15]

A Gift from the Sea That Could Save Your Life[16]

In his book *Sharks Don't Get Cancer,* Dr. William Lane says that the reason sharks don't get cancer is that shark cartilage contains certain proteins that prevent the development of blood vessels. A tumor cannot grow without creating a network of blood vessels around itself for nourishment. (This process is called angiogenesis.)

---

[15]*Shark Liver Oil, op. cit.*
[16]From *Sharks Don't Get Cancer* by I. William Lane and Linda Comac © 1992. Published by Avery Publishing Group, Inc., Garden City Park, NY. Reprinted with permission.

Researchers reasoned that since cartilage is without blood vessels, something in the cartilage was keeping blood vessels from forming and could be used in humans to keep new blood vessels from forming around tumors. Without blood for nourishment, a tumor shrinks and dies.

In the mid-1970s, scientists at MIT succeeded in preventing the formation of new blood vessels around tumors in lab animals with an extract of calf cartilage. The tumors stopped growing. Further research was thwarted due to the short supply of cartilage. Only small amounts of it exist in calves and other mammals.

These researchers then turned to sharks, whose skeletons are composed entirely of cartilage. Research on shark cartilage had already been started by Carl Luer, Ph.D., a biochemist in Florida. He found that sharks failed to develop cancer even when exposed to massive amounts of highly carcinogenic chemicals.

Several studies have confirmed the tumor-shrinking power of cartilage, especially shark cartilage, according to Dr. Lane. For example, at the Institut Jules Bordet in Brussels, under the direction of Dr. Ghanem Atassi, 40 mice received grafts of human melanoma. Half received no treatment. Half received daily doses of whole dry shark cartilage given by mouth. Tumors in the untreated animals doubled in size in 21 days, while the tumors in the animals that had received the shark cartilage decreased 17 percent.

Tests on Humans[17]

Dr. Lane reports on the experimental work of various doctors using shark cartilage, among them Ernesto Contreras, Sr., M.D., and his two sons, Ernesto, Jr., and Francisco, who are also medical doctors. Together they run the Contreras Hospital in Tijuana, Mexico. Dr. Lane approached them, asking if they would try shark cartilage on some of their terminal patients. They agreed to treat ten cancer patients free of charge, all of them in the late stages of their disease with little chance of surviving even 6 months.

---

[17]*Sharks Don't Get Cancer,* by I. William Lane and Linda Comac, *op. cit.*

"The initial plan," says Lane, "called for four months of cartilage treatment to be administered to 10 patients. Dr. Ernesto Contreras, Jr., elected to treat the chosen patients with 30 grams of the cartilage material daily in the form of a water suspension. For female patients, half the daily dose would be given via retention enema and half would be introduced into the vaginal body cavity. Male patients would receive 2 retention enemas. These methods of treatment would allow the protein of the shark cartilage to be quickly absorbed into the system."

Pain Relief, Shrinking Tumors, and Two "Miracle Cures" Claimed[18]

Eventually eight patients were involved in the study, one having dropped out, and one having died early. Of these "hopeless" cases, in seven patients there was a reduction in tumor size of 30 to 100 percent, and two "miracle" cures, says Lane:

> A 48-year-old woman with a Stage III inoperable locally advanced uterine and cervix cancer with invasion to the bladder. Earlier doses of radiation had not helped. She had considerable pain. Following 7 weeks of shark-cartilage therapy, the pain was largely gone and the tumor 80 percent smaller. After eleven weeks, there was a complete (100 percent) reduction in tumor size.

> A 62-year-old female with bone metastasis to the right sacroiliac from a previously treated uterine cervix cancer. The metastasis developed in an area that had been previously radiated. After 9 weeks of shark-cartilage therapy, the tumor was at least 80 percent smaller. At eleven weeks, all signs of the tumor were gone, and the patient was considered cured.

---

[18]Lane and Comac, *op. cit.*

A 36-year-old female with a Stage IV peritoneal carcinoma from a colon primary cancer. Exploratory surgery had confirmed the diagnosis of inoperable cancer, and the patient had been given little chance of survival. After 7 weeks of shark-cartilage treatment, she needed an operation to remove an abscess, during which the tumor was found to be 80 percent smaller, and what was left had gelatinized. At eleven weeks, the patient was tumor-free and was considered by the doctors to be a "miracle cure."

Lane cites many other cases in his book, including many who failed to respond to treatment, or improved initially and then had relapses. But certain facts emerged: *"Absolutely no toxicity was noted at any dosage level. In each case, use of shark cartilage significantly reduced pain. This may be one of the most important findings in the study. Pain reduction seems to be the first effect of shark cartilage."*

He tells of a medical doctor in the United States who, after reading about shark cartilage, began giving it to cancer patients, watching their progress and checking for side effects. This doctor soon discovered that high-level doses of shark cartilage—up to 120 grams—brought amazing results. "He has worked with over 110 patients," says Lane. "MRI and CAT scans reveal that at least 15 of Dr. Martinez's patients are basically tumor-free. Others are showing a reduction in tumor size." Dr. Martinez was preparing a paper on it for scientific journals.

Ailments Most (and Least) Likely to Be Affected[19]

"Breast, cervical, prostate, central nervous system, and pancreatic cancers are among the most heavily vascularized cancers and therefore potentially the best targets for shark-cartilage therapy," says Lane. "Cancers such as lymphoma, Hodgkins, and leukemia are less likely to be affected by shark cartilage since new vascularization is rarely involved in their development."

---

[19]Lane and Comac, *op. cit.*

Dosage[20]

In all these clinical trials, 100 percent pure shark cartilage was used. "The data seem to indicate that with Stage III and Stage IV tumors, approximately 1 gram of shark cartilage per 2 pounds of body weight should be used on a daily basis," Lane says. "When possible the material should be administered as a retention enema, but it can be administered orally if necessary. . . . Most tumor reduction has been seen with oral/rectal administration. Doses should be spread throughout the day to keep the level of active protein in the blood fairly constant. . . .

"Lower dosages given in the early stages of cancer or as a preventative measure seem to be effective when administered orally . . .

"For oral administration, mix the cartilage in a vegetable juice such as tomato or carrot, or in beef juice, or in fruit nectar. To prepare a retention enema, mix 15 grams (3 level teaspoons) of shark cartilage powder in two-thirds of a cup of body-temperature water. Women might prefer to take at least one dose as a water suspension introduced into the vaginal cavity, especially in the case of vaginal, cervical, or uterine tumor. . . .

"Preliminary results indicate that some reduction in tumor size will be noted within six weeks after the start of treatment," says Dr. Lane, "and major tumor reduction will be noted within eleven weeks. When tumors are less life-threatening, the dosage level can be lowered; evidence indicates that dosage can be reduced up to 60 percent."

Πot a Substitute
for Qualified Medical Care[21]

Shark cartilage, says Lane, "is largely inert and non-toxic and can therefore be used in conjunction with other therapies. *I want to make it crystal clear, I am not suggesting that conventional medical approaches be replaced by shark-cartilage administration.*

I do believe that shark cartilage can and probably should be used along with conventional approaches."

---

[20]Lane and Comac, *op. cit.*
[21]Lane and Comac, *op. cit.*

Effect on Other Conditions[22]

"Tumors and metastases are not the only conditions that can be controlled by shark cartilage," says Lane. "Once shark cartilage is in a person's system, its anti-inflammatory and antiangiogenic characteristics begin to work on a variety of diseases.

"Its effects on arthritis, psoriasis, and enteritis have already been demonstrated, and its probable effects on diabetic retinopathy, neovascular glaucoma, and macular degeneration have been discussed in a number of scientific journals."

One study using shark cartilage was conducted in 1988 by Dr. Serge Orloff, one of Europe's leading arthritis experts. He administered dried shark cartilage to humans, giving them 9 grams of cartilage daily for 4 weeks followed by 4.5 grams daily for an additional extended period.

100% Pain Reduction[23]

One of Dr. Orloff's patients was a 49-year-old woman with painful degenerative arthritis in her knees and low-back pain due to a chronic disk problem. Her pain decreased by 50 percent after the first 2 weeks of treatment and then by another 50 percent after 6 weeks of treatment. She reported that she could bend both her knees and her back while doing her daily chores and that she felt renewed strength in her muscles.

Spine Straightens[24]

In a clinical study in Panama, a 42-year-old man with rheumatoid arthritis was bedridden with intense pain and deformity in the large joints. For 25 years he had been treated with analgesics, salicylates,

---

[22]Lane and Comac, *op. cit.*
[23]Lane and Comac, *op. cit.*
[24]Lane and Comac, *op. cit.*

nonsteroidal anti-inflammatory drugs, gold salts, immunosuppressants, and corticoids. Then he began receiving shark-cartilage capsules—one capsule per 11 pounds of body weight for 21 days, then four capsules per day for the next 21 days.

After 3 weeks, doctors noticed that his spinal column had straightened and his pain had completely disappeared. He now says, "I am able to move my arms and legs without pain; my walk has improved; I am more agile. I feel like working; I'm not tired and my constipation and gastritis have improved."

He continues to take four capsules of shark cartilage along with 5 milligrams of prednisone and sulindac in isolated form every 48 hours.

Dosage[25]

According to Lane, researchers have found that shark cartilage is successful in reducing pain in approximately 70 percent of osteoarthritis cases and 60 percent of rheumatoid arthritis cases. Dosage: 1 gram of dried shark cartilage for every 15 pounds of body weight (or one 750 mg capsule per 11 pounds of body weight)—divided into three equal doses, 15 minutes before each meal—per day for 21 days.

"Generally speaking, users experience pain relief within 16 to 18 days," he says. "If major pain relief is not observed after 30 days of continuous and correct use, the cartilage will probably not work with your system or problem."

Once pain relief is noticed, the dose is decreased to 2 grams for each 40 pounds of body weight (or one 750 mg capsule per 30 pounds of body weight). This may be consumed all at once or divided into two equal doses, says Lane.*

---

[25]Lane and Comac, *op. cit.*

Note: Glucosamine sulfate—a food supplement that has become extremely popular in recent years because of its effectiveness in relieving crippling arthritic stiffness, better than drugs in many cases—*is a natural constituent of cartilage.* It seems to work best at a dose of 500 mg three times daily. *Unlike drugs, glucosamine sulfate stimulates cartilage repair and is free from side effects.*

Caution[26]

Dr. Lane cautions that "anyone who has recently suffered a heart attack needs to rebuild blood vessels" and therefore "should not use an angiogenesis inhibitor for at least 3 months or as advised by his or her doctor . . . A pregnant woman who is building a blood network to feed the developing embryo should not use shark cartilage. Women who are attempting to conceive should also avoid taking shark cartilage."

"The Water of Life" for Arthritis

Years ago, a doctor reported the effects of sea-brine therapy on his 97-year-old father-in-law, who was senile and completely crippled with arthritis. He had to be lifted out of bed and could not feed or dress himself. On this doctor's advice, he was given 1 teaspoonful of concentrated sea water daily for 4 months.

Suddenly he began to perk up. He got out of bed one day, hobbled into the kitchen, and began fixing breakfast. He'd had an arthritic hip for over 20 years and would yell if anyone touched his right leg even gently. But now he crossed his legs to put on his shoes, and let the right foot hit the floor without a peep. After being senile and crippled for many years, he began to get up every morning without help, walk to the bathroom, wash, and come in for breakfast.

Reportedly, the only new item in his food or drink was the daily teaspoonful of sea water, the kind sold in health-food stores, concentrated to ten times the usual ocean strength.

---

[26]Lane and Comac, *op. cit.*

CHAPTER · 1 0
A BIBLE FOOD
THAT WIPES OUT
ARTHRITIS PAIN

The miracle healing powers of fish—a food blessed by Jesus—as revealed in Chapter 9 would be incomplete without the startling facts about codfish and its amazing curative oil. For generations given to babies to prevent malformed bones, this oil can do much more.

＋ Its rich vitamin-A content protects the heart and lungs from viruses, bacteria, and infections; repels and retards cancer of the stomach, intestines, cervix, and prostate gland; and lowers cholesterol without the side effects of drugs used for that purpose. Its vitamin-D content makes it important to nerve health, normal heart action, and sugar metabolism.

＋ This oil is also healing to various skin conditions, such as varicose leg ulcers, wounds, burns, and sores. It forms a protective, nonirritating layer over a wound and acts powerfully to stimulate rapid tissue healing.

One doctor claimed to have successfully treated his psoriasis patients with cod-liver-oil capsules. A lifelong sufferer claimed her psoriasis suddenly went into remission after taking one capsule daily for a month.

Miraculous Relief for Arthritis

But cod-liver oil's most famous use is for arthritis. It has been known to relieve arthritis at least since the 1700s.

As early as 1766 in England, physicians recommended cod-liver oil to treat chronic rheumatism and gout. By the mid-1800s, cod-liver oil was routinely prescribed for those diseases as well as for other diseases of the joints and spine.

During World War I, Dr. Ralph Pemberton began using cod-liver oil to treat over 400 arthritic patients—most of whom were helped—at the University of Pennsylvania. His conclusion was that cod-liver oil was effective in eliminating the pain, stiffness, and swelling of chronic arthritis. He reported his findings in *Studies on Arthritis in the Army Based on Four Hundred Cases,* which appeared in the *Archives of Internal Medicine* (March 1920).

Rapid and Astonishing Results

In an article in the *Journal of the National Medical Association,* Charles A. Brusch, M.D., and Edward Johnson, M.D., obtained rapid and astonishing results in relieving arthritis and rheumatism with a partial fasting or cleansing diet. The main points of this plan are the taking of cod-liver oil on an empty stomach and the restriction of all water intake to a single portion taken 1 hour before breakfast.

These doctors tested 98 patients, and found 92 showed major improvement in their arthritic symptoms and wonderful changes in their blood cleanliness. Cholesterol levels were normalized, even though this controlled fasting plan allowed eggs, butter, and milk. One diabetic patient gave up taking insulin. Blood pressure also normalized.

These doctors also stated: "We felt these [rapid] improvements were primarily due to the cod liver oil and unusual arrangements for liquid drinking intake. . . . We obtain our results in 3 to 6 months' time. A wholesome diet alone would perhaps take 6 to 36 months to produce 50 to 75% of our results at best."

Unlocking Fused Bones!

But what if the bones are actually fused? For a long time, even doctors who prescribed cod-liver oil for arthritis drew the line when it came to advanced cases such as this. It remained for Giraud W. Campbell, D.O., to discover how this could be done, as revealed in his book, *A Doctor's Proven New Home Cure for Arthritis* (Parker Publishing Company, 1972).

Dr. Campbell says this method—involving cod-liver oil—has cured hundreds of sufferers, regardless of age or condition. In all cases, heat and swelling in the affected joints was eased within 1 week. Pain was relieved—in most cases eliminated—in two weeks or less. Normal movement was restored in almost all cases in 3 weeks or less. X-rays revealed progress in the restoration of damaged bone structure in 3–6 months.

Wheelchairs and crutches were tossed aside. The only cases to whom he cannot guarantee relief, he says, are those who have had extensive gold or drug therapy, which sometimes permanently alters the body chemistry, and advanced spinal arthritis if not caught within the first 5 years. Even so, spectacular relief is reported in many such cases, and further bone degeneration is halted. Even the agony of weather changes can be a thing of the past, he says.

Not only are pain and inflammation relieved, bone structure is improved, says Dr. Campbell. And he offers X-rays showing kneecaps unfusing, compressed vertebrae regenerating, and bony overgrowth reduced and absorbed, which medical doctors consider impossible. "Those that are bed-ridden . . . in the acute inflammatory state . . . show the most dramatic response," he says. "In from 3 to 10 days their pains cease, and repair sets in."

Dr. Campbell gives the following cases:

A woman said: "I found myself a cripple, unable to walk without pain. I tried several doctors, aspirin, gold injections, cortisone drugs—nothing seemed to help. I kept getting continually worse, endured constant pain and had to be pulled from a chair, helped at every step." After 4 years of suffering, she tried this method and said: "Within three weeks I was without pain and could go to work feeling my old self again . . . jump out of bed and feel alive. I am now able to stand up straight, move about without pain, get a good night's sleep and do housework. I enjoy life again."

Mrs. A. S., 65, began to experience pains and stiffness in her arms and legs. Her doctor called it arthritis (rheumatoid) and treated her for 1 month. Then he sent her to a specialist, who referred her to another specialist, who gave her 6 months of treatment and sent her to a medical center for cobalt treatment (another 6 months). No cure, they all said. With this method, she said: "I am able to arise in the morning, make my own bed, walk up and down stairs, go out to dine, visit friends and go shopping . . ."

Walter M. said: "I was in agony. Something was wrong with my spine in the region of my shoulder blades. I had visited medical men . . . and I could not obtain relief. The neurosurgeon prescribed traction . . . which did not ease my pain . . . I could not sleep in bed . . . I had to sleep in an upright position at the dining room table." With this method, in two weeks he could once again sleep in comfort."

Mrs. G. W., 42, was in such pain she could not stand the pressure of bedsheets, and she'd been bedridden 6 months. Even her jaw was in pain. With this method, in two days her pain was gone, without medication or aspirin. In two weeks she was walking and housecleaning. Her hands no longer bothered her. After 6 months, you'd never guess she had arthritis.

One man said shortly after his Army service, he began experiencing pain in his lower back and shooting pains down the back of his legs. Doctors gave him no relief. He could hardly move and was in constant agony. He spent 4 years going to a VA hospital, with no relief. Then he tried an arthritic specialist for 9 years, with all kinds of medications and injections. He grew steadily worse. His spine practically fused solid. Then he heard about this method. In two weeks, 50 percent of his pain vanished. He was able to walk better, and gradually straightened up. Years of agony vanished!

"Arthritis can be cured," says Dr. Campbell. "While a search for a cure for arthritis goes on, *hundreds, for a fact, are being cured,"* he emphasizes. "While scientists theorize about the high white blood cell count or the low red blood cell count, hundreds of arthritic sufferers are emerging from their ordeal with a normal blood count. While scientists are debating over bacteria, viruses and mycoplasma, the disease is abating [with this method] . . . While new salicylates, like aspirin, are perfected to relieve those whose lives are destined to be plagued by arthritic pain, *that pain is gone forever within seven days* for those who eat in a special way . . . While patients are being injected with [drugs], with ACTH and with gold . . . others are injecting themselves with delicious nutritional foods and enjoying *permanent cure* . . . [with] no need for aspirin or other pain relievers in a week or 10 days . . . a gradual restoration of damaged bone . . . return to a normal life without arthritic pain."

How to Regain Normal Use of Joints in 7 Days!

Dr. Campbell says the following diet will relieve all types of arthritis, including osteoarthritis, rheumatoid arthritis, or any other type of arthritis—in 7 days. Many facets of this program have been known and used for centuries. Fasting, for example. Moses, Elijah, and Jesus each fasted for 40 days. You, however, are only required to fast for 1 day with this method.

Day No. 1

Breakfast—none

Lunch—none

Dinner—none

Stay away from food completely for 1 full day. Drink at least four 8-ounce glasses of water.

Day No. 2

Breakfast— Unsweetened grape or prune juice
              Bananas

Lunch—   Fresh beef liver, preferably raw or lightly sauteed
              Mixed green salad, oil-and-vinegar dressing
              Bowl of blueberries or other fruit in season

Dinner—   Raw vegetable plate (green peppers, celery, tomatoes, etc.)
              Raw fruit salad (shred apples, figs, grapes, bananas, etc., but not citrus fruits).

Take 1 tablespoon of cod-liver oil, twice a day.

Day No. 3

Breakfast— Blended raw fruits
              8 ounces raw certified milk

Lunch—   Fresh fillet of ocean fish, lightly sauteed
              Raw cauliflower or other raw fresh vegetable
              8 ounces certified milk with 1 tablespoon powdered brewer's yeast and 1 tablespoon blackstrap molasses

Dinner—   Fresh (or kosher) beef liver, lightly sauteed with onions
              Mixed green salad
              Melon, or other fruit in season

Take 2 tablespoons of cod-liver oil, twice a day.

Day No. 4

Breakfast— Prunes or prune juice
              8 ounces raw certified milk

Lunch—   Veal kidneys, lightly sauteed
              Mixed green salad
              8 ounces raw certified milk with 1 tablespoon powdered brewer's yeast and 1 tablespoon blackstrap molasses

Dinner—   Halibut steak (or other seafood), broiled
            Raw spinach salad
            Half avocado
            Strawberries or other fruit in season
            8 ounces raw certified milk

Take 1 tablespoon of cod-liver oil, twice a day.

Day No. 5

Breakfast— Cantaloupe half or other raw fruit in season
            8 ounces raw certified milk

Lunch—   Half avocado, sliced tomatoes, and watercress
            8 ounces raw certified milk with 1 tablespoon
            powdered brewer's yeast and 1 tablespoon black-
            strap molasses

Dinner—   Fresh beef liver patties, as rare as you can eat
            them
            Mixed green salad
            Rhubarb
            8 ounces raw certified milk

Take 1 tablespoon cod-liver oil, twice a day.

Day No. 6

Breakfast— Unsweetened grape or prune juice
            Veal kidneys, lightly sauteed
            8 ounces raw certified milk

Lunch—   Shrimp salad
            Cantaloupe half or other raw fruit in season
            8 ounces raw certified milk with 1 tablespoon
            powdered brewer's yeast and 1 tablespoon black-
            strap molasses

Dinner—   Large chef's salad including raw peas, raw string
            beans, and other uncooked vegetables and greens
            Plums or other raw fruit in season
            8 ounces raw certified milk

Take 1 tablespoon of cod-liver oil, twice a day.

Day No. 7

Breakfast— Sliced bananas
8 ounces raw certified milk

Lunch—   Lightly broiled filet of sole
Carrot sticks and watercress
Grapes
8 ounces raw certified milk

Dinner—   Lightly sauteed sweetbreads
Raw vegetables mixed in blender
Honeydew melon or other raw fruit in season
8 ounces raw certified milk

Take 1 tablespoon of cod-liver oil, twice a day.

During all 7 days:

1. Drink only when thirsty, and then only raw fresh fruit or raw fresh vegetable juice, or raw certified milk or water.

2. Take an enema daily until charcoal or corn test shows no further need. (Purchase charcoal tablets at a health-food store. Take six at the end of an evening meal. They color your stool black. The entire black charcoal should be eliminated the following morning. In arthritis, it usually takes 4–7 days for the black to disappear. The next night instead of charcoal eat one or two ears of corn for dinner. Swallow some of the kernels whole. The following day, these should appear in the stool. If not, take a warm-water enema.)

3. Continue this diet until heat, pain, and swelling disappear.

4. Add one food from the allowable lists per day after heat, pain, and swelling disappear.

ALLOWABLE FOODS

VEGETABLES

Asparagus
Beans, lima
Beans, navy
Beans, pole
Beans, string

Mushrooms
Okra
Onions
Parsley
Parsnips

Beans, wax
Beets
Beet tops
Broccoli
Brussels sprouts
Cabbage, red
Cabbage, savoy
Cauliflower
Carrots
Chives
Corn
Cucumbers
Eggplant
Endive
Escarole
Horseradish
Kohlrabi
Kale
Leek
Lettuce

Peas
Peas, black-eyed
Peppers, green
Radishes
Rice, brown
Rice, wild
Rutabagas
Salsify
Scallions
Spinach
Squash, banana
Squash, butternut
Squash, golden
Squash, Hubbard
Squash, summer
Squash, Zucchini
Swiss chard
Tomatoes
Turnips
Watercress

FOWL

Cornish hen
Duck
Goose
Range chicken
Squab
Turkey

MEATS (Veal)

Chops
Cutlets (not breaded)
Veal, breast of
Veal roast

MEATS (Beef)

Chopped beef
Flanken
Ox tails
Roasts (all kinds)
Shank meat
Short ribs
Steaks (all kinds)
Stew beef

MEATS (Pork)

Chops (all kinds)
Head cheese
Pigs knuckles
Roasts (all kinds)
Sausage (homemade)
Spareribs

MEATS (Lamb)

Chops (all kinds)
Lamb patties
Lamb, roast leg of
Lamb shank
Lamb stew

MEATS (Organ)

Brains
Heart
Kidney
Liver
Sweetbreads
Tripe (cattle only)

SEAFOOD

Bass, striped
Clams
Cod
Concha
Eels
Flounder
Fluke
Halibut
Lobster
Oysters

Pompano
Mussels
Salmon (fresh)
Scallops (bay)
Scallops (deep sea)
Sea bass
Shrimp
Smelts
Tuna (fresh)
Whiting

FRUITS

Apples, Baldwin
Apples, golden
Apples, northern spy
Apples, red
Apples, Rome
Apricots
Bananas
Blackberries
Blueberries
Boysenberries
Cherries
Cortlands
Currants
Figs
Gooseberries

Grapes (any)
Loganberries
Melons (any)
Mulberries
Nectarines
Peaches
Pears, Bartlett
Pears, sickel
Plums
Prunes
Raspberries
Rhubarb
Russets
Strawberries
Winesaps

NUTS

Almonds	Hazel nuts
Brazil nuts	Hickory nuts
Butternuts	Peanuts
Cashews	Pecans
Chestnuts, Chinese	Walnuts
Filberts	Walnuts, black

SOUPS   *SEEDS*

Barley (unpearled)   Pumpkin
Lentil   Sesame
Lima bean   Sunflower
Marrowbone
Navy bean
Split pea

Foods to Be Permanently Avoided

1. Flour of all kinds, whether it is whole wheat (unless grown without artificial fertilizers and poisonous sprays), white flour, corn flour, rye flour, soy flour, etc.

2. All flour products, such as bread, toasts, cakes, pies, cookies, crackers, buns, crullers, doughnuts, spaghetti, macaroni, noodles, pizza, etc.

3. Coffee, tea, cocoa, liquor, beer, wine, colas, carbonated beverages, and all so-called "soft drinks"

4. Sugars, candies, ice creams, and artificial sweeteners

5. Jellies, jams, and marmalades

6. Canned or processed foods such as Jello®, custard, pudding, and prepared mixes

7. Frozen fruits

8. Any food manufactured or adulterated by man, such as prepared breakfast cereals or semi-prepared ones like quick-cooked oatmeal

You may be able to cheat from time to time and get away with it. But you should always be on your guard for adverse symptoms or flare-ups and immediately go back to this program, says Dr. Campbell.

In Dr. Campbell's list of allowed foods, you'll notice you get your B vitamins from liver, Brewer's yeast, and blackstrap molasses (iron too); you get your calcium from fresh vegetables; your A and D vitamins from cod-liver oil; and your iodine from fish. In his book, *An Eighty-Year-Old Doctor's Secrets of Positive Health,* William Brady, M.D., states: "If you ask me about 'rheumatiz' [that's what he calls all forms of arthritis], I'll tell you it is a degeneration of the joint tissues due to nutritional deficiency . . . and that *it is chiefly a calcium, vitamin D, iodine and vitamin B deficiency. There is no more to tell about the nature and cause of insidiously developing joint disability of long standing . . .*

"This is not something I picked out of the air. It is a conviction that came from a professional lifetime of study . . . I am not promoting any remedy or cure. I merely recommend a regimen, a way of life to prevent, relieve . . . perhaps even cure the 'rheumatiz.' This last claim I hesitate to make. But I am emboldened to speak of cure by numerous reports I have received from victims who declare they really are cured and back at their jobs."

The main difference between Brady's program and Campbell's is that Brady, an M.D., ignores most food sources of these nutrients (he does recommend 1-1/2 pints of milk, cod-liver oil, and plain wheat daily). He suggests you get your calcium, vitamins D, B-complex, and iodine from high-potency tablets, at your local health-food store. He makes no mention of what foods to avoid, or internal cleansing. While users no longer required aspirin or pain relievers after 10 days, there is no real difference between being chained to one type of pill or another, an aspirin or a calcium tablet. Except for the fact that if you can't stand the taste of cod-liver oil Dr. Campbell says it's okay to use cod-liver-oil capsules, and he does recommend Brewer's yeast (a concentrated protein), Campbell's program uses only food as medicine.

A Vitamin in This Oil Protects against Viruses, Bacteria, Infections

Vitamin A, found in abundance in cod-liver oil, is used by the body to ward off fevers and infections. In studies at Michael Reese Hospital and at Northwestern University in Chicago, in 1955, children suffering from rheumatic fever showed low blood levels of vitamin A. The same effect was noticed in pneumonia patients. Any fever seemed to decrease sharply the amount of vitamin A in the body.

In 1967, a London physician, Dr. Max Odens, told of his experiences giving vitamin A to patients suffering from chronic bronchitis. He had begun giving the vitamin to 17 patients in the early 1950s. Some 15 years later, all of them were alive, the eldest age 79. All had shown considerable improvement.

In 1973, Dr. Benjamin E. Cohen of the Massachusetts General Hospital told a meeting of the American Society of Plastic and Reconstructive Surgeons that vitamin A strengthens the ability of laboratory animals to fight off infection. He told how he had inoculated mice with 3,000 units of vitamin A, an enormous amount for such a tiny animal. He had then injected the mice with deadly bacteria. Another group of mice that had not been given the vitamin A also received the bacteria.

The non-vitamin-A recipients all died of infection after 24 hours. The mice that received the vitamin developed severe infections for the first 3 hours. But at the end of 5 hours, the infections seemed to have disappeared. No more bacteria could be cultured from their blood.

Many different types of bacteria were tested. In all cases, those animals fortified with large amounts of vitamin A resisted the infection much better than did the non-vitamin-A recipients.

In 1975, Eli Seifter of the Albert Einstein College of Medicine injected pox virus into two groups of mice. One group had been given five to ten times its usual daily requirement of vitamin A. The other had received the normal amount present in the usual laboratory diet. The vitamin-A-fed mice developed fewer pox lesions, and those they did develop cleared up faster than did those that the control animals developed. The mice that received the vitamin also suffered less fever than did the control group of mice.

Dr. Seifter concluded that vitamin A is "very protective" and enhances the body's ability to immunize itself against attack.

Effect on Cancer

In 1942, vitamin A was given to an animal undergoing radiation for a tumor, by researchers at the Anderson Hospital and Tumor Institute of the University of Texas. As a result, the amount of radiation needed to control the tumor was reduced by 25 percent. The more time the animal had to absorb the vitamin A, the better it was able to resist the tumor. (*Journal of the National Cancer Institute,* 48, 1942)

In 1967, Dr. Max Odens found that cancer-causing substances applied to the neck of the uterus would not cause cervical cancer if vitamin A were added to them. He noted that although cancer cells grown outside the body could be induced into prostate glands, this did not happen when the carcinogen used to induce the cancer was supplemented with vitamin A.

In 1968, Dr. Umberto Saffioti, a pathologist at Chicago Medical School, told a conference at MIT that of 113 hamsters exposed to high dosages of benzypyrene, a known carcinogen found in tobacco smoke, 60 of them had previously been given substantial amounts of vitamin A. The other 53 had not. Of the 53 animals that had not received the vitamin, 16 developed lung cancer. *Of the 60 animals that had received vitamin A, only one developed any cancerous tumors.*

In addition to protecting the lungs, vitamin A also tended to protect the fore-stomach, the gastrointestinal tract, and the uterine cervix from cancer, in other tests on laboratory animals, according to Dr. Saffiotti.

The Saffiotti report resulted in a flood of additional research throughout the seventies, all of it favorable, on the immunizing power of vitamin A against cancer.

Dr. Raymond J. Shamberger of the Cleveland Clinic Foundation, following a series of experiments with vitamin A on lab animals, flatly concluded that "vitamin A, when administered [externally or internally] retards the growth and inhibits the induction of benign and malignant tumors."

Not only did vitamin A seem to protect lab animals from induced tumors, but when they did develop malignancy, their tumors developed much more slowly than they did in non-vitamin-A-protected mice and regressed about twice as fast, according to a research team from Albert Einstein College of Medicine, in 1973.

Vitamin A was found to inhibit the growth of cancer in all cases, in tests with lab animals at Vanderbilt University, the National Cancer Institute, the National Institute of Allergy and Infectious Diseases, and MIT.

In tests on humans in Norway, 8,278 males were divided into two groups, those whose vitamin A intake was low and those whose vitamin A intake was relatively high. The results of the 5-year study were reported by Dr. E. Bjelke of the Cancer Registry of Norway in 1975. *The low-vitamin-A group was responsible for nearly three quarters of all the lung cancer in both groups combined.*

Vitamin A can be taken in daily amounts ranging up to 25,000 units, according to one expert. Cases of vitamin A overdosages are very rare, he says, pointing out that there are over 50,000 units in a normal serving of carrots, and that Eskimos eating their normal diet consume 200,000 to 300,000 units of vitamin A a day. Dr. G. H. Whipple, who received a Nobel prize for his discovery that liver stops the progress of pernicious anemia, once put his patients on a diet of raw liver three times a day over a long period of time. He never reported noticing any signs of vitamin overdosage, and if he had it could have been easily corrected by simply reducing the dosage.

Natural vitamin A, derived from fish oils, actually gives you a complex of vitamins, believed by some to be more effective and less toxic than synthetic vitamin A. Among those rare cases of overdosage of vitamin A, there are no cases where such overdose occurred as the result of taking this vitamin in its natural form, according to one expert.

Vitamins in This Oil That Lower Cholesterol

For 10 years, Dr. F.C.H. Ross used vitamins A and D in treating certain patients. On studying the records of these patients, he noticed that those treated with these vitamins had shown reduced incidence of heart trouble. He theorized that the reason might be that these vitamins somehow lowered cholesterol.

In order to check this, the effects of vitamins A and D on coronary heart disease were observed over 5-1/2 years in 136 patients, with 271 patients serving as controls. The controls received medication with no vitamins A or D added.

The capsules used contained 6,000 units of vitamin A and 1,000 units of vitamin D and were given three times a day for anywhere from 6 months to 5 years.

Only eight patients—5.8 percent—of the group treated with vitamins A and D developed coronary heart disease, while 43 patients in the untreated group—15.8 percent—developed heart problems.

In 13 patients, serum cholesterol was reduced an average of 30 milligrams per milliliter after 2–4 weeks on this vitamin A and D combination. In contrast, the untreated group of patients showed no real change in their average cholesterol levels over the same length of time.

Dr. Ross and his associate Dr. A. H. Campbell wrote, in the *Journal of Australia* for August 19, 1961: "In Australia and America, owing to changing food habits, there has been a definite fall in vitamin A consumption per head in the last 20 or 30 years. . . . It is of interest also that in underdeveloped countries such as New Guinea with a low incidence of coronary heart disease, the vitamin A intake is high. . . . Of course, the fat-poor diet may be equally important in such groups. But the Eskimos, who are reputed to have a fat-rich diet with a low incidence of coronary heart disease, have a high vitamin A intake from fish and marine animal livers."

Wipes out Common Cold

Dr. Irwin C. Spiesman, M.D., of the University of Illinois College of Medicine, studied the effects of vitamins A and D on the common cold, as reported in *Archives of Otolaryngology* in 1961. He wanted to know if any reduction in the incidence of colds could be due to intake of one or the other, or both, of these vitamins. He studied 54 "chronic or frequent cold sufferers" who had five to seven colds, with high fever, lasting 1–2 weeks, sometimes requiring bed rest, every winter.

These patients were divided into three groups. Group 1 received only vitamin A; Group 2 received only vitamin D; Group 3 received both vitamin A and D.

None of the patients who received either vitamin A or D alone were helped. Of those who received both vitamins, 15 percent were completely free of colds in the second and third year of the 3-year study and experienced a marked reduction of colds during the first year. Of those that received both vitamins, 80 percent showed significant reduction in both the number and severity of the colds. The number of colds dropped from seven to three a year, and the average duration was 5 days with little temperature elevation.

+ + +

Vitamin A is a fat-soluble vitamin. It dissolves in fat, and it can be stored in the body. People who have had a serious illness or infections are almost certain to be short of vitamin A; anyone who suffers from any stomach, liver, or intestinal disorder probably lacks vitamin A; taking mineral oil for long periods of time destroys vitamin A. Experiments at Columbia University showed that animals who receive far more than the recommended daily requirement of vitamin A live longer and are freer from the symptoms of old age. Vitamin A was also found to be protective against cataracts in a study of 50,000 female nurses, ages 34–59, over a 10-year period.

A lack of vitamin A causes night blindness, sensitivity to glare, and difficulty reading in dim light. It is necessary for skin health, fighting colds and infections, preventing kidney stones and good growth and dental health in children.

The richest sources of vitamin A are liver, milk, eggs, and liver oils from cod and halibut.

The Twin Miracle in This Oil

The other vitamin for which cod-liver oil is famous is vitamin D. It is the reason cod-liver oil is given to babies, to prevent the crooked bones of rickets. Vitamin D is important for adults, too. It protects the thyroid gland. Some types of arthritis have been improved or cured with vitamin D. Some eye diseases improve when vitamin D is given. Children who suffer from myopia (nearsightedness) have shown a lack of either calcium or phosphorus in their blood, neither of which can be absorbed without vitamin D. Vitamin D is important to nerve health, normal heart action, and normal clotting of the blood, for the same reason.

If there is a shortage of vitamin D in your diet, there will be a shortage of phosphorus, without which sugar is not burned efficiently. This means that energy-supplying sugar will be lost in the urine and the feces. Lack of vitamin D may be a reason why so many people seem to lack energy.

Fish-liver oil is the richest source of vitamin D. It is a good source of vitamin A as well, and can be obtained in capsules.

CHAPTER 11
STRANGE JUICE MEDICINE REVEALED BY THE BIBLE CLAIMED BY MANY TO HEAL AILMENTS QUICKLY

A land of wheat, and barley, and vines . . . *Deuteronomy 8:8*

Take thou also unto thee wheat, and barley, and beans, and lentils, and millet . . . and put them into one vessel, and make thee bread thereof . . . And thou shalt eat it as barley cakes . . . *Ezekiel 4:9 and 12*

Wheat is specifically mentioned in the Bible 52 times. So much wheat was produced that the growing season was used like a calendar to reckon time. *Wheat* and *corn* mean the same thing in the Bible. Luke 6:1 refers to Christ's disciples plucking ears of *wheat,* rubbing off the grains in their hands, and eating them.

Jesus Christ used the planting of wheat in one of His most important stories—the parable of the sower: he who plants seed in good ground is like "he that heareth the word, and understandeth it; which also beareth fruit, and bringeth forth, some an hundredfold . . ." (Matthew 13:18–30).

Great Biblical events have been associated with wheat. Gideon was threshing wheat at the time of his call (Judges 6:11); Ornan was doing the same when he saw an angel of God (1 Chronicles 21:20). Wheat symbolized eternal life.

✦   ✦   ✦

Ann Wigmore is credited with bringing the amazing healing power of wheatgrass juice to the attention of millions of people throughout the world through her books, lectures, and the free emergency health care she gave to hopelessly sick and dying people who had been declared incurable by doctors.

She claimed that wheatgrass juice is an effective treatment for ailments such as high blood pressure, some cancers, obesity, diabetes, gastritis, ulcers, pancreas and liver problems, fatigue, anemia, asthma, eczema, hemorrhoids, skin problems, halitosis, body odor, and constipation. Wheatgrass juice contains abscisic acid, she says, even small amounts of which proved to be "deadly on any form of cancer" in lab animals. *It also contains laetrile, which, she says, "has shown the ability to selectively destroy cancer cells, while leaving non-cancerous ones alone."*

Wigmore came to the United States in 1917, at the age of 8, from a small, war-torn village in Lithuania, where her grandmother, an expert on herbs and natural healing, ran a makeshift hospital for wounded soldiers.

She spent the next 10 years in Middleboro, Massachusetts, working long, hard hours, in her father's bakery, under harsh conditions, without pay, without schooling, and without any kind of social life. She learned to read and write from a retired schoolteacher she met on her delivery route.

Defies Doctors; Avoids Double Amputation with Strange Medicine

At 18, as a driver for her father's bakery, she was severely injured when her horse-drawn delivery wagon overturned. She woke up in a local hospital, both her legs broken. When swellings began to appear above the casts, it was discovered gangrene had set in. The doctors decided that both her legs would have to be amputated below the knees, or she'd die. In Europe, she had seen many soldiers with gangrene saved by her grandmother without need of amputation. She had also seen many taken to city hospitals, who then came back minus arms and legs. She refused—against her father's orders—to let them amputate. She was taken home by ambulance, where her parents refused to help her. An uncle brought her food daily on his way to work and carried her out into the yard for some sunshine. She could not move, and the pain was terrible as the gangrene spread.

Remembering what her grandmother would do, she decided to eat everything green she could find. Her uncle refused to bring her herbs, fearing that she might poison herself with them. But he brought her flowers every morning, which she *ATE* after he left. By reaching down beside the bench where she lay, she was able to fill her stomach with ordinary grass, which her grandmother believed held every nutrient required for human health. This food was fresh from the earth, raw and unprocessed. She had her uncle carry her to different places in the yard, under the pretext of wanting more sun. In this way, she was able to supply her body with fresh grass each day.

After several weeks, a friendly neighbor who was a doctor stopped by to say hello. On examining her legs, he removed a small sample of the gangrenous material, which he placed in a small container and left. The next day, he returned, puzzled and pleased. He asked if she had been taking any medication and was surprised to learn that the only things she had been taking into her body were grass, flowers, and leaves. The doctor said nothing but told her unbelieving father he thought she was getting well. She continued to improve. Her wounds had turned pinkish. The pain had almost vanished. The doctor returned a third time, bringing with him the young doctor who had attended her in the hospital. There was no question that a healing was taking place.

In a few months, her wounds were completely healed. She agreed to return to the hospital for an examination. X-rays showed that the bones had knitted firmly. All signs of gangrene had vanished. The doctors were speechless.

(The leaves and green parts of plants have been used for centuries to accelerate wound healing. Among the ancients, the greenest plants were chosen for health remedies.)

"And Build My Temples"

Not long afterward, Wigmore left home, for good. She found work in Brockton, first as a factory worker, then at a restaurant, then as a hospital attendant.

She liked hospital work, liked the idea of helping others. There she met her future husband. She became a volunteer charity worker, wanted to become a minister, but her priest just laughed at the idea of a woman minister. Nevertheless, every few months—against her husband's wishes—she'd visit a Midwestern Bible college, with a view to becoming a minister. *A Voice kept telling her, "Become a minister and build My temples." But how?*

Upon returning from one of these trips, she found herself locked out of her home. Penniless, with only the clothes she was wearing, she sought the help of a friend and was able to find work caring for an invalid woman, on Cape Cod. Each week she drove 40 miles to Boston, where she taught a Bible class and attended a series of health lectures given by a medical doctor—a renowned surgeon—which taught her the scientific reasons why her grandmother's herbal treatments had so often worked. Through these meetings, she met the publisher of *The Natural Health Guardian,* for which she became a feature writer, then editor.

"Now the exact meaning of . . . 'and build My temples' was clear," she wrote. Jesus needed no lofty buildings in which to teach. "His congregations were wherever He could find them. . . . His methods seemed to me warm, friendly, and intimate. . . . No longer need I ponder about the mythical lofty [temples of brick and stone]. No. I would do my utmost . . . to enable the soul to dwell in a disease-free palace by the teaching of natural, everyday health procedures. . . ."[1]

---

[1]From *Why Suffer?* by Ann Wigmore and the Hippocrates Health Institute, Inc. © 1985. Published by Avery Publishing Group, Inc., Garden City Park, NY. Reprinted by permission.

The Secret of Manna

Living alone in Boston, in a furnished room, working for this magazine for very little pay, Wigmore was literally starving. The simple meals she was able to fix at home, on a small electric hot plate, did not contain sufficient nourishment. Her weight dropped from 123 to 114. People at work were beginning to notice the thinness in her face. In her biography, *Why Suffer,* she writes:

I realized that here was a situation I must remedy . . . I opened my Bible to the Book of Nehemiah in the Old Testament. There, in Chapter 9, verse 21, I read: "Yea, forty years didst thou sustain them in the wilderness, so that they lacked nothing; their clothes waxed not old, and their feet swelled not." . . .

The Israelites had wandered into a section of the Arabian desert where there was no opportunity for farming, no fruit of any kind . . . nothing apparently but brambles and barrenness, yet they had sustained themselves healthfully for forty long years . . .

I found allusions to "manna from heaven," but . . . I could not picture it coming out of the sky in showers. No, the manna which had enabled the wanderers to exist in such a wonderful fashion clearly was [already] in that wilderness at the time of their arrival . . . the leaders [must have had] a sort of awakening . . . a comprehension that some type of vegetation . . . previously regarded as useless, was actually a life-sustaining form of nourishment.

A search through the libraries disclosed that there were many varieties of plants indigenous to arid countryside that brought forth, at some season of the year, a whitish flower or leaf which might easily conform with the descriptions of manna as set forth in the Old Testament.

. . . these investigations turned my attention to weeds and the more I studied, the more I became convinced that they were the simple explanation of the Biblical manna. . . .

In these vagrant [plants] I believed I had come upon a source of nourishment that would solve my particular problem of malnutrition.[2]

She decided to concentrate her efforts on a few easy-to-recognize weeds that grew everywhere. In vacant lots, close to where she lived, she found a large variety of vegetation. "These hardy growths," she says, "were fighting for life against huge odds and the books told me they were loaded with nutrients. *In due time, after days of trial and error, I brought together a drink that brought vigor to my muscles, weight to my body, and alertness to my mind.*"

Bible Passage Leads Her to Miraculous Juice Medicine

Finally, one evening, she opened her Bible to the Book of Daniel in the Old Testament, at the Fourth Chapter, Verses 31 and 32. Here she read that the dissolute King, Nebuchadnezzar, was instructed by a voice from Heaven to go into the fields and "eat grass as did the oxen." He followed this advice and in time regained his crown and his physical health.

This sparked her interest in grasses as food. Out of hundreds of samples of grass seed she received from people all over the world who read *The Health Guardian* she noticed one that grew twice as tall and thick as all the others—wheat grass. This simple food, she soon discovered, was capable of mending shattered health and extending life spans.

The Healing Miracles of This Bible Juice Medicine Unfold

At the suggestion of a well-known New England medical doctor, she began testing the green chlorophyll juice of wheatgrass on ten elder-

---

[2]*Why Suffer?* op. cit.

ly patients who were ill beyond the aid of drugs or surgery. Each day she would bring freshly made wheatgrass juice to their homes.

Many of these patients were so weak and emaciated they were confined to bed and could not even stand without assistance. She listened to their problems and explained to each one that where there was life there was hope—not only for improvement, but possibly for permanent relief from pain.

"I saw them every day," she writes, "giving each one a drink of freshly made wheatgrass juice and watching the amazing results. . . ."[3]

ℿultiple Sclerosis, Emphysema, Arthritis, and Cancer Victims Find Relief

One of these people was a multiple sclerosis patient. "This little woman had existed miserably in bed for months," writes Wigmore. "I began furnishing her regularly with wheatgrass juice. Within a month this sufferer was out of bed, taking short walks, and for the first time in years visited a beauty parlor," saying her prayers had been answered.

Another patient was a stooped, elderly man in the throes of emphysema. Often gasping for breath, he felt certain he would die in a matter of months. "Here again," writes Wigmore, "the wondrous combination of the nutrients in the wheatgrass and a new outlook seemed to work a miracle. The unfortunate man straightened his body for the first time in many years and began to walk unassisted. As he glowingly expressed it, 'A new force seems to be welling up inside of me. It is wonderful.' "

"Just a few blocks away," Wigmore continues, "in a dismal room, the wheatgrass juice drink was being taken regularly by an arthritis sufferer, a middle-aged man with badly swollen ankles, knees, and elbows. He was unable to leave his quarters [and was] without friends, undernourished, his body afflicted with almost unendurable spasms of pain. Yet the regular drinks of wheatgrass, coupled with a fresh vegetable meal each evening, brought startling results in a few weeks. . . .

---

[3] *Why Suffer? op. cit.*

"Thus, one morning he joined me on the daily wheatgrass route. [It turned out that he knew the man with emphysema. They had worked as professional musicians together before ill health had forced them both to retire.] When he met the multiple sclerosis victim he clasped her hand with a shout of delight; she was another old friend of the musical days. . . . In time, the concert pianist afflicted with emphysema, the soprano with multiple sclerosis, and the arthritic basso pledged the remainder of their lives to aid others. . . .

"Of the dozens of individuals with whom I worked during those twelve busy months, most had not worked steadily for several years. Yet . . . I learned that three had found regular employment, many had part-time jobs, and not a single one remained bedridden."[4]

In addition to drinking wheatgrass juice, these people agreed to follow a diet consisting of vegetables, fresh fruits, sprouts, baby greens, sea vegetables, and sprouted seeds, nuts, and grains, all eaten raw and prepared in tasty combinations.

How to Enjoy the Juice of This Bible Healing Plant at Home

Wheatgrass is available in tablet form, or as a powdered drink mix, from the following companies (who are in no way connected with the author or publisher of this book):

Pines International, Inc.
POB 1107
Lawrence, KS 66044
1-800-MY PINES or 913-841-6016
(Wheatgrass in tablet, powdered, or bulk form.)

Wakunaga of America Co., Ltd.
23501 Madero
Mission Viejo, CA 92691
California phone number: 1-800-544-5800
Nationwide: 1-800-421-2998

---

[4] *Why Suffer? op. cit.*

(This company markets one of the finest wheatgrass/barley grass powdered juice drinks available today. Called Kyo-Green, it consists of organically-grown young barley and wheatgrass, with kelp, unpolished [brown] rice, and Bulgarian chlorella, a mineral-rich algae.)

But there is nothing difficult about growing your own wheatgrass at home. It can be done quickly, easily, at little or no cost.

For instructions on growing wheatgrass indoors, see *The Wheatgrass Book* by Ann Wigmore (Avery Publishing, 1985). All you really need is a place to store your seeds, topsoil, and peat moss; a place to soak the seeds (usually near a sink); and a place where the trays full of sprouting seeds can get some indirect sunlight. The juice can be extracted with an ordinary meat grinder. The only expensive item you may want to get—because you don't have to grind it by hand—is an electric juicer.

For instructions on sprouting, which can be done without soil, see Appendix B, at the end of this book. Unlike wheatgrass, which is too fibrous to be eaten—and can only be juiced—sprouts are delicious and can be eaten by themselves, added to salads or sandwiches, or they too can be juiced. The nutritional value of sprouts is much higher than at any other time in a plant's life.

Doses

Never drink an entire 8 ounce glass of wheatgrass juice at one sitting. The concentrated cleansing effect of that much juice can make you queasy. Drink it in small amounts—1 or 2 ounces each time—throughout the day, preferably on an empty stomach or near-empty stomach. Up to 4 ounces a day, or every other day is sufficient. These 1- or 2-ounce drinks can be taken straight or mixed with other juices.

Many Ailments Helped

Ann Wigmore says that the people she treated with wheatgrass juice were struggling with a variety of ailments, from cancer to rheumatism. Yet in not a single instance, where the regimen was followed, was there a failure to improve.

The diet she recommends, along with wheatgrass juice, consists of simple, uncooked foods, such as fresh vegetables, greens, fruits, sprouted seeds, grains, beans, and nuts, along with pure liquids such as fresh vegetable juices, fruit juices; and "green drinks" made from a variety of sprouts, greens, and vegetables are nutritious, yet light on digestion.

"In my years of working with this simple diet," she says, "I have observed that after following such a diet for a number of weeks, many people notice the disappearance of nagging problems they had lived with for months or years. Blocked sinuses open up, sleep is deeper and most restful, aches and pains are relieved, excess weight is quickly shed, the eyes become brighter, and facial stress disappears."[5]

Testimonials[6]

Many people wrote to Ann Wigmore, telling of their experiences using wheatgrass juice. The following are some testimonials that appear in her book, *Be Your Own Doctor:*

> Mrs. R. M. says that a friend, knowing that her husband was troubled painfully with arthritis, told her about wheatgrass juice. "We were so impressed," she says, "that we had an indoor garden of wheatgrass growing within two days. My husband began taking it as soon as it was five inches tall. We cut down our eating—trying to follow your simple diet. The results were miraculous. Getting up in the morning no longer meant massage and groans. After just seven days on your therapy, he was able to tie his own shoes without help. Within two weeks, on two drinks a day, morning and evening, his pains and the swollen redness about the knees disappeared."

---

[5] *Why Suffer? op. cit.*
[6] From *Be Your Own Doctor* by Ann Wigmore © 1982. Published by Avery Publishing Group, Inc., Garden City Park, NY. Reprinted with permission.

Mrs. G. A. says that for many years she had suffered from asthma. Every so often her husband would have to rush her to the hospital in an ambulance where she would stay in an oxygen tent. She seemed to be allergic to everything. A friend got her started on wheatgrass juice. In 3 weeks, her asthma "completely disappeared." Her allergies "seemed to have vanished." Her friends told her she looked 20 years younger, and she returned to work once more. Her doctor warned her that she would have asthma again. But she says in 3 years it has not returned, and she has a "new life."

Mrs. N. S. says, "Even as a child, I seemed to have high blood pressure. My face was always flushed, and the least exertion sent my heart pounding." [The stress of raising a family just seemed to make it worse. Her sister suggested she try wheatgrass juice. In a short time, she had three indoor boxes of wheatgrass sprouts growing.] "Two weeks later," she says, "my doctor said my pressure had fallen 37 points and the following week 17 more. So the danger is passed and has been for over half a year. I cannot thank you enough."

Mr. H. L. B. says, "Eleven months ago, I had diabetes; my circulatory system was so bad, my tear glands weren't functioning; my digestive organs were shot. I was spending between sixty and seventy dollars per month on drugs and vitamins and getting worse. My doctor, a good physician and very dear old friend shook his head and said, 'There's nothing more I can do.' Even though I did not speak of it, I was giving up." Then a neighbor told him about wheatgrass juice, and how it helped so many of her friends. She gave him a box of wheatgrass, and showed him how to grow it and juice it. He started immediately. "Within 3 weeks, my blood sugar was normal," he says. "Soon after, my other problems showed tremendous improvement. . . . Today I am happy, healthy, and 74 years young."

Mrs. P. M. says, "My husband has been a victim of emphysema for several years. Lately, he could only take a few steps at a time. Then he would have to stop and gasp for air. I do not believe he would have lived very long if it were not for wheatgrass. I could only raise enough for one good glassful each day. However, within a month he became a new man. The shortness of breath was gone, and today he helps with everything, lifts, lugs, and works all day."

Ms. H. G. says she was determined to see what wheatgrass juice could do for her. "I took a glassful once a day. After about a month . . . I began to notice that my hair was coming in thicker and, strange to say, was the color it used to be when I was a girl. This was indeed surprising as I had been getting much gray hair in the past ten years."

J. R., a leukemia victim, says, "I have been taking wheatgrass regularly. I have one box inside as well as two outside the house. It is doing very well. But here is the good news. After all my discouraging trips to the hospital and things continually getting worse, hope at last arrived. Last Friday I had a blood test and my blood count is normal. I don't know how long this will last, but I shall continue taking the wheatgrass regularly. . . . According to medical science there is no cure for this disease. My blood count now seems to prove that somebody is mistaken."

Mr. J. Y. says, "I had been a victim of Parkinson's disease for many years. It first appeared when I fell over backwards . . . and was taken to the hospital where the diagnosis was made. When I was released, I believed I was well again. Then, however, the trembling came to my left hand and spread to my right foot. Fortunately my aunt in Washington sent me [information about wheatgrass juice]. I will have been on the therapy for 2 full months next Monday, and all my shakes have gone. It was like being born again. Unbelievable!"

Mrs. J. N. says, "I am doing fine on the wheatgrass [juice]. I have 6 children and they are all taking the drinks. . . . I can see that the children are more alert and energetic. . . . For me it has been God-send indeed. My weight, when I started, was a pudgy 197 pounds. Within 6 weeks, without being hungry a single day, I brought my weight down to 165."

A. O. says, "My ankles were swollen out of shape and pained like an ulcerated tooth. I put them under a sunlamp in the evening, but that didn't seem to help. I rubbed them with salves and I had them massaged. Still the swelling would not go. Then I started the wheatgrass as you suggested, two drinks a day and a poultice of the pulp at night. In 3 nights, there was a marked difference. The redness vanished, and the swelling began to go down. The pain disappeared. Within two and a half weeks they were back to normal."

Mrs. R. D. says, "I am trying to prevent an operation for a fibroid tumor in the uterus. I am following your simple diet. I eat only raw foods and am taking my wheatgrass [juice] regularly. I nearly bled to death three months ago. However, since I have been taking the wheatgrass, the bleeding has completely stopped. I am 48 years old. The reason I am writing to you is that when my doctor examined me three days ago, he was surprised. The tumor had been reduced tremendously. He tells me to continue and that an operation will evidently be unnecessary. God bless you."

Mrs. C. T. G., a victim of uterine cancer, says, "I went to the Brookline Hospital [in 1970] and had a D&C, which is a scraping of the uterus [and] had an unfavorable result. The doctor advised this operation because I had been hemorrhaging about every six weeks. The report came back that I had early cancer of the uterus and the doctor wanted to have the uterus removed. I . . . wrote my doctor that I would put the surgery off until June because I was going to try another method. He wrote back saying that I probably would not be around in June." [She came to Ann Wigmore for help, and was placed on the wheatgrass juice program.] "After four weeks, I reported to the doctor and had another test, which he was not too happy about because . . . the hospital reports from the Brookline Hospital for Women . . . did say that I had cancer of the uterus. He told me to either follow his advice or change doctors. Then I got the letter afterwards concerning the most recent report which is as follows: 'Dear Mrs. G.— This is to notify you that the cancer smear taken recently at the time of your office visit was reported as normal. This comes as good news. Best wishes as always.'"

Claims Her Arthritis and Colitis Healed with This Secret, Hair Color Returns

"I, myself, have lived primarily on sprouted seeds, beans, grains, and nuts for more than two decades," says Wigmore.

"Not only have I healed my body of colitis [a form of intestinal irritation and bleeding] and arthritis. . . . I have also achieved a greater level of vitality and health than I had even as a child—and I am no child at 77. And my hair has returned to its natural brown color, too!"[7]

Average Weight Losses of 4 to 15 Pounds per Week

Wigmore says that one of the most satisfying discoveries she made was the dramatic weight loss obtainable while using wheatgrass and following the living-foods diet, which consists of vegetables, fresh fruits, sprouts, baby greens, sea vegetables, and sprouted seeds, nuts, and grains, all eaten raw, and prepared in tasty combinations.

"Wheatgrass," she says, "helps dieters by speeding up blood circulation and the metabolic rate, and by enhancing digestive powers, thereby melting fat in the body." She cites work by Edward Howell, M.D., showing that measurements of the enzyme content of body fat in people weighing 300 pounds or more revealed a deficiency of fat-splitting enzymes.

---

[7]From *The Sprouting Book* by Ann Wigmore © 1986. Published by Avery Publishing Group, Inc., Garden City Park, NY. Reprinted by permission.

"Even if you are not a heavyweight," says Wigmore, "chances are that if you want to reduce, the enzymes in wheatgrass juice and raw foods can help you."

"At the Hippocrates Institute,"[8] she continues, "I have never stressed weight loss because it is as natural to wheatgrass and the living foods diet as swimming is to a duck. Nevertheless, among our guests at the Institute, the average weight loss per week is between four and fifteen pounds. I am convinced that the rich supply of enzymes in wheatgrass and live foods is the deciding factor."[9]

A Miracle Ingredient in This Bible Food for Women's Problems

Wheat germ is the richest source of vitamin E in nature. Vitamin E is an essential vitamin, meaning your body needs it and can't produce it. It is essential to the health of the blood vessels, heart, lungs, nerves, pituitary gland, and skin. It has proven of therapeutic benefit in many conditions. Here are some examples:

✦ *Lumpy breasts*—doctors tell us that the great majority of breast lumps that come and go are neither cancerous nor precancerous; they simply reflect changing hormone levels. The best policy, of course, is to rely on your physician's advice. But it *is* interesting that vitamin E seems to have helped many women with lumpy breasts and other problems.

Robert London, M.D., directory of obstetrical and gynecological research at Mount Sinai Hospital in Baltimore, Maryland, says that vitamin E can relieve fibrocystitis of the breasts (*Ob. Gyn. News*, December, 1976). Out of 12 menstruating women with fibrocystic breast disease, ten improved in 2 months on 600 I.U. of vitamin E daily. It seems to stimulate increased adrenal hormone secretion. No

---

[8]Now known as the Ann Wigmore Foundation, 196 Commonwealth Avenue, Boston, MA 02116, tel. (617) 267-9424.

[9]From *The Wheatgrass Book* by Ann Wigmore and the Hippocrates Health Institute, Inc. © 1985. Published by Avery Publishing Group, Inc., Garden City Park, NY. Reprinted with permission.

cure is claimed, but he says that it certainly seems to relieve lumps, sores, and tenderness of the breasts, and no harmful side effects have been found.

+ *Leukoplakia cured*—Mrs. F. A. says, "About five years ago, my mother, who was 80, developed leukoplakia inside and outside of her vaginal area. Her family doctor treated her with hormones, salve, etc. After a few weeks, she became worse. I then took her to a specialist who treated her to no avail. Finally, they informed me there was nothing else they could do.

"The specialist said her system had dried out resulting from a complete hysterectomy performed 35 years earlier. (At that time, the doctor did not prescribe hormones.) After 8 or 9 months, mother was in so much misery with her raw, burning area she could not sit, stand or walk in comfort.

"By the grace of God, I began thinking about vitamin E. I went to a health food store and got a bottle of vitamin E and gave her 200 units a day. After a few days she felt better. I was happy that she had relief, but was afraid to hope for recovery. In about a month's time her misery was completely gone. Mother is now 85 and doing very well."

Epilepsy, Paralysis, Blindness Miraculously Healed

In *Summary* (June 1961), Dr. Alfonso del Guidice, of the National Institute of Public Health, Buenos Aires, Argentina, says that in cases of nerve-caused eye ailments treated with vitamin E—the vitamin most plentiful in wheat—he has had "brilliant results" with myopia (nearsightedness), nystogmus (involuntary rapid eye movements), strabismus (crossed eyes), cataract, paralysis, and epilepsy. Every patient improved.

"Generally we have begun treatment with 200 to 300 milligrams of vitamin E daily, increasing over a period of as long as 6 months, doses approximating two grams daily," depending on the age of the patient. "Vitamin C was also given in doses of 500 to 1500 mg. daily. Relief seemed permanent."

Reported cases:

A girl, 3, was suffering from epilepsy (resulting from a bad fall). At the age of 2, she had her first seizure, lasting 4 minutes, with unconsciousness, spasm, and frothing at the mouth, followed by a violent headache lasting 6 hours. For 90 minutes she was unable to speak. After that, she was nervous, restless, had crying spells, and wet the bed. Vitamin E was started as the only treatment. In 3 months she had no more convulsions, and in less than a year she stopped her bed-wetting and became friendly and normal.

A 9-month-old boy was diagnosed as epileptic. He had convulsions several times daily during which his eyes pulled to one side, his neck became rigid, and he lost consciousness. He was nervous and restless. Drugs and sedatives did not help. Then he was given vitamin E only. In 5 months, he had no more convulsions and slept peacefully.

A girl, 12, was mentally retarded and violent. She shouted and cried all the time, was unable to speak properly, could not understand questions or manage her toilet functions. This had been going on 6 years. No treatment helped. In a little over a month on vitamin E, she suddenly improved, became quiet, sat correctly, and ate by herself by the end of the year.

A girl, 5, was paralyzed in both legs, and retarded. She could not speak. All treatments had failed, since birth. After 7 months on vitamin E she began to walk and talk clearly. Four months later, she could even run!

A man, 23, suffered nerve-caused blindness. His eyes were normal, but he could not see. Eight years of treatment had failed. In less than 2 months on vitamin E, he could see the fingers on a hand almost 7 feet away, and recognized people 10 feet away, with his left eye. With his right eye he saw a little less, but he could now dress and feed himself, travel alone, and walk through city traffic!

A girl, 10, born with cataracts on both eyes, was totally blind. She could not see light, even after an operation on her right eye. She was extremely quiet and depressed. After 6 months of vitamin E, she became extremely cheerful, and could see light! The cataracts were disappearing. Her right eyeball was now clearly visible!

A boy, 10, born with cataracts on one eye and defects in both eyes, was also retarded. Vitamin E was begun. He became brighter and was more alert, the cataracts disappeared, and vision in both eyes improved. All this started immediately.

A child, 10, born with cataracts on both eyes (both operated on unsuccessfully), started taking vitamin E. In 8 months, she could see small objects at a distance!

Amazing Improvement from Muscular Dystrophy

We are told* that 25 children afflicted with the crippling and wasting disease known as muscular dystrophy were given wheat-germ oil daily, plus vitamins C and B. Every child improved under this plan, and there was one complete recovery. In another experiment, 151 patients with various nerve-muscle disorders were given wheat-germ oil. Their progress was followed for 12 years:

In five (three children and two adults) out of 25 patients with progressive muscular dystrophy, symptoms were arrested and moderate to marked improvement occurred.

Three out of five patients with menopausal muscular dystrophy showed remarkable improvement. (Other than the wheat-germ oil, these patients were not placed on any particular diet.)

---

*"Experiments with Wheat Germ Oil," *Journal of Neurology, Neurosurgery and Psychiatry* (London, May 1951).

Cerebral Palsy Healed

A 7-year-old boy, Tommy, was suffering from cerebral palsy, which caused spastic paralysis of his arms and legs (wild, jerky movements) and affected his speech. The doctor shook his head: no cure for cerebral palsy. Tommy was due to be fitted for a back brace to support his withered muscles.

Meanwhile, someone suggested wheat-germ oil, which has been known to bring relief in cases of cerebral palsy. A month later, when Tommy came in for his brace, it didn't fit. His withered muscles had firmed up.

Later, a snapshot of Tommy was sent to the doctor to show his amazing progress. The photo showed this boy whizzing by on a bicycle, for he was so healthy he could run and play like any normal child. Yet every day on TV we are told that cerebral palsy is incurable.

Horrible Cases of Shingles Healed

A. N. reports: "A couple of years ago I showed my chest to my M.D. and he gravely informed me that I had a severe form of shingles. They were all around my back and chest and refused to be ignored. They'd run you wild. I promptly stocked up on high concentrations of the B vitamins as well as all other vitamins, especially E and a big bottle of E liquid—the oil to be applied liberally over all red spots on my chest and back. Two weeks later I kept my appointment with the doctor and cheerfully removed my shirt. He gaped in utter amazement and disbelief. He said, 'I *never* saw anything like that before! What in heaven's name did you put on it?' When I told him vitamin E oil, he sneered. Needless to say, I soon healed up."

Wasp and Hornet Stings Quickly Relieved!

Mrs. M. G. reports: "Wheat germ oil is a sure cure for stings. Last summer a wasp stung my brother. He decided to try wheat germ oil and discovered it relieved all pain as soon as it was applied. Hornets stung my arm and hand. I rubbed wheat germ oil on and instantly the pain left—no swelling. Try it. It is a miracle how quickly it relieves and cures stings. It is also good for frostbite and chapped hands and fever blisters."

CHAPTER 12

THE SACRED MEDICINAL DRINK THAT SAVED THOUSANDS, PREVENTS BLOOD CLOTS, RELIEVES PAIN, AND MELTS FAT OFF ARTERY WALLS

"I am the true vine," said Jesus, whose first miracle was the changing of water into wine. His last act was the introduction of the sacrament of wine. He specifically mentioned wine as a healing food in the story of the Good Samaritan: ". . . and bandaged his wounds, pouring in wine and oil."

Red wine is a proven and powerful healer. There is no question that the Bible and its writers recognized its actions on the human body, especially on the functions of the heart and circulatory system, on the gastrointestinal tract, and on the central nervous system.

Wine was used as an antiseptic to clean wounds (Luke 10:34). As an anesthetic, it induced sleep and took away pain ("they have beaten me, and I felt it not: When shall I awake?"—Prov. 23:35). On the dining table it improved digestion and appetite ("Drink no longer water, but use a little wine for thy stomach's sake and thine often infirmities."—Tim. 5:23). Priest-healers used it as a stimulant for weak hearts ("And wine that maketh glad the heart"—Ps. 104:15), to strengthen the heartbeat, and improve respiration. For centuries before pills, people used it as a natural tranquilizer ("Let him drink, and forget his poverty, and remember his misery no more."—Prov. 31:6–7)

A Heart Medicine Revealed by Angels

German herbalist Maria Treben says no Christian household should be without a remedy called "heart wine"—revealed in a vision to the Abbess Hildegard von Bingen, a German mystic and herbalist who lived in the twelfth century. She entered a Benedictine convent at the age of 8, and became head abbess at the age of 37. She was regarded as a saint in her time, and many high church officials, including Pope Eugenius III, became convinced that she was a true prophetess of the Lord.

She claimed to have received a series of visions showing new ways to use medicinal herbs, revealed to her by God or His angels. These visions were recorded on scrolls of parchment that can still be viewed by scholars. In one of these visions, an angel appeared to her and told her about a mixture of herbs called *Heart Wine*. Writing 800 years later . . .

. . . *a German medical doctor is quoted as saying: "When your heart troubles you, take 1, 2 or even 3 more tablespoonfuls of this wine a day, and all pains in the heart, caused by a change of the weather or excitement, will disappear as if blown away. You need not be anxious or afraid, because you cannot do any harm. Not only for slight pain in the heart, but also for cardiac weakness and real heart trouble, this parsley-honey wine will do you a great service, maybe even bring about a recovery."*

To make it, ten fresh parsley stems with leaves are put into 1 liter (about a quart) of pure wine, and 2 tablespoons of wine vinegar are added. This is simmered for 10 minutes on low heat, taking care not to let it spill over, because it foams. Then 300 grams (about 10-1/2 ounces) of pure honey are added and everything is low boiled for 4 minutes. While still hot, it is strained, and placed in a bottle that has been thoroughly cleaned by wiping with alcohol and drying, beforehand, and that can be covered tightly. The sediment that forms is harmless and can be consumed with the honey.

You can use red or white wine, but the proper sequence must be followed. The honey is added after the first boiling, and then the whole mixture must be boiled again.

Reported case:

One person writes: "I want to tell you that I have prepared the wine and that I have obtained amazing results. Ten years ago I was operated on and told that I have a weak heart and therefore will always have pain, nothing could be done about it and I would have to accept it. But thanks to the wine all my complaints have vanished. After taking the parsley-honey wine for 2 months I do not feel weak anymore."

Sacred Medicinal Drink Has Penicillin Power

In telling the Jews of antiquity to use wine as an antiseptic, the Bible was prescribing an ingredient that is still the most common antiseptic of modern medicine: alcohol. But there's something more to wine's germ-killing powers than that.

Every test of wine shows the same thing. Wine kills cholera germs in 30 seconds to 10 minutes, *E. coli* bacteria in 25 to 60 minutes, typhoid in 5 minutes to 4 hours. The germ killer in wine was long thought to be alcohol. But even *without* alcohol, it still kills bacteria. A French scientist in the 1950s found that *polyphenols* in wine kill bacteria in much the same way as penicillin does.

Even *diluted with water (4 to 1) it has the same potency in 15 minutes as five units of penicillin per millimeter.* Of all juices tested, freshly squeezed apple juice, commercial grape juice, and wine were the strongest.

Kills Viruses Pencillin Can't Touch

What's more, unlike antibiotics, which can kill bacteria but can't touch viruses, red wine stops them dead. In tests in the 1970s virtually none of the viruses tested survived 24 hours' contact with grape extract. Grape juice and red wine showed strong antiviral activity against poliovirus, herpes simplex virus, reovirus (which causes meningitis, mild fever, and diarrhea), and influenza viruses. Red wine was even more antiviral than grape juice itself.

One day when one of the researchers had a cold sore, he dabbed a little freeze-dried red wine concentrate on it. "The pain disappeared instantly," he said, "The lesion shriveled up; no scab appeared. And that was the end of it."

Since the phenols in wine knock out herpes simplex, you can get rid of a cold sore by dabbing a little wine residue on it. It clears up cold sores and instantly takes the pain away.

Risk of Hepatitis Nearly Eliminated

If you drink wine at the same time you ingest food contaminated with disease-producing viruses or bacteria, you are less likely to become ill, says one expert. Tests have shown that wine consistently kills *salmonella, staphylococcus,* and *e. coli* bacteria, the most common causes of food poisoning, and almost eliminates the risk of hepatitis from eating raw contaminated oysters.

(Wine has no effect, however, on the deadly *Vibrio vulnificus* organism found in raw oysters. Only cooking destroys it.)

Saves Thousands of Lives during Cholera Epidemic

Wine saved countless lives during the cholera epidemic of Paris in the late 1800s. A French physician, noting that wine drinkers showed more resistance to cholera, advised the public to mix wine into their water for protection. Science confirmed it. Wine did, indeed, kill cholera germs, and this was equally true of red or white wine, full strength or mixed half and half with water. Mothers began soaking fish and fruit in wine, in order to kill the bacteria in them.

Free of Genital Warts

Keri C., 38, a social service case worker, was troubled with genital warts that had recurred after surgical removal. Her doctor told her they were caused by a virus. When she read that grapes kill viruses pencillin can't touch, she bought some 100 percent pure grape juice and started drinking it. She also used a syringe to inject some of it, once daily, into her vagina. The next time her doctor examined her, he was surprised to find her cervix and vagina totally free of warts.

Good for the Heart

All alcoholic beverages in moderation seem to discourage heart disease, but wine appears better than beer and hard liquor in doing so. This is because

1. Alcohol relieves stress and contains antioxidants that prevent damaging free radicals from forming. (Free radicals are said to be the cause of most diseases, aches, and pains.)
2. Alcohol boosts good HDL cholesterol, which melts damaging fat off artery walls and carries it off to the liver where it is broken down— in effect destroyed—and sent out of the body. There is no difference between red and white wine in this respect.
3. But red wine contains an anticlotting medicine—called resveratrol—that prevents blood clots from forming.

Studies consistently show that the risk of heart disease falls with one or two drinks a day. In one study, two-drink-a-day drinkers were 40 percent less likely than nondrinkers to be hospitalized for heart attacks.

But alcohol in excessive amounts—as the Bible cautions ("Moab also shall wallow in his vomit"—Jer. 48:26)—is dangerous and can lead to poisoning and even death. Your risk of death from all causes, including cancer, rises with three drinks a day. Three to five alcoholic drinks a day increased death rates 50 percent, according to one study. The maximum *safe* amount of alcoholic drinks per day is two.

An Anti-clotting Medicine from the Bible

Frenchmen have one third as many heart attacks as American men do, even though the French indulge in fatty foods and have cholesterol and blood pressure as high as American men. This is thought to be due to the French habit of drinking wine, especially red wine, *with* meals.

French health authorities suggest that red wine consumed along with fatty meals *counteracts* the fat. Fatty foods tend to make the blood more sluggish so it tends to clot and to plug arteries. Red wine thwarts that process.

Cornell University scientists say that the anti-clotting medicine in red wine is a chemical agent in grape skins—called reservatrol—a chemical that has an anti-clotting effect when consumed by humans.

You get this chemical when you drink grape juice or red wine. Grapes found in supermarkets contain very little of it, because of chemicals used to prevent fungal infections.

White wine has very little of the anti-clotting medicine because in making white wine, the resveratrol-rich skins are discarded. But in making red wine, the crushed grapes are left to sit in the skins to ferment.

Home-grown grapes *do* contain resveratrol. It takes a pound of home-grown grapes to get as much resveratrol as there is in 2 cups of red wine.

How This Sacred Medicinal Drink Relieves Angina Pains

An effective concoction used by some doctors in Japan to relieve the chest pains of angina calls for a raw egg to be mixed with two-thirds cup each of sake or wine and canned apple juice. This concoction is then brought to a boil and taken internally after it has cooled a while but is still quite warm. An average of 3 cups per day for 3–4 days is taken.

Pure grape sugar has an immediate effect in strengthening weak heart muscles, according to Dr. Alfred Vogel.

A Bible Plant Seed for Hardening of the Arteries, Diabetes, Eye Problems, Varicose Veins

Grape-seed extract is a rich source of one of the most powerful and beneficial groups of plant flavonoids—the procyanidins, or PCOs for short. These flavonoids exert many health-promoting benefits.

Their most celebrated effect is their ability to rid the body of dangerous oxidants and free radicals, which are thought to cause aging and every chronic degenerative disease including heart disease, arthritis, and cancer.

PCOs are *50 times* more powerful than vitamin C and vitamin E, in terms of antioxidant action, and they provide incredible protection to the cells against free-radical damage.

PCO extracts are mainly used in the treatment of vein problems including varicose veins, disorders of the retina including diabetic retinopathy, and macular degeneration. In tests, people who were given 200 mg per day of PCO extracts showed considerable improvement in vision, over a 5–6-week period, compared to those who took a placebo or received no treatment at all.

Grape seed and pine bark are excellent sources of procyanidins, but PCOs extracted from grape seeds have emerged as the preferred source in Europe. A daily maintenance dose of either grape-seed extract or pine-bark extract—available at health-food stores—is 50 mg. When used for therapeutic purposes, the dose is usually increased to 150 to 300 mg.

PCO extracts reportedly have no side effects.

Helps Boost Estrogen Level for Women; Fights Osteoporosis

Boron, a trace mineral found in grapes, may help prevent osteo-porosis or bone thinning in older women, by maintaining higher levels of estrogen. New research shows that boron dramatically *raises* blood levels of estrogen, the hormone that prevents calcium loss and bone deterioration in women.

In tests, boron caused the most active form of estrogen, estri-adol 17B, to *double,* reaching levels found in women on estrogen replacement, according to researchers at the U.S. Department of Agriculture.

Researchers found that postmenopausal women on low-boron diets tend to lose calcium and magnesium, but that all it takes to pre-vent this loss is 3 mg of boron daily, easily available in food. The best sources of boron are apples, pears, peaches, and *grapes.* As an added bonus, boron boosts brain power and mental alertness and dramatically protects against tooth decay.

Credits His Remission to the Juice of This Bible Plant

As one researcher has noted, it seems likely that many of the phe-nolics in red wine turn off cancer and generally protect body tissues. Scientists say that certain phenolics, especially the ones called caffe-ic acid, ellagic acid, ferulic acid, and gallotanic acid, prevent cell changes that lead to cancer in animal studies.

Ogden K., a retired photographer, had been diagnosed with a malignant tumor in his abdomen. The doctors wanted to do surgery and give him massive doses of chemotherapy and radiation, but he refused. Instead, he went on a fast for several months, subsisting mostly on grape juice and a fruit-and-vegetable diet. He stated that his tumor began going into remission within a week after starting the grape juice and raw-fruits-and-vegetable diet. He stayed on this juice therapy until X-rays showed that the cancer was totally gone. "I felt great and had more energy than I've had in years," he says. "I felt like a kid all over again. My mind was sharp, my energy levels incredible and I slept like a log!"[1]

A Bible Food Cure

In 1928, in her book, *The Grape Cure,* Johanna Brandt wrote: ". . . as long as I can remember I suffered from gastric trouble, bilious attacks and stomach ulcers. . . . I was [often] conscious of a gnawing pain at the left side of my stomach. . . .

"I was persuaded by my doctor to go into the General Hospital . . . for an X-ray examination. Many plates were taken, and a noted surgeon pronounced his verdict—the stomach was being divided in two by a vicious, fibrous growth. An immediate operation was recommended as the only means of prolonging my life. This I refused. . . .

"The three years that followed were years of great suffering, but . . . in 1925 . . . I accidentally discovered a food that had the miraculous effect of healing me completely within six weeks. . . . a method that may cure almost any disease. . . .

". . . on January 21, 1928, my article (called "The Grape Cure") appeared in *The New York Evening Graphic.* This article created widespread interest . . . I was overwhelmed with correspondence and visits . . . The many heart-breaking appeals for help could not be ignored. . . . I simply related my experiences and described the procedure I had adopted. People treated by my methods recovered. They in turn told relatives and friends—always with the same results. . . ."

Reported results:

One young woman had six operations on her rectum and the base of the spine. Nothing could relieve the excruciating pain in her spine. A doctor had said she would never be able to sit

---

[1]John Heinerman, *Heinerman's Encyclopedia of Healing Juices,* 1994.

properly. After beginning the grape cure, large amounts of pus and intestinal worms drained from her system. She was transformed from sickness to vibrant health; she looked and felt years younger.

A middle-aged woman from New York, the mother of a large family, was constantly vomiting, day and night. Just a few grapes were given at a time. Within 24 hours the vomiting stopped. The desperate strain on her stomach and bowels was relieved, but she was so weak she fell into unconsciousness. Her legs, which had begun to swell, were wrapped in grape compresses. Overnight, no trace of swelling was left in her legs, and her stomach was now so normal and strong that her incessant demand was for "Food!"

External wounds were treated with grape poultices or compresses. (A poultice is made by spreading crushed grapes between layers of soft cloth and applying to affected area; a compress is made by dipping a soft cloth in 2:3 diluted grape juice, applying and renewing as frequently as possible). The grape juice seemed to absorb into the wound, says Mrs. Brandt, cleansing and eliminating poisons. No scabs or crusts formed. Healthy new pink tissue appeared.

"I have seen *teeth* . . . loose in their pus-filled sockets, become steady and fixed within a few weeks, the gums free of pyorrhea . . ."

Diabetes: "This method has been particularly successful with diabetes," says Mrs. Brandt. "The grape sugar is believed to be an organic solvent which neutralizes the sugar deposits in the blood."

Gallstones: "Gallstones have been reported dissolved while the patients were [on the grape diet] treatment for other diseases."

Cataract: "The same may be said of cataract of the eye [that they have been reported dissolved on the grape diet]."

Sinus: "Amazing results" are reported for treatment of nasal catarrh, sinus trouble, and the like, using diluted grape juice several times a day in nasal douches.

"Grapes apparently *dissolve hardened mucus* adhering to the walls of the stomach and intestines," says Mrs. Brandt. The grape juice appears to dislodge this accumulation and act as a flush, carrying it to the rectum, where it is eliminated.

One case was that of a woman who was said to be suffering from *double lobar pneumonia, leakage of the heart, bleeding of the kidneys,* and other complications. She was told that she could live but a few weeks. A European doctor was called in on the case. He had seen the effects of the grape cure in Austria. He ordered her to be fed on unsweetened grape juice, 1 spoonful at a time, gradually increasing the quantity and intervals between until the required results were obtained. "Remember," he said, "this is the same as a blood transfusion. Grape juice makes blood." She immediately began to regain strength and later claimed to have no kidney trouble and that her heart was sound.

Two years later, she was also able to ward off the flu with grape juice and claimed to have finally rid her system of the "pneumonia bug for all time."

On the grape diet, says Mrs. Brandt, "the senses become abnormally acute; dim eyes brighten; faded hair takes on new gloss; the lifeless, hopeless voice becomes vibrant, magnetic, and the complexion clears."

The method was as follows:

1. *Preparation:* To prepare the system for a change of diet, the best way is to fast for 2 or 3 days, drinking plenty of pure, cold water and taking an enema of a quart of lukewarm water daily with the strained juice of one lemon therein.

   By this short fast, complications may be avoided; the stomach is cleared of poisons and fermenting accumulations to a certain extent; and the grape can begin its work more quickly, says Mrs. Brandt. The preliminary fast has the advantage of giving the patient a keen relish for the first grape.

2. *After the fast:* The patient drinks one or two glasses of pure, cold water the first thing in the morning.

3. *First meal:* Half an hour later the patient has his or her first meal of grapes. Wash them well. (Chew the skins and seeds thoroughly, says Mrs. Brandt, and swallow only a *few* of them as food and roughage. If there is an ulcerated condition of the stomach or bowels, seeds should not be swallowed, she cautions.)

4. *Time:* Starting at 8 A.M. and having a grape meal every 2 hours till 8 P.M., this would give seven meals daily. This is kept up for a week or two, even a month or two, in chronic cases of long standing, but no longer, under any circumstances.

5. *Variety:* Any good variety may be used—purple, green, red, white or blue. Hothouse grapes are better than none, and the seedless varieties are excellent. The monotony of the diet may be varied by using many varieties. Different varieties contain different elements so it is advisable to use as many kinds as one can get. Some like them acid, others like them sweet. The best time is when the grape season is at its height, says Mrs. Brandt.

6. *Quantity:* This varies according to the condition, digestion, and occupation of the patient. It is well to begin with a small quantity of 1, 2, or 3 ounces per meal, gradually increasing this to double the quantity. In time about half a pound may safely be taken at a meal, says Mrs. Brandt. A minimum of 1 pound should be used daily, while the maximum should not exceed 4 pounds. Patients taking larger quantities at a meal should allow at least 3 hours for digestion and should not take all the skins. Invariably, the best results have been effected when grapes have been taken in small quantities.

7. *Enjoyment:* "Loathing for grapes may indicate the presence of much poison in the system and the need of another short fast," says Mrs. Brandt. "The rule in such cases is to abstain from every form of food, drinking an abundance of cold water. Unless patients can eat the grapes with perfect enjoyment, they are better off without them. Skip a few meals. Let Nature regulate this matter. We hear of over-zealous relatives forcing grapes

down the throats of unfortunate patients. This is a great mistake. (Always remember that grapes are nourishing and maintain life in the body while the cleansing process is going on.) Loss of strength is due to the presence of poisons in the system. The patient continues to weaken under the grape diet and under the complete fast, until the poison has been expelled. Then, without a change of diet . . . the patient returns to strength and in some cases even puts on weight. . . .

First Stage

Mrs. Brandt speaks of four stages in the grape cure:

"It is safe to say that the first seven to ten days on grapes only would be required to clear the stomach and bowels of their ancient accumulations," says Mrs. Brandt. "And it is during this period that distressing symptoms often appear [gas, pains, dark stool, and constipation—for which a teaspoon of olive oil just before eating is recommended]. Nature works thoroughly. She does not build on a rotten foundation. Purification of every part of the body must be complete. . . . When this point has been reached . . . and it may last from two weeks to two months—it is advisable to go on to the second stage."

Second Stage

This is the gradual introduction of other fresh fruits, tomatoes, and sour milk or cottage cheese. "We do not expect anyone to live on grapes forever," says Mrs. Brandt.

"Grapes still form the main food and are always taken as the first meal in the morning at 8 A.M. But now, during the day, some other fresh fruit may be used instead of grapes. An endless variety presents itself—a slice of melon, an orange, a grapefruit, an apple, a luscious pear, the scarlet strawberry, the golden apricot. . . . Only one kind of fruit to be taken at a meal but something different every day.

"After a few days a glass of sour milk or buttermilk, yogurt, or cottage cheese may be taken instead of grapes for supper. Patients who dislike milk should take a ripe, finely mashed banana, or some other nourishing fruit.

"After a week or ten days, every other meal may consist of different varieties of fruit, or sour milk, taking them, for example, in the following order:

8:00 A.M. Grapes

10:00 A.M. Pear, banana, or peaches

12:00 Noon Grapes

2:00 P.M. Sour milk, buttermilk, or cottage cheese

4:00 P.M. Grapes

6:00 P.M. Oranges, grapefruit, plums, or apricots

8:00 P.M. Grapes.

"At this point some patients crave for something savory. The sweet fruits begin to pall. There may even be a positive aversion to grapes, in which case they should be omitted altogether and the other foods taken every three hours. One or two sliced tomatoes with pure olive oil and a little lemon juice may safely be included in this diet."

(Extreme care must be taken not to eat heavy foods until the completion of the four stages.)

Third Stage

The raw diet: "This includes every food that can be eaten uncooked—raw vegetables, salads, fruits, nuts, raisins, dates, figs and other dried fruits, butter, cottage cheese, sour milk, yogurt and buttermilk, honey and olive oil.

"Begin the day as usual with cold water [as much as desired] and grapes or some other fruit for breakfast, but instead of sour milk for lunch, have a substantial salad of raw vegetables. Reduce the number of meals, as raw vegetables require longer to digest.

"It is surprising to some people to find that nearly all the vegetables can be used raw—young green peas and string beans, celery, tomatoes, cucumbers, lettuce, sprigs of cauliflowers, squash, shredded cabbage leaves, grated carrots, turnips, beets and parsnips, finely chopped onion and spinach.

"After the light fruit diet, it is wise not to start out too soon with a large variety of vegetables. Choose two or three of the above-named as a foundation for your salad and mix them with lemon juice and olive oil. Try different varieties the following day and watch the combinations of flavors. . . .

"Above all things, this noonday meal should be made palatable. Patients who have been used to animal food crave for something stimulating. There can be no objection to adding one or two savory ingredients to this salad—some finely chopped nuts, grated cheese, sour cream, or a good homemade mayonnaise made of eggs, lemon juice and olive oil. In some cases, a finely-chopped hard boiled egg maybe included in the salad."

Time to Digest

"Give this meal more time to digest than is required for raw fruits, especially if nuts, dates, raisins or other dried fruits have been added to it. The supper should consist of sour milk or fruit, or a highly nourishing and digestible dish may be made of ripe bananas mashed, with sour cream.

"Sufficient stress cannot be laid upon the importance of raw [foods]. . . . Raw foods digest more easily than cooked ones, and pass through the system far more rapidly. The result is that they have no time to decompose in the alimentary canal. There is no undue fermentation, no fear of toxic poisoning.

"Therefore patients are strongly advised to abstain from every form of cooked food during the full period of treatment. . . .

Fourth Stage

The mixed diet. "At this stage, there is sometimes a recurrence of the old trouble, and the patient—sadder and wiser for the experience—is glad to go back to the raw diet. But if the disease has not been very deep-seated and the cure complete, the following is recommended," says Mrs. Brandt:

1. A fruit breakfast, one kind only
2. A cooked lunch
3. A salad supper

For breakfast, eat plentifully of any of the juicy fruits that may be in season. Make a strict habit of this and observe it for the rest of your life if you want to be healthy. Your cooked meal should be a dry meal, says Mrs. Brandt. No soups, no liquids of any kind. No raw salad. No fruit either fresh or cooked.

Your cooked meal should consist of steamed vegetables, beginning with one kind at a time, following the grape cure. If results are good, take two or three varieties at a meal.

If you are not a vegetarian, indulge in a piece of baked, broiled, or steamed fish occasionally, with a baked potato. Or this meal may consist of fish with stewed tomatoes, or any of the green vegetables steamed and baked. An infinite variety of savory dishes may be made by mashing one of the green vegetables with steamed potatoes, mixing with egg, covering with bread crumbs and pats of butter, and baking this to a rich brown in the oven. Leftovers of the cauliflower, carrots, cabbage, parsnips, steamed lettuce, spinach, baked onions, and so forth, lend themselves especially to this form of cooking.

Watch the effects of the cooked meal, and with the first sign of discomfort return to the raw diet.

Use the Juice, Too

Mrs. Brandt says unsweetened, unfermented, bottled grape juice can take the place of whole grapes during the winter months or whenever grapes are not available:

"It has been found that the patient can get along almost as well on grape juice as on whole grapes. . . . Raisins have been taken . . . to supply bulk, with good results. For instance, a glass of grape juice on arising, two hours later a cupful, more or less, of raisins; and either grape juice or raisins at two-hour intervals [for the rest of the day]. They should not be taken at the same meal. The raisins may be eaten dry, or they may be soaked in ordinary cold water for several hours, and the raisins and raisin water taken for one meal. [Use *un*-sulfured raisins.]

"When neither whole grapes nor unsweetened juice could be procured, patients have taken only raisins and raisin water instead of grapes and grape juice. The raisins should be eaten at 2-hour intervals, the same as grapes."

"Will It Really Help Me?"

Ask your doctor. He or she is the right person to supervise your case. "The grape is a powerful natural solvent," says Mrs. Brandt. "Certain growths, ulcers, abscesses and fibrous masses seem to be dissolved by the powerful chemical agents in grapes. Diseased tissues and fatty degenerations, every form of morbid matter, is apparently broken up into minute particles and thrown into the bloodstream to be carried to the organs of excretion, the bowels, kidneys, lungs and skin.

"You would be amazed if you could visualize the rapid changes which take place in the body during the grape cure. The effects are almost magical. Science may never discover in the laboratory the secret of the grape, but it is far more potent than most people imagine."

CHAPTER + 13
THE "METHUSELAH" PLANT: HE USED IT AND LIVED IN THREE CENTURIES

And the Lord spake unto Moses saying, "Command the children of Israel that they bring unto thee pure *oil olive* beaten for the light, to cause the lamp to burn continually . . ." *Exodus 27:20*

And went to him, and bound up his wounds, pouring in *oil* and wine . . . *Luke 10:34*

And at night He went out, and abode in the mount that is called the Mount of *Olives. Luke 21:37*

Olive oil is the most important food in the Bible, where it is mentioned more than 200 times and is the symbol of goodness, purity, and—especially—long life. It is one of the few specific foods mentioned by Jesus as a healing food, as reported by Luke the physician in the third Gospel.

The olive tree grows slowly and attains a great age. Some of the original trees at Gethsemane—which was an olive orchard at the foot of the Mount of Olives—have been there since the time of Christ, or at least spring from the original roots. For even though the

Romans tried to destroy the orchard in A.D.70, it is almost impossible to kill the roots, from which many new sprouts arise. Jesus spent His last night before the Crucifixion in the Garden of Gethsemane, waiting and watching for the dawn. Afterward, He ascended to heaven from the Mount of Olives.

What Strange Power Does This Oil Possess?

Why have olives always been regarded with such reverence and awe? Ramses II, who ruled Egypt between 1300 and 1200 B.C., supposedly downed olive oil for every complaint. Ramses III attempted to plant an olive grove in honor of the sun god Re, near the temple at Heliopolis. Olive oil was used at coronations, employed in sacrificial offerings, and as fuel, food, and medicine for the body.

The ancient Hebrews regarded olive oil as the key to long life and rejuvenated mental powers. Often attaining lifespans of 100, 200, 300 years or more, they not only consumed olive oil, but virtually all of them—male or female, rich and poor alike—used oil embrocations daily. According to the Psalmists, the oil directly penetrated the body when rubbed on, relieving aches and pains, restoring strength.

Today we know that olive oil—which *can* be absorbed by the skin—protects veins and arteries, guards against dangerous clots, lowers high blood pressure, normalizes low blood pressure, and, according to Dr. Ancel Keys, *helps ward off death from all causes, including cancer.*

"The Pain in Every Joint Was Gone"

"I was not taking my medication for arthritis," says one woman, "even though I have had this disease for over 10 years. I recently started drinking olive oil. I took approximately 6 tablespoons a day (during the day) for two weeks. Then I took one tablespoon a day for two weeks.

"The pain in every joint was gone. I stopped this procedure feeling maybe the arthritis had been arrested, as happens in some cases. After 3 weeks, the pain started to return. I knew it must have been the olive oil that relieved my pain . . .

". . . so I started taking 3 tablespoons a day. I kept this up for one week, then discontinued the dosage. After 2 weeks the pain, though only slight, was returning. I began taking 3 tablespoons just one day a week, and I find it lasts one week and I have no pain for this period."

Oldest Woman Ever in Guinness Book of World Records Attributes Long Life to this Plant

On August 4, 1997, CNN-TV announced: "Jean Calment died today at 127—the oldest person ever documented in the Guinness Book of World Records." She attributed her long life to olive oil, and a single glass of port wine before meals, and plenty of chocolate in between. She took up fencing when she was 87, smoked until recently, and remembers seeing the famous impressionist painter Vincent van Gogh in her father's art supply store, when she was 14.

Keeps the Heart Healthy, Arteries Clean, Lowers Blood Pressure

People in Mediterranean countries—Greece, Italy, Spain, and southern France—who are heavily dependent on olive oil in their diets are only half as likely to die of heart disease as are Americans. And yet the diet of these people is not low-fat.

In fact, they eat *more* fat than Americans do. But about three-fourths of all their fat comes from olive oil. They eat very little animal fat. In a 15-year study, only 38 out of 10,000 residents of Crete died of heart disease, compared to 773 Americans.

Olive oil protects your heart and arteries three ways:

1. It reduces bad LDL cholesterol in the blood.
2. It raises the level of good HDL cholesterol.
3. It keeps blood platelets from sticking together and forming clots.

Other oils such as corn, soybean, safflower, and sunflower lower *both* good HDL and bad LDL. Olive oil is even better than standard low-fat diets in reducing cholesterol. When subjects ate 41 percent of their calories in fat, most of it from olive oil, their bad LDL cholesterol sank more than when they ate a diet with half as much fat.

In one study, volunteers took three-fourths of a tablespoon of olive oil twice a day for 8 weeks in addition to their regular diet. Olive oil contains oleic acid—a dominant fatty acid that discourages clotting. As a result, their platelet-clumping scores took a dive.

As for lowering blood pressure, a study at Stanford Medical School of 76 middle-aged men with high blood pressure showed that the monounsaturated fat in 3 tablespoons of olive oil a day could lower systolic pressure about nine points and diastolic pressure about six points. Even more remarkable, a University of Kentucky study found that just two thirds of a *single tablespoonful of* olive oil daily lowered systolic pressure about five points and diastolic pressure four points in men.

The Secret of Longevity

As if this were not enough, the most fanatical olive-oil lovers among these people *were least likely to die of cancer or anything else!* Using artery-protecting "mono" oils—such as olive, canola, almond, or avocado—as the major source of fat was the only dietary factor, according to Dr. Keys, that warded off death from all causes—which is why olive oil has always been known as the longevity food.

Specifically, countries in which olive oil is a major source of fat in the diet tended to have more reduced risk of breast, prostate, ovary, and colon cancer.

The antioxidants in olive oil may help retard aging by keeping cells alive longer, as well as fight off attacks that cause cells to become disorganized and more cancer-prone.

The Man Who Lived in 3 Centuries

Goddard Ezekiel Dodge Diamond, who lived to 120—the same age as Moses—attributed his long life to olive oil, which he used in food and for external applications for aches and pains, and to the distilled water he drank. In 1899, he wrote a book about it, called *The Secret of Long Life: Or How to Live in Three Centuries,* stating:

"If I live until May 1, 1900, I will celebrate my 104th birthday. . . and am now in the enjoyment of as good health as when in my 30s, 40s or 50s. . . . There is not a pain disturbing my body; not a joint ailing from rheumatic twinges . . . not a sign of heavy hearing; not so much as a dimmed vision . . .

"Most people desire to know how to grow old gracefully, but my limited experience has taught me that it is a more desirable thing to grow old in the enjoyment of every faculty unimpaired . . . or what is better, not to grow old at all . . ."

Sight and Hearing Restored

"Not until I was nearly 40 did I [experience] sickness. . . . At that time I had what was known as the black measles, in its worst form. The result of this sickness was impaired sight and hearing. . . .

"After 3 years my eyes were very painful, water running from them and a film gathering over them. My hearing was quite dull and growing worse. . . . I recalled . . . reading of the Hebrew Kings, how they were anointed with oil, and how oil was used as a means of healing. . . ."

"I resolved to use the best oil I could get . . . I applied it first to the eyes. Just two or three applications were made before decided improvements appeared . . . Sore places healed . . . water ceased to flow so profusely . . . the film [was] less troublesome.

"The change was so great that I resolved to use [olive] oil for the loss of hearing. I used [the] oil freely about the ears externally, and put drops of oil into the ears, holding it there with bits of cotton balls.

"In a very short time my sight and hearing were entirely restored. I did not leave off treating them because they appeared to be free from infirmity, but have kept them well oiled for 60 years, and they have never failed me whenever called into service."

Overcomes Stiffness in Spine, Hips, Shoulders, and Knees

"Not until I was past three score years did I again feel the effects of infirmity. . . . Up to that time I had never felt signs of rigidity of bones or joints, and knew not that the machinery was running down.

"One day I jumped from a wagon to the ground and my joints did not respond with the usual rebound. I was startled and surprised. Resuming my place in the wagon, I leaped to the ground again, as a proof trial. The proof was there, for not only did the knees refuse to rebound, but the backbone creaked and cried out in pain.

"I was humiliated and gave way to tears and general lamentations. . . . my senses at once sought for a remedy. The cure of failing sight and hearing by the use of [olive] oil externally led me to believe that the same remedy might apply to hardening bones and rigid joints. . . .

"I resolved to begin the practice of oiling every joint and such portions of the physical frame as might be subject to the rigid and hardening processes of old age. . . . My age at that time was about 65 years."

"How I Used the Oil"

"Having secured such oil as to me was best, I began by first preparing the skin to receive it. To this end the ordinary tub bath was discarded, and the sponge bath put into practice [using] tepid water. I use a wet and soaped towel, which I pass over the body, rubbing every part as thoroughly and as rapidly as possible. Rinsing the towel and wringing as dry as can be done, I apply it again thoroughly, finishing with a coarse dry towel. . . .

"Turning a little oil into the hollow of the hand I apply it to the joints, on the inside especially—that is, under the arms, in elbows, in rear of knees, on the insteps and in the groins. After that upon the shoulders, spine, hips, knees, bottom of feet [even the head if desired]. Rub . . . until the oil is absorbed [and can't be seen]. Then off to bed . . .

"This practice I began and have kept it up, sometimes both morning and evening, for the past 60 years for the eyes, and nearly 40 years for the bones and joints. This should not seem strange to anyone."

The gardener knows he must enrich the soil if it is to remain useful and productive. The body also requires enriching, he says.

"It has been suggested to me," says Diamond, "that olive oil is expensive, and that bathing in it is beyond the reach of the average man. I do not bathe in oil. The amount I use upon each occasion will not exceed a tablespoonful."

Doing Somersaults at 100, Bicycling at 108, Dancing with a Teenaged Girl at 110

Apparently it worked so well that when Diamond was past 100, he was able to do gymnastics that few young men could equal. At the age of 108, he was riding a bicycle and walking 20 miles a day. He attended social events, and when he was 110 he danced most of the evening, on one occasion, with an athletic girl of 16.

In April 1896, a photographer named John R. Hodson agreed to make a life-sized portrait of Capt. Diamond on his 100th birthday. Naturally expecting so old a gentleman, he covered the skylight so as not to hurt his eyes and set out an easy chair for him. But he said when Diamond appeared at his door: "I was dumbfounded! Here was a man standing straight as a young prince, moving with an elastic, sprightly step, and with a bright, youthful twinkle in his eye! . . . *He is erect, square shouldered, and has a military bearing.*"

Capt. Diamond also submitted to a physical examination by Dr. Frederick William D'Evelyn, a graduate of Edinburgh University, who was the head of St. Luke's Hospital in San Francisco. The doctor's report—dated March 22, 1898—was as follows:

Goddard Ezekiel Dodge Diamond [was born in] Plymouth, Mass., May 1st, 1796. Lived nearly all his life in the United States . . . Has had very little illness in his life. Yellow fever once; pneumonia once. Has been asphyxiated twice from charcoal fumes. Met with numerous accidents; bones broken, left shoulder dislocated. Height 5'6-1/4".

Present weight 141 lbs. Nine years ago he weighed 225 lbs. Reduced himself by diet. . . . Keeps the same weight. No difficulty breathing. Can lie in any position. . . . No palpitation. Visceral functions normal. Virility good. Pulse regular in rhythm, tension slight, easily compressible, irregularly intermittent . . . Pulse rate 76. Respiration regular . . .

Vision good; reaction of pupils normal; range of vision somewhat shortened reading a 10-foot chart short at 8 feet. Physical appearance good, resembling a well-preserved man of 78. Absence of wrinkles; face slightly flushed; condition of skin in all parts of body excellent, except over abdomen . . . owing to great reduction in weight.

Hair grey, not bald. Chest well formed . . . 36 inches . . . expansion very limited . . . Abdominal 34 inches. Thigh firm, 16-1/2 inches. Arm 9-1/2 inches. . . . Legs are firm . . . calf 13 inches; absence of all varicosity. Blood . . . morphology of red cells almost normal. . . . Kidney reaction—very fair. . . . albumen, none; large excess of bile; urates abundant . . . Appetite always good; digestion excellent. . . . Uses olive oil external and internal . . .

The doctor's report includes a photo of a pulse tracing, and concludes: "The physical examination of Capt. Diamond reveals a remarkable preservation of tissue integrity and functional activity. . . ." *The doctor feels, however, that Captain Diamond's "proposed walk from San Francisco to New York," including mountain climbing, would be too much for a man of 102.*

Extra-Strength Oil

Diamond preferred to use the highest quality olive oil he could find. To him that meant pure, unadulterated olive oil, from the first—not the second or third—pressing. Today, this is called extra virgin olive oil, extracted by crushing and pressing the highest quality olives, which contain the most potent, disease-fighting chemicals. Diamond regarded California olives as the best.

"What I Eat and Drink"

Diamond claimed that for 50 years he faithfully did certain things. First, he always breathed the freshest air possible, "long, deep draughts," and never smoked.

Second, he ate no flesh foods after the age of 56. He believed that humans were originally intended to eat only vegetation—fruits, vegetables, nuts, and seeds.

"When we eat meat," said Diamond, "we are eating the product of the earth second-hand. The vegetation has been eaten by the animal and a large part of it converted into bone and tendon . . . and we eat only what is left." Meat eating, he said, produces too much uric acid, resulting in conditions such as rheumatism, headaches, and various nervous conditions.

Third, he believed in chewing his food thoroughly, to ease digestion, and in using whole wheat instead of white flour which he said produces constipation.

Fourth, he used no stimulants, even though the Bible encourages the use of wine as food, in moderation, and as medicine. He never used tobacco, tea, or coffee. "None of these things contain food," he said.

Fifth, he drank no unboiled water, "unless it be distilled," and drank distilled water whenever possible. He believed that mineral salts—held in solution in natural spring water—when released into the body are finally deposited in all the tissues, cells, and organs, where they build up "in such quantities that by constant use up to the middle of life a man has taken into his system enough calcareous matter to form a pillar of solid chalk, marble or salt, not unlike Lot's wife," producing stiffness, rigidity, old age, and decrepitude.

His daily menu included a cup of hot water—he tried to drink 3 cups of hot water daily—oatmeal or farina with milk, boiled codfish with potatoes, coarse bread and butter, two poached eggs, applesauce, and fruit in season *for breakfast*. He seldom ate lunch. A typical supper would include a cup of hot water, vegetable or rice tomato soup, coarse bread with butter, sweet potatoes, beans, hot milk, and fruit in season.

An All-Purpose Miracle Remedy?

Over the centuries, olive oil has been used to loosen the bowels, stimulate bile flow, soothe mucus membranes, induce urination, soften skin, and calm the nerves. It is found in folk remedies for cancer, chills, diarrhea, earache, fever, high blood pressure, low blood pressure, malaria, goiter, toothache, tumors, wounds, genital warts, polyps, sclerosis of the liver, spleen, and uterus; and tumors of the ear, fingers, neck, and stomach.

Algerians still chew olive leaves for toothache and mouth sores caused by too much tobacco. They also use it for baldness, cough, earache, fractures, gonorrhea, hemorrhage, hernia, impotence, liver congestion, skin diseases, sprains, and stones. In Lebanon the oil is used for burns, colds, constipation, and stomach ache.

Are there any factual bases for these wide-ranging uses?

Controlling Adult-Onset Diabetes

Olive oil significantly lowered the blood-sugar levels of most adult-onset diabetics and reduced their daily insulin needs, according to a study at the University of Texas Southwestern Medical Center at Dallas.

This—together with the fact that olive oil prevents and reverses deadly buildup of cholesterol in heart, veins, and arteries—may help millions of diabetics avoid the many serious complications of this disease.

Unlike standard low-fat, high-carbohydrate diets that doctors normally prescribe for adult-onset diabetics, which are so tasteless most patients can't stay on them, the olive-oil diet is much easier to follow because it's so close to what people normally eat.

With this method, olive oil is used for frying foods and as a salad dressing and wherever else a cooking oil is needed. It's 75 percent polyunsaturated, which makes it far healthier than other fats.

If you have adult-onset diabetes, you should check with your doctor first before using this method, to determine if it's safe for you.

How This Bible Healing Food Relieved Gall-Bladder Problems

If you've ever had a gall-bladder attack, you know how painful it can be, especially if stones have formed. *To prevent painful gall-stones from ever forming, if your doctor says you have a lazy gall-bladder, you can usually get it into action by taking 1 or 2 table-spoons of olive oil before each meal, says one doctor.* This starts the flow of bile before the rest of the food enters the stomach. You may get some indigestion at first, but you should see marked improvement within 2 weeks.

Olive oil has been found to cause strong, healthy contractions of the gallbladder, greatly favoring complete emptying, and can be regarded as a good gall-bladder tonic, according to the October-December 1962 issue of *Minerva Dietologica*. It also seems to melt gallstones. In 1893, an experiment was reported in which a gallstone lost 68 percent of its weight when immersed in pure olive oil.

If your doctor has determined with X-rays that your gallstones are small enough to be passed without getting stuck, an old folk remedy for passing them—occasionally recommended by doctors—is to mix half a cup of olive oil with half a cup of lemon or grapefruit juice, stir, drink, and go to bed. You may experience nausea. In the morning, drink something hot and you may pass the stones from your bowels. It sometimes helps to fast for 2 days, drinking apple juice at 2-hour intervals and then drink the olive-oil–lemon-juice mixture on the second night. This is said to dissolve small stones and cleanse the bladder too.

Reported cases:

M. C. writes: "A number of years ago a complete physical by a very reputable clinic showed I had gallstones . . . there were five of various sizes. Through friends . . . I learned how to get rid of them. For three days drink good organic apple juice. Do not eat or drink anything else, except at the end of the second and third day drink a half-cup of olive oil with a half-cup of apple juice. The gallstones passed on the fourth day. Several years later I had X-rays . . . and the doctor reported no signs of gallstones."

D. R. writes: "My sister was scheduled for surgery after being told she had gallstones. A relative advised her to wait and try the juice of half a lemon placed in a small wine glass and float four tablespoons of olive oil on top to take one hour before breakfast each day. She did this for about six months and found no need for surgery."

Medical anthropologist John Heinerman says: "For the complete removal of gallstones [olive oil] seems to have worked for several thousand people across the U.S. and Canada . . . I've personally interviewed about 125. . . . In every single instance, the treatment with some slight variations here and there always seems to have met with success."[1]

Earlier Medical Findings

Dr. A. E. Osborn, director of a children's hospital in Glen Ellen, California, writing in the epilogue of Capt. Diamond's book, gives the results of his experiments in treating various diseases with olive oil:

1. "Two years ago measles swept through the hospital. Over 60 patients were down at the same time. Lacking the proper hospital facilities . . . we were obliged to treat them in the regular sleeping dormitories. . . . My invariable treatment was to . . . give them a thorough hot water sponging . . . followed immediately and repeatedly every few hours with copious [applications] of warm olive oil, well rubbed in . . . [plus] a generous diet . . .

"All recovered nicely, notwithstanding the extremely delicate condition of many previously. The mainstay of the treatment was the oil (no drugs being used) . . . Whenever the skin became dry and hot the oil relieved it and brought to the patient a sense of relief . . . followed by sleep, from which they awoke refreshed.

2. "In scarlet fever the frequent [applications] of hot olive oil [were] particularly effective in sustaining the patient and [avoiding] many dangerous complications. From personal trials . . . I am convinced that of any single remedy in this disease, olive oil is the most valuable and potent."

3. A retarded boy, 6 years old "contracted pneumonia; both lungs involved . . . Previous history bad, a strong syphilitic taint being well-rooted in a [tubercular] constitution." The child refused all food except bread and milk and a little well-cooked potato. His digestion was poor. "In addition to regular treatment, gave olive oil

---

[1]*Heinerman's Encyclopedia of Fruits, Vegetables and Herbs,* West Nyack, NY: Parker Publishing Company, Inc., 1988.

internally on bread, well salted, and externally to body and limbs, by hand rubbing . . . followed by wrapping. . . . He recovered from the pneumonia."

4. "Other cases have demonstrated the superiority of olive oil over cod liver oil in consumption [tuberculosis], which again I am aware is saying a great deal. . . ."

"My experience warrants me . . . to assume the following conclusions:"

"Olive oil stands unrivalled . . . as a remedy in most and probably all wasting diseases, where it relieves the stomach, rests overtaxed digestive organs, lubricates inflamed alimentary tracts, [halts] further congestion . . . and restores . . . worn-out or broken-down tissue.

"It exerts a distinctive influence upon the liver and, apparently, also upon the kidneys. The benefits to be derived from olive oil in liver derangement are not at all [imaginary]." It gives the liver a rest, he says.

"The chief value of olive oil in fevers lies in its ability to be rapidly absorbed through the skin. . . . In all cases it will reduce the temperature of the body, which means a saving of vital importance. On account of its chemical constitution, it is especially adapted for the feeding of fevers . . . as it is so readily absorbed by the skin . . ."

This is true, he says, in cases of measles, scarlet fever, malaria, and typhoid fever.

"I am continuing to use and to advocate the use of olive oil in . . . nervous diseases characterized by great [loss] of power and the progressive waste of nerve tissue . . . The usual way of applying it is by massage . . . once to thrice daily. With paralytics the operations of massage are most valuable. With epileptics [applications] of oil immediately followed by sufficient bed rest to induce the best results."

Another physician, Dr. P. C. Remondia of San Diego, California, writing in the epilogue of Capt. Diamond's book, gives the following uses of olive oil:

As a vermifuge: "Olive oil is one of our safest vermifuges. In the case of children, it should be given in ounce doses, and frequently repeated. It is harmless, as it does not provoke active purging, and if the child's stomach does not reject it, it will often do its work without any additional drug. In cases of tapeworm, it has often carried away [all of it] simply by its weight and volume."

Bladder and kidney affections: "In cases of severe pains located in the region of the kidneys, olive oil taken internally, in medium dose, has often proved beneficial in granting prompt relief. It has also been used with success in cases of painful urination, strangury [a slow and painful discharge of urine, drop by drop], and in cases of what is popularly termed gravelly urine."

In intestinal affections: "Simple diarrhea, dysentery, colicky pains, flatulence or constipation, have all been relieved by the prompt and generous use of olive oil [particularly with children]. There is nothing that will act more energetically in a case of imprisoned intestinal gases [or] accumulation of feces . . . than a large dose of olive oil . . .

Fluid retention (edema): "Olive oil, taken both internally and by [external application], has often given great results in cases of dropsy [swelling from fluid retention], either abdominal or general."

Burns and wounds: "Olive oil, in connection with an equal part of lime water, makes an excellent application to burned surfaces, relieves pain and promotes repair; have used it so mixed, in burns, scalds, powder wounds, and in skin abrasions. In powder accidents involving the eyes this makes a soothing and protective application."

An antidote to poison: "Olive oil has been given with success in cases of mushroom poisoning, being liberally mixed with powdered charcoal. In general, it may be said that olive oil is a safe and efficacious antidote in many cases of poisoning . . ."

Absorbed by Her Skin
It Lowers Her Cholesterol

One woman claimed that soaking her feet for 10 minutes every day in a hot foot bath prepared with shavings of castile soap reduced her blood cholesterol. She said, "I know it sounds crazy, but it worked—it really did! The drop in cholesterol was confirmed by a doctor." Castile soap is made with pure olive oil, which has been found to reduce cholesterol by as much as 26 percent. In one study where olive oil was widely used, out of 1,215 men, only four cases of heart or artery disease were found in 6 years.

A Famous Remedy for Constipation

One of the mildest laxatives is olive oil (one tablespoon at bedtime). Constipation is often relieved in long-standing (20-year) sufferers with this simple method. In enema form it is often used to relieve fecal impaction or blockage.

Ulcers Healed

"To relieve heartburn, indigestion and ulcers," says John Heinerman, "just mix together 2 tablespoons of pure virgin olive oil with the white of one raw egg. Then take internally several times a day to experience rapid relief."[2]

One doctor reports that he treats his ulcer patients with olive oil. He relates how a friend of his is able to eat an astonishing

---

[2] *Heinerman's Encyclopedia of Fruits, Vegetables and Herbs, op. cit.*

amount of the hottest Mexican sauces—after taking this oil. Some medical men believe that olive oil contains vitamin U, a substance that is believed to have a healing influence on ulcers.

Bursitis Cured

In one reported case, Mrs. R. B. says: "My husband had arthritis for several years and at one time got a bad case of bursitis in his right shoulder and was unable to raise his arm. To relieve the soreness I started massaging the shoulder and upper arm daily with hot olive oil, using slight manipulation while massaging. This helped and gradually he got the motion back in his shoulder and hasn't been bothered with bursitis since."

St. Vitus' Dance Cured

An 11-year-old girl began to act strangely and was diagnosed with St. Vitus' Dance, a nervous disorder marked by spasmodic movements of limbs and facial muscles and by lack of coordination. Her mother learned from the other children that the girl had been in the habit of eating a certain weed whenever she went near where it grew. Olive oil was then given to the girl, two or three times a day, in tablespoonful doses. It was also applied to her skin, where it reportedly turned green as it absorbed the poison through the pores. The olive-oil treatment was continued, both externally and internally, with no other remedies. The child recovered both her physical and mental powers, and there was never a trace of any recurrence.

Relief for Earaches and Inner Ear Infections

In an effort to find an alternative to antibiotic drugs that a pediatrician had prescribed for his children, one man came up with a simple remedy for the earaches and inner-ear infections they had been having.

He squeezes the contents of one vitamin E capsule (400 units) and one garlic-oil capsule into a clean glass container. He adds 13 drops of olive oil (with an eyedropper) to these ingredients and mixes them all together thoroughly. Then he sets the container in a soup bowl filled with "very warm" water, where he allows it to sit for 1 minute, testing until it's warm enough to bear without scalding. With the child's head tilted sideways, he places an equal number of drops in each ear.

He says this remedy also relieves ringing in the ear, but advises against using it if there is a purulent discharge, or if the eardrum has ruptured.

Emergency Relief for Burns

John Heinerman claims olive oil is "terrific" for ulcers and burns. He says severe burns on the surface of the skin can be effectively treated with just olive oil and egg whites, when nothing else is available. As proof, he cites a painful scalding he received when boiling hot liquid sprayed the entire inside of his right forearm. A mixture of virgin olive oil (two cups) and whites of six fresh eggs—beaten together— was brushed onto the wound with a clean basting brush (sterilized under extra hot water). This was covered with a dressing of loose, light gauze, from elbow to wrist and changed again the next day.

"In less than a week, I was completely recovered and required no medical attention whatever," he says. "Surprisingly, no scars remained . . ."[3]

Helps Tighten Loose Skin

A famous cosmetician claims olive oil can help tighten loose, sagging skin around the face and throat. Just take two egg yolks and beat them thoroughly in one-half cup of olive oil. Brush on face and

---

[3]*Heinerman's Encyclopedia of Fruits, Vegetables and Herbs, op. cit.*

throat and allow to set for 10 minutes. The whites of the eggs are then beaten and layered over the first dressing. This is left on for about a half hour, then rinsed off. The skin appears tightened and wrinkle-free.

Secret of Wrinkle-Free Skin

Most of the medicinal uses of olive come from its oil. But in Greece, the *juice* is used by women to keep their skin virtually wrinkle-free. They merely rub the juice of green olives, which is bitter and astringent, on the skin of the face, throat, hands, wrists, and forearms, in quick circular motions, patting the skin briskly from time to time. This keeps the skin tight enough so that there is nothing loose enough to sag or wrinkle. Additionally, daily intake of olive *oil* with meals keeps skin soft and resilient. The juice should be used only externally, due to its highly bitter taste.

Olive juice may be obtained from fresh or pickled olives by removing the pits and running them through a juicer, adding water if the juice becomes too thick. (Pickled olives should be soaked first to remove the salt.) This can then be stored in your refrigerator in a covered container and a little bit used each morning to rub on your skin.

Drinking olive juice is not advisable due to its extremely bitter taste. This is particularly true if the juice is from pickled olives, which can aggravate high blood pressure. In Indonesia, this bitter juice has been successfully used in small doses for expelling intestinal worms.

CHAPTER · 14

HOW SOME OF THE MOST FAMOUS BIBLE FOODS FIGHT AIDS, ALZHEIMER'S, PARKINSON'S, AND MORE

During their 40 years of wandering in the barren desert, the Israelites were often discouraged, and wanted to turn back. To their leaders, they complained, "You have led us out here in the desert to die . . ." In this atmosphere of discontent, when Moses' brother Aaron was appointed High Priest, they questioned his authority.

Moses prayed for guidance and was instructed by God to have each family bring a rod with the name of the head of the family carved on it. On the rod of the house of Levi, Moses carved Aaron's name. The rods were all presented in the great tent, or tabernacle, and the next day, when Moses went into the tabernacle, the rod of Aaron had sprouted. It budded and blossomed and bore ripe almonds.

The word for almond in ancient Hebrew means "gift from God." The miracle of the rod that sprouted almond blossoms can still be witnessed to this day. If the tip of a branch of an almond tree is placed in water or wrapped in a wet cloth, it will sprout blossoms virtually overnight.

The almond tree is the first in the Holy Land to flower, producing its lovely pink blossoms from bare and apparently lifeless branches as the first sign of spring, renewed life, and the wakening of Creation. Jews still carry rods of almond blossoms to the synagogues for great festivals.

There are two principal forms of almond—sweet almonds and bitter almonds. Sweet almonds are valuable as food and also as medicine. Bitter almonds must be used with caution, because they contain cyanide, a poison.

Stomach and Intestinal Pains Ceased in Minutes

Centuries ago it was discovered that when a tablespoonful of crushed almonds was slowly simmered in milk or thin hot barley gruel for about 30 minutes and then given to someone with indigestion, their stomach or intestinal pains ceased in a matter of minutes.

Relief for Stones, Gravel, Kidney, and Bladder Problems

"Blanched and beaten into an emulsion with barley-water (see page 000), Sweet Almonds are of great use in the stone, gravel, strangury and other disorders of the kidneys, bladder, and biliary ducts," says Maude Grieve in *A Modern Herbal.*

Set Your Aging Clock Back 20 Years with This Do-It-Yourself Face Lift

Ninon de L'Enclos was a great French beauty who, at 90, was still so physically alluring that young men fell hopelessly in love with her! Her face was as smooth and free of wrinkles as it had been at 20! (This is a well-documented fact.) Louis XIV declared that she was the marvel of his reign.

Authentic pictures of Ninon de L'Enclos at ages ranging from 50 to 85 show a clear, smooth face, with youthful rounded contours, a smooth throat, and symmetrical neck.

Ninon taught her intimate friends the secret. One of them, Saint Evremond, at the age of 89, was still so handsome that young girls swooned over him. Her secret was revealed in a French pamphlet published in 1710. The author, Jeanne Sauval, was her personal attendant for almost half a century. It is said to be the only successful method for removing wrinkles, aside from plastic surgery.

The secret was an ointment that contained 4 ounces of almond oil, 3 ounces of lard, and 1 ounce of spermaceti (a waxy substance obtained from sperm-whale oil). Onion juice was added, and then the mixture was melted, stirring until cool, and scented with rose-water. For lard you can use olive oil, or any vegetable shortening. For spermaceti you can use chopped or shaved candlewax. You can squeeze the juice out of a piece of onion with an ordinary hand-held garlic squeezer. Stir over heat until melted, adding a teaspoonful of rosewater. Allow to cool, and bottle it for storage and future use. Apply once a day to forehead, face, and neck, whenever convenient, as at bedtime. Cover the pillow with something to prevent staining. Wipe off a few hours later, or upon awakening, with cotton balls soaked with rubbing alcohol. Then use any gentle commercial skin cleanser and toner or moisturizer.

Fun to Eat, Good for the Heart

Eating almonds may reduce cholesterol. Dr. Gene Spiller, director of the Health Research and Studies Center in California, tested a group of people with high cholesterol by giving one group 3-1/2 ounces of almonds to eat each day for 3–9 weeks. Two other groups got equal amounts of fat from cheese or olive oil. All ate identical amounts of fruits, vegetables, and whole grains. Those who ate almonds experienced a drop in cholesterol 10 to 15 percent greater than the cheese eaters, and slightly better than the olive-oil group. His conclusion was that almonds and olive oil, both of which contain monounsaturated fat, are good for the heart and are useful for bringing down cholesterol, but should be used sparingly because they're high in calories.

Laetrile

Controversial Anticancer Substance Found in Bible Food

The bitterness in the bitter almond is due to the presence of the gly-coside *amygdalin,* which has been used in cancer chemotherapy since 1845 . Its other name, which most people are more familiar with, is *laetrile.*

Laetrile was said to release hydrocyanic acid into the body, which destroys cancer cells, leaving normal cells intact. The evidence for and against laetrile is strong.

For example, there is only one place in the world that is cancer-free, and that is the Hunza region of Pakistan, the only place where apricot pits are an important part of the diet. An oil extracted from the pits is used by the Hunzas as their main cooking oil. In New Mexico, the Pueblo Indians, whose cancer rate is unusually low, drink a beverage made from the pits of apricots, peaches, and cherries, all three of which contain amygdalin, the substance from which laetrile is made. In the early 1970s, a writer doing research among the Pueblo Indians began drinking this beverage. He told *Prevention* magazine that within 3 days, a couple of benign skin growths on his arm began to shrivel up. In a week, they were completely gone. Friends of his who also drank the beverage had the same experience. And the drug does seem to work on some patients. A medical doctor in Palo Alto, California, says he saved his own mother's life with laetrile. In 1976, a 4-year-old child suffering from a growth on the base of his spine (esonophilic granuloma), with the potential for turning cancerous, was given small amounts of laetrile daily by his mother, a registered nurse, who rejected her doctor's recommendation for radiation and surgery. Within 2 months, X-rays showed no sign of the growth.

One advocate of laetrile, Hans Nepier, M.D., a cancer specialist, of Silbersee Hospital in Hanover, Germany, says that it is an important bone-cancer therapy, although it does not work for everybody. He says it works only when the body's natural defense mechanisms are operating. He calls the banning of laetrile in the United States "the greatest and most depressing tragic comedy of modern medicine."

On the other hand, most medical and scientific organizations regard laetrile as worthless. In various tests by the National Cancer Institute, the Food and Drug Administration, and other health agencies, laetrile failed to show any benefits. One study examined the case histories of 12 patients of a Mexican physician. Of the nine patients whose records could be obtained, six had already died, and one still had cancer which had spread since using laetrile. No tests were approved or done by the FDA on human beings.

Dr. Dean Burke, a biochemist and former head of the NCA's cytochemistry division, said that tests on animals showed laetrile to have a deterrent effect on cancer. He resigned over this controversy. In his book *The Treatment of Cancer with Herbs* (Orem, UT: BiWorld Publishers, 1980, pp. 171–82), John Heinerman says that in tests done by Dr. Kanematsu Sugiura at the Sloan Kettering Institute in New York City, laetrile "had a definite inhibitory effect on lung cancer" in test animals, but that officials at the Institute informed the press that "all the tests with laetrile had turned out to be negative . . ."

Dr. Harold W. Manner, former chairman of the Department of Biology at Loyola University in Chicago is quoted by Heinerman as saying that the cyanide in laetrile "is not a poison when it is part of a complete chemical complex"—meaning the bitter almond itself—and that cancer patients could safely take small amounts of bitter almonds, up to ten per day, without suffering serious consequences. "Almonds could do no more harm than chemotherapy or radiation does, and probably a lot less," said Dr. Manner, in an interview with Heinerman.[1]

Manner resigned his teaching post, and opened the Manner Clinic in Tijuana, Mexico, which Heinerman says has helped hundreds of people recover from different types of cancer in the past decade. Cancer treatment with laetrile is, of course, illegal in the United States. But, reportedly, many health-conscious people eat small amounts of almonds daily, to safeguard against cancer, or as informal, unofficial therapy for existing tumors they may have, along with standard medical care.[2]

What shall we make of all this mass of conflicting evidence? In his book *Cancer: How to Prevent It* (Prentice-Hall, 1978), Dr. George E. Berkley says, "A few conclusions can be drawn. Firstly, Laetrile probably does no one any harm. Even some of its fiercest opponents do

---

[1]John Heinerman, *Heinerman's Encyclopedia of Nuts, Berries and Seeds,* West Nyack, NY: Parker Publishing Company, Inc., 1995.

[2]Heinerman, *op. cit.*

not claim that it can do any damage to the human body. Secondly, Laetrile . . . may help some people overcome the disease. Thirdly, Laetrile . . . a substance found in apricot pits . . . is chemically identified as nitriloside [and] can be found in many other foods.

"Foods rich in Laetrile-like nitrilosides include many fruits, such as apples, cherries, cranberries, prunes, plums, pears, lemons, and limes. . . . They also include many legumes, such as kidney beans, chick peas, and lentils . . . and many whole grains, such as millet and buckwheat. . . . Almonds, sweet potatoes, lettuce, and linseed have also been identified as nitriloside sources. Sorghum contains quite a bit of nitriloside, although molasses, which is like sorghum . . . contains none. . . . Mung bean sprouts and alfalfa sprouts supply especially large amounts of this possibly anti-carcinogenic substance.

"Keeping these facts in mind, you would do well to partake heavily and heartily of these nitriloside-containing foods [because they contain] many other nutrients that promote better health and increased resistance to malignancy. . . ."[3]

A Delicious Way to Eat It

A delicious way to get almonds in your diet is to prepare an almond salad by combining 2 cups of grapefruit segments with one-half cup of chopped dates and a cup of shredded almonds. An attractive appearance is made by arranging the ingredients on lettuce leaves, with green pepper rings spread over the leaves and with the grapefruit and dates in equal proportions placed on the pepper rings and the shredded almonds sprinkled over all. Oranges or tangerines may be substituted for, or combined with, the grapefruit. Figs may be substituted for, or combined with, the dates. Watercress could be substituted for the lettuce. Or slices of avocado or other fruits such as apples or pears could be added or substituted, depending on what is available. Whole almonds may be substituted for shredded almonds.

---

[3]George E. Berkley, Ph.D., *Cancer: How to Prevent It & How to Help Your Doctor Fight It,* Englewood Cliffs, NJ: Prentice-Hall, Inc., 1978.

Michael the Archangel's Healing Plant for Women

Angelica's reputation as a cure for every conceivable ailment goes back many centuries. Surprisingly, modern scientific research has confirmed a great many of these beliefs.

In Christianity, this plant is held sacred because it blooms on the day of Michael the Archangel, hence its Latin name, *Angelica Archangelica*. It seems to guard the health of women especially, but for both sexes it seems to normalize the heartbeat, protects against ulcers, inhibits tumors, abdominal pain, anemia, migraines, nephritis, shingles, and even acts as an all-purpose sex enhancer.

In the Orient, where it is called *dong quai*, angelica has been used for centuries by herb doctors to treat many female problems, such as premenstrual tension, cramps, weakness, dysmenorrhea (profuse bleeding between periods), menopausal symptoms (especially hot flashes, vaginal spasms and dryness), and to assure easy delivery.

Angelica's essential oil relaxes the smooth muscles of the uterus and intestines. This confirms its historical use in the treatment of uterine cramps and intestinal spasm.

Reported cases:

"I never had cramps . . . or flooding, so I thought that the menopause would be a cinch. But when it came . . . All my female organs seemed to be sore . . . I lost a lot of sleep . . . a painful spasm of the vagina would awaken me. . . . I had a medical examination, but everything checked out just fine. I was given some tranquilizers [but the spasms got worse]. One of the women I worked with suggested I consult [an] herbalist. . . . Due to the severity of my case he advised me to take two capsules [of Angelica] three times a day until my spasms had stopped and my organs were no longer sore and then to keep taking only one capsule twice per day . . . throughout menopause until it was over. [It] worked beautifully. My symptoms were gone within a week."—Mrs. M. L.[4]

---

[4]Richard Lucas, *Secrets of the Chinese Herbalists,* West Nyack, NY: Parker Publishing Company, Inc., 1977.

"Since I began taking capsules of [angelica], my menopausal symptoms have improved beyond belief. For the first time in years I have no rheumatism aches and pains, no hot flashes, and no weepy spells of depression. The improvement is so noticeable that friends have asked what I have done to bring about such a transformation!"—Miss M. J.[5]

More Startling Facts

Angelica is also used in the treatment of abdominal pain, anemia, injuries, arthritis, migraine headache, and many other conditions. It has a long history as a remedy for diabetes, hypertension, cancer, angina pectoris, nephritis, and shingles.

+ Angelica's pain-relieving action was 1.7 times that of aspirin in one study. That, combined with its smooth-muscle-relaxing ability, could explain its reputation for relieving cramps, headaches, and arthritis.

+ The Chinese say that angelica—called *dong quai*—does for women what ginseng does for men: it's an all-purpose sexual and reproductive tonic. Typically, 3–6 teaspoons of powdered root are added to a pint of boiling water. Dose: 1–3 cups a day. (Since it can cause uterine contractions, do not take it if you are pregnant.)

+ Angelica seems to normalize the heartbeat, greatly reducing incidents of arrhythmia (irregular heartbeat), according to recent studies. It contains at least 14 anti-arrhythmic compounds. It inhibits clumping or clotting of the blood and increases blood flow to the heart, brain, and extremities. It has significant blood-pressure-lowering action, an effect largely due to its ability to dilate (widen) blood vessels. It contains 15 compounds that act like the widely prescribed anti-angina drugs known as channel blockers.

---

[5]Richard Lucas, *Magic Herbs for Arthritis, Rheumatism and Related Ailments,* West Nyack, NY: Parker Publishing Company, Inc., 1981.

+ A 1990 study found that angelica has anti-ulcer effects. Two components of this herb "significantly inhibited acid secretion and the formation of stress-induced gastric lesions."

+ A 1991 Japanese study found that two extracts of angelica may be useful in preventing cancer. It induces the body to produce interferon and has exhibited anti-tumor activity.

Herbalists generally recommend two capsules of the powdered plant two or three times a day for severe symptoms, less in more moderate conditions. Since it tastes somewhat like celery, the capsules may be opened and sprinkled on hot soups or broth, thereby adding to their flavor.

Thousands of Women Use This Plant for Relief of Menopausal Rheumatism

All over America, women are talking about a remarkable new way to get incredible relief from the agonies of menopausal rheumatism, all-day, all-night relief that seems permanent in many cases. After years of discomfort, many now claim they are completely pain free, thanks to angelica.

Reported cases:[6]

"After suffering much misery from menopausal rheumatism and wasting good money on the doctor's fees and pills with not the slightest relief, I tried [angelica]. In a short time, there was a marked reduction in the rheumatism pains. Now, two months later, I consider myself completely cured. I was also happily surprised to find that I have not had any more of those aggravating hot flashes since taking [angelica]. I plan to continue . . . until I am completely over menopause."—Mrs. D. S.

_____

[6]Richard Lucas, *Magic Herbs for Arthritis, Rheumatism and Related Ailments,* *op. cit.*

"[Angelica] has worked wonders for me. I feel like a new woman. I had 'change of life' rheumatism, which bothered me so much at times that I could not rest comfortably, either sitting, standing, or in bed. After taking [angelica] capsules, the super kind [prepared from the root tops of several angelica plants rather than just one], for several weeks, I am now free of pain."—Miss T. W.

"I want to tell you about a woman who was advised by a friend to try [angelica] for menopausal rheumatism. Not only did she soon feel ever so much better, but after a few months, she no longer needed to take estrogen."—Miss V. B.

"For three years I suffered with menopausal rheumatism. Then a friend showed me a letter in a newspaper column where [angelica] was mentioned for the relief of rheumatism that occurs during the change of life. I insisted on trying it. Before long, the pain vanished and has not been felt since."—Mrs. S. E.

∏ew Treatment for Psoriasis Revealed in Ancient Tablets

I asked my friend Bob why he was rubbing figs on his elbows. Expecting the punch line of some joke, I was surprised when he said it was a technique used by the ancient Egyptians to get rid of psoriasis. They worshipped Ra, the sun god, from whom all manner of blessings flowed. To heal various skin afflictions, they would rub the area with certain plant juices, and would then expose themselves to the sun's healing rays. We now know that some of the plants they used, such as figs, contained psoralens, which are chemical compounds that photosensitize the skin.

This technique actually has a counterpart in modern medicine, called UVA photochemotherapy, used in serious cases of psoriasis. First, a drug is given that contains psoralen. Then the patient sits in a box that delivers ultraviolet A rays to the body.

To get a natural version of this, you would consume plants that contain psoralens, such as angelica tea, celery, figs, parsley, or parsnips—all of which just happen to be Bible foods. You could have just one, or mix several in a soup or salad, or juice them and then spend a short time daily in the sun, or under a sun-lamp, for ultraviolet light. Only the area involved need be exposed, such as elbows, knuckles, knees, or lower back, to minimize the risk of overexposure. If you notice any irritation, stop using the therapy. Always obtain your doctor's okay before self-treating.

Bob said it seemed to be clearing up his psoriasis, and no matter how strange the method, you can't argue with success.

A Bible Food Aphrodisiac and a Remedy for Parkinson's from the Book of Daniel

The clear message of the Bible is that beans are a miracle source of health. Esau was willing to sell his birthright for a bowl of pottage—lentil soup.

> And Esau said to Jacob, Feed me, I pray thee, with that . . . red pottage, for I am faint. And Jacob said, Sell me this day thy birthright. . . . And Esau said, Behold, I am at the point to die . . . and he sold his birthright unto Jacob. Then Jacob gave Esau bread and pottage of lentiles . . . *Genesis 25:30, 34*

Daniel refused to eat the king's meat, but instead asked only for pulse to eat and water to drink. Pulse, in Biblical days, referred to broad beans, such as fava beans and lentils. Daniel knew that the best way to maintain a clear mind and a strong body was to steer clear of the king's rich food and drink.

Daniel purposed in his heart that he would not defile himself with the portion of the king's meat but instead asked, "Give us pulse to eat, and water to drink . . . And at the end of ten days their countenances appeared fairer and fatter in flesh than all the children which did eat the portion of the king's meat." (Daniel 1:8)

Beans reduce the rise in blood sugar after meals, and delay the drop in blood sugar later on, which would certainly guarantee a clear mind.

Beans contain plant estrogens. They also contain PIs (protease inhibitors) that interfere with cancer-producing enzymes. PIs help prevent the growth of tumor cells. According to medical anthropologist John Heinerman, "PIs prevent radiation-induced cancer and enhance tissue resistance to invasion by tumor cells. If people consume adequate amounts of PIs in the form of beans and grains, they can then be protected against cancer at a variety of sites."[7]

Beans also reduce cholesterol: 1-1/2 cups of dried lentils or kidney beans a day can lower total cholesterol by 19 percent due to their lecithin and fiber content. *The American Journal of Clinical Nutrition* for October 1983 cites studies that show beans can definitely lower serum cholesterol and triglyceride levels in the body substantially, so much so that they should be eaten more frequently to keep too much fat from accumulating in the blood.

Fava beans are our best food source of L-dopa, the drug used for Parkinson's disease (to control trembling and rigidity). L-dopa is used by the brain to make a chemical called dopamine. While no one is suggesting that fava beans can replace a sufferer's current medication, they might prove helpful in the early mild stages of this disease, if your doctor approves.

L-dopa, which is abundant in fava beans, also stimulates strong, healthy erections in men. Reportedly, 8–16 ounces of fava beans might be just enough to relieve male potency problems.

Amazingly, fava bean *sprouts* contain ten times as much L-dopa as unsprouted ones. See sprouting instructions in Appendix B.

Fava beans—all beans, in fact—are rich in lecithin and choline, which increase concentrations of acetylcholine in the brain and

---

[7]John Heinerman, *Heinerman's Encyclopedia of Fruits, Vegetables and Herbs*, West Nyack, NY: Parker Publishing Company, Inc., 1988.

improve memory in laboratory animals. People with Alzheimer's are often lacking in acetylcholine, which plays a key role in thinking and reasoning. Researchers have tried feeding high-choline and high-lecithin foods to people with Alzheimer's, with initially encouraging results.

Black-bean juice is used in Japan to correct constipation caused by eating too much white bread and refined foods and to calm hyperactive children, according to John Heinerman. To make it, 2 tablespoons of cleaned black soybeans are boiled in 2 quarts of water for 10 minutes, then simmered until just 1 quart of water remains. Some kelp is added to season before the broth is strained. Dose: 1 cup of juice three times a day.

As previously mentioned, cancer treatment with laetrile is illegal in the United States, but many people eat small amounts of foods that contain it, as a safeguard against cancer, or as informal, unofficial therapy for existing tumors they may have, along with standard medical care. Foods rich in laetrile-like nitrilosides include many legumes, such as kidney beans, chick peas, and lentils. Mung bean sprouts supply especially large amounts of nitrilosides. Legumes and grains are highest in nitriloside content when they are in the sprouting stage.

The Bible "Wonder Cure" for Diabetes

If I had diabetes, I would eat lots of beans. The *Indian Journal of Medicinal Research* for February 1987 reports that beans have a significant effect in lowering blood sugar levels in diabetics. Dr. Paavo Airola says:

> Juices for the treatment of diabetes are: green beans, nettles, cucumber, celery, watercress, lettuce, onions, garlic and citrus juices. [Note that eight out of nine of these are Bible healing foods, discussed in this book on pages 22, 35, 57, 257, 303, 309, and 363.] . . . Bean skin tea is considered by many biological doctors to be a natural substitute for insulin and extremely beneficial in diabetes. The skins of the pods of green beans are

very rich in silic acid and certain hormonal substances which are closely related to insulin. One cup of bean skin tea is equal to at least 1 unit of insulin. The recommended dose: 1 cup of bean skin tea morning, noon and evening (Waerland system).[8]

Kidney-bean-pod tea has permanently cured diabetics. (This is the water in which the pods—not the beans—have been cooked.) Around 1900, Dr. Ramm, of Preetz, Germany, reported that diabetics who had taken this treatment 12 years previously—and had stopped using it—stayed cured. Others whose sugar returned were able to find relief again by using it.

Dr. Ramm said that the bean-pod water must be freshly made and taken the same day as it is prepared. If more than 24 hours old when used, he reported, it causes diarrhea. Only the pods are used. They should be garden-fresh and used immediately. Boil 2 ounces of sliced pods in 4 quarts of water, slowly, for 4 hours. Then filter the liquid through fine muslin and store in a cool place for 8 hours. After 8 hours, strain again with muslin—slowly and carefully (too many fibers in the fluid can cause intestinal upset). It is then ready. Dose: 1 glassful every 2 hours. Used this way, said Dr. Ramm, the remedy is completely harmless. The length of time involved was 3–4 weeks, during which a strict diabetic diet was advised.

Caution: **As with all remedies in this book, a doctor's permission is required before self-medication may be tried.** You may have a condition, such as juvenile diabetes, that makes this method totally inappropriate for you. It may be incompatible with the medication you are taking and which your doctor feels you should not stop taking. He may not think it safe for you to depend on this method as the sole means of treating this disease. It might lower your sugar too much. Only your doctor knows for sure. Discuss it with him or her. For more details on the best treatment for various kinds of diabetes, I recommend *The Best Treatment* by Isadore Rosenfeld, M.D. (1992), now a Bantam paperback, which

---

[8]Paavo Airola, N.D., *Health Secrets from Europe,* West Nyack, NY: Parker Publishing Company, Inc., 1970.

gives an excellent discussion of this and many other ailments from a doctor's point of view. Besides being authoritative, it's easy to understand and fun to read.

Kidney Blockage, Stones and Gravel, Rheumatism, and Gout Disappeared

This tea has also brought remarkable permanent cures for kidney and bladder trouble. All this was discovered by Dr. Ramm, as mentioned previously, around the turn of the century. As reported by Rex Adams in *Miracle Medicine Foods* (Parker Publishing Company, Inc., West Nyack, NY, 1977):

Dr. Ramm had been treating a woman for dropsy (accumulation of fluid in the tissues) following a valvular disease of the heart. Nothing worked. Suddenly, while making his rounds one day, he discovered that her swelling was gone. She told him she had accidentally drunk a glass of kidney-bean water, and began passing large amounts of crystal-clear urine— it happened every time she tried it. After 3 weeks of this her dropsy was gone!

Just to make sure, she continued drinking the kidney-pod tea for a few weeks, then stopped. The condition never returned. Dr. Ramm said she was as healthy as a woman can be. Dr. Ramm tried it on other patients. In all cases of heart disease and other ailments, large quantities of clear urine were passed and long-standing cases of dropsy were cured in a matter of days and stayed cured!

He found that kidney blockage of long duration was completely cured with bean-pod water and that bleeding from any part of the urinary system was quickly halted. Stones and gravel were rapidly dissolved and did not return. Diseases of the bladder and ureter were cured. Rheumatism and gout vanished. Even some cases of diabetes were cured. He said this remedy was completely harmless and could be used indefinitely with excellent results.

In some cases, the kidney-bean water caused nausea, in which case Dr. Ramm gave it in enemas instead (a half pint with a teaspoon of salt, every 2–4 hours), and the results were just as good as the drink. In fact, the enema seemed to halt the convulsions of uremia, releasing large amounts of water.

Reported results:

Mrs. B. D. writes: "I developed kidney trouble six weeks [ago]. The doctor kept giving me antibiotics but my kidney trouble wouldn't clear up. I went to the third doctor and he told me to come back for tests and X-rays. He found a kidney stone and diabetes. My sugar count was 326. He said I must have an operation if the stone didn't move. . . . When I got home . . . I started taking the bean pod tea. I drank a quart a day. Two weeks later when I went back to the doctor, my stone was gone and my sugar count was 128. He said, 'You're well.' I no longer had a stone nor diabetes. He was as surprised as I. At no time was I given any medication for diabetes."

Mr. D. S. writes: "My wife has had kidney problems for years . . . I [prepared a liquid from the kidney bean pods] taking care to strain and re-strain the fluid, since any extra particles of suspended matter might play havoc with a weaker digestive system. After [letting it stand 8 hours], I told my wife to consume an 8-ounce glass every hour. She said the stuff tasted awful and made a lot of faces, but you know what? The concoction worked. Her urine appeared crystal clear after she drank the juice, and she has reported no kidney pain or problems in the kidney area since."

Mrs. T. D. writes: "I had dropsy for several years and was taking dropsy pills for swelling and fluid. . . . Then I started cooking these red kidney bean pods, boiling them (and drinking the water). . . . I began the treatment according to directions. I did not have to wait long for results. Seems I passed large quantities of urine real often (and some gravel). I continued taking the bean water for about 2-1/2 weeks and within two weeks I had no sign of dropsy. The swelling had left my legs and ankles. The fluid above my stomach had also left."

Miss K. B. writes: "My urethra had been swollen for years. I've been to Duke Hospital and my own hospital and another one. They cut and treated, but nothing helped. I planted the beans and drank tea made with them for three weeks, and I've never had such results. It took out the swelling all over the body and it was equal to a good laxative. . . . Several swollen friends are going to plant some. . . . [They] are desperate and glad to hear about it."

Official Flower Seeds of Holy Land Cure Nerve Pain Overnight

Black pepper is such a common spice in the Holy Land that at one time it was declared the state's official flower. Its existence in Biblical days has recently been demonstrated by scientists examining the mummy of Ramses II. One of the ingredients used in the preservation of his body was black pepper. Peppercorns were found lodged in his nostrils and abdomen.

George P. Wood, M.D., states: "The combination of black pepper and the white of an egg has never been known to fail in curing a case of neuralgia [nerve spasms]. A lady of affluence . . . who had been a victim of neuralgia for nearly a year and had been treated in vain by the best medical skill obtainable, when almost in despair was told that . . . black pepper and the white of an egg would cure her in a single night.

"She applied it as directed and the next morning said she felt almost like a new person. For the first time in months every particle of pain was gone, and to her great surprise never returned."

Dr. Wood's instructions: "Wet one side of a piece of cotton cloth with the white of an egg. Sprinkle over it the best quality of black pepper until the egg is colored almost black, then bind it over the affected parts. When the disease is in the head, bind it on the temple and another small application (without the pepper) in back of the ear. One application will effect a cure."

Dr. S. Asada, a Japanese physician, declared that the remedy when applied as directed would cure any case of neuralgia in one night. "I have cured numerous cases with it," he said, "and never failed in a single instance, whether it was a recent case or one of years' standing."

Blessed (Holy) Thistle

Thistles are abundant in Palestine. Between Nazareth and Tiberias, one researcher was amazed to find the earth covered with immense tracts of these plants. Little wonder then that they appear so frequently in the Scriptures. The Emperor Charlemagne once found his army threatened with destruction by an epidemic of bubonic plague. He was informed by an angel that if he would shoot an arrow from his crossbow into the air, it would fall upon a plant that would cure the disease. The arrow fell on a thistle of the species since known as Blessed Thistle, Holy Thistle, or Our Lady's Thistle, *Cnicus benedictus* L.

Herbalists have ascribed many virtues to the thistle. It was regarded at one time as having near supernatural powers:

+ One writer relates the case of a woman whose breasts were wasted by a cancer to the very ribs, and yet was cured by washing them with the distilled water of Blessed Thistle (*Centaurea benedicta*), and sprinkling them with the powder of its leaves.

+ Another writer relates that he saw the putrid and hollow ulcers of a man, who had all the flesh of his legs consumed to the bone and who had tried all other medicines in vain, cured by the following recipe: Take the bruised leaves of this plant, and boil them with some generous wine, then add some melted lard; let them boil a little more, and then put in some wheat flour, stirring it about all the while with a spatula, till it comes to the consistency of an ointment, which is to be laid warm upon the ulcers twice a day.

Compounds in this herb reportedly have anti-HIV activity. In modern research, cell cultures have shown cytotoxicity against cancer cells using extract of Blessed Thistle, as well as antitumor activity in mouse cancer (sarcoma). A powdered extract of the herb has been applied externally for skin cancers with varying success.

In-vitro studies with extracts of Blessed Thistle have shown considerable antibacterial and anti-yeast activity against *Candida albicans*. Blessed Thistle is used by herbalists to increase the flow of milk in breast feeding. For this purpose the warm tea is given to mothers. It also reputedly breaks up blood clots, relieves jaundice, stops bleeding, increases appetite, and lowers fevers.

Blessed Thistle contains a volatile oil and a bitter principle known as cnicin. Grieve's *Modern Herbal* states: "In large doses, Blessed Thistle acts as a strong emetic, producing vomiting with little pain and inconvenience. Cold infusions [teas] in smaller drafts are valuable in weak and debilitated conditions of the stomach, and as a tonic, creating appetite and preventing sickness. The warm infusion—1 ounce of the dried herb to a pint of boiling water—in doses of a wineglassful, forms in intermittent fevers one of the most useful diaphoretics [perspiration inducer] to which employment can be given. The plant was at one time supposed to possess very great virtues against fevers of all kinds. . . . It is said to have great power in the purification and circulation of the blood, and on this account strengthens the brain and the memory."

Dosage

Add 1/2 ounce of the leaves to 1 pint of water. Boil water separately and pour over the plant. Steep for 5–20 minutes, depending on how strong you want it. Drink hot or warm, 1–2 cupsful per day.

The Bible Food Said to "Heal a Man of His Sickness with a Complete Cure"

Cabbage is not usually mentioned as a Biblical food, but it was. The original Hebrew version of Numbers 11:4–5 reads:

> "Who shall give us flesh to eat (*sir habosar*)? We remember the fish which we ate without cost (*dogo chinom*) in Egypt, and the melons (*avatichim*), cucumbers (*kischooim*), cabbage (*chotzir*), onions (*b'tzolim*), and garlic (*schoomim*)."

Current translations of Romans 14:2 read: ". . . who is weak, eateth herbs." But a translation from the original Greek, in *Biblical and Talmudic Medicine* (Germany, 1911), the exhaustive and definitive life work of Julius Preuss, M.D., translated into English and edited by Fred Rosner, M.D. (Sanhedrin Press, NY, 1978), reads: *". . . he who is weak should eat cabbage."*

In the Talmud, the 39 books of Biblical commentary dating from the first century A.D., we find cabbage listed as one of several foods that *"heal a man of his sickness with a complete cure"* (cabbage, mangold, chamomile, fish).

"Diseases Very Grave That Other Remedies Could Not Heal"

Cabbage has been described as "the bread and butter of therapeutics . . . the doctor of the poor . . . the providential physician," by Dr. Blanc, a French physician. In his *Notice on the Medicinal Properties of the Cabbage Leaves,* he describes a hundred examples of the healing benefits of cabbage, choosing diseases "very grave, that other remedies could not heal."

"Let unbelievers try it!" he says. "Nothing could be simpler. As a remedy [cabbage] is fast, safe, and easy. You can see the results with your own eyes."

Jean Valnet, M.D., a leading authority on natural medicine, says that he has often used cabbage leaves in a wide variety of diseases, and that it has seldom failed to bring about a healing. "Cabbage therapy," he says, "has indeed stood the test of time."

Asthma—Cabbage contains at least four anti-asthmatic substances (so does sage, and onion has five). An old folk remedy for asthma and bronchitis is to sip a broth prepared by cooking 2 ounces of cabbage for 1 hour in a pint of water to which 2 ounces of honey have been added.

Ulcers—Raw cabbage juice contains considerable amounts of two compounds with anti-ulcer activity, glutamine and S-methylmethionine. In Dr. Garnett Cheney's 1949 study of people with ulcers who were given raw cabbage juice as a treatment, 95.9 percent were pain-free in 2 weeks, 81 percent were symptom-free in 1 week, and 66 percent were pain-free in 4 days. Their diet consisted of cooked vegetables, vegetable soup, and stewed meats, avoiding fried foods and dairy. All patients were required to drink 1 quart of fresh raw cabbage juice daily, in four or five doses. You may achieve the same results with more pleasing taste, by mixing it with carrot juice, or by having cabbage soup.

Osteoporosis—Cabbage ranks highest in boron content among all leafy vegetables—and boron raises estrogen levels in the blood, thus helping to preserve your bones and ward off osteoporosis.

Edema—Cabbage relieves edema (swelling from water retention) because of its high potassium content. One method is to juice one whole cabbage, and one whole pineapple, mix them, and drink this in small amounts throughout the day. Make sure you're near a bathroom when you use this method, as it drains out pounds of water.

Arthritis—A time-tested folk remedy for arthritis, including back pain, is to drink two glasses of cabbage juice daily. Another traditional method is to steam a few cabbage leaves until they are limp. Massage a little olive oil on the painful area. Then place some warm—not scalding hot—cabbage leaves on the area. Cover with a towel. Repeat an hour later with new cabbage leaves.

Boils—To get rid of a boil, another old remedy is to place a crushed cabbage leaf on it, and leave it there till the boil opens, releasing the pus, and thereby relieving the pain. (A slice of onion reportedly has the same effect.) Clean the area with a little lemon juice or other disinfectant, and place a bandage over it.

Intoxication—An ancient folk remedy to prevent inebriation is to eat some raw cabbage just before attending a party, and you won't get drunk. Cato the Elder, a Roman statesman, is credited with this bit of advice: "If you wish to drink heavily at a banquet, dip some cabbage in vinegar and eat as much as you wish. The cabbage will keep you from getting drunk, and you can drink as much as you wish."

Hangover—To prevent a hangover, drink as much water as possible before going to bed to counteract the dehydrating effect of liquor; the following morning, have some cabbage soup.

Dr. Valnet says cabbage leaves may be applied externally in the treatment of leg ulcers, eczema, and chronic or infected wounds. This sometimes causes a temporary flare-up, he says. When this happens, apply for an hour or two, separated by intervals of 6–12 hours, for a few days. If acutely inflamed, replace the cabbage leaf applications with virgin olive oil or sweet almond oil. When the irritation has subsided, resume cabbage leaf therapy.

To prepare the leaves, simply wash them under running water, or soak them for a few minutes in water to which lemon has been added. Cut away the center rib of each leaf. Then crush the leaves with a rolling pin or bottle. The juice appears at the surface of the leaves, ready for application. Cover with a thick cloth and continue for several hours, overnight if necessary. If cabbage leaves are to be applied to ulcers with swollen irritated margins, soak the leaves for a half-hour in olive oil. This will soothe inflamed tissues, as well as combat infection and aid healing.

When treating lumbago, joint pain, or other afflictions of the nerves or bladder, poultices of cabbage leaves bring rapid relief, says Dr. Valnet. Boil two to four cabbage leaves and two whole chopped onions with 3 or 4 handfuls of bran and a little water. When the water evaporates, put the poultice on gauze and apply hot for 1–2 hours, or overnight. This mixture, he says, although it sounds old-fashioned, is highly effective.

Never apply heat to a painful abdomen, he cautions. Only a doctor can diagnose and treat abdominal pain. Heat may be harmful in a case of appendicitis or infection of an ovary.

Dr. Vanet recommends external applications of cabbage leaves for chapped skin and chilblains; skin contusions; wounds of various kinds; leg ulcers due to varicose veins; gangrene of the extremities; burns, shingles, eczema, cold sores, acne, skin eruptions of syphilis; inflammation of blood vessels and lymph channels; hemorrhoids; various types of infections including abscesses, vein infection, boils, anthrax, and felons; various types of neuralgia including lumbago and sciatica, dental pain, and facial neuralgia; gout pain; renal colic; headaches including migraine; stomach, bowel, bladder, and liver disorders; respiratory diseases including colds, bronchitis, pleurisy, and asthma; animal bites; tumors.

Reported cases:

About 1880, a cart driver in a small French village fell off his wagon and—as frequently happened in those days—a wheel rolled over his leg. Doctors arranged for his leg to be amputated the next morning. But the parish priest advised the patient's mother to cover his injured leg with cabbage leaves. With this simple dressing in place, the man was able to sleep all night. When he awoke, his family and one of the doctors noticed that he could move his leg. The cabbage leaves were removed to reveal a leg without swelling, with improved color. Eight days later, completely well, the man returned to work.

Mr. Z, a watchmaker, suffered for a year with painful eczema of both hands, preventing him from working. The lesions were acutely inflamed, and the fingernails were separating, about to fall off. Applications of cabbage leaves twice daily for a few days brought relief from pain, and clear fluid drained onto the dressing. With continued treatment, Mr. Z was healed within 2 months.

In 1875, Mr. S, age 75, suffered arteriosclerotic gangrene of the lower right leg and right foot. The skin was black and the front of the lower leg was decayed. Following the local application of cabbage leaf dressings, the skin changed from black to brown to red and then returned to its normal healthy color.

Nearly a century later, a New York City doctor reported a case of an elderly man suffering from a peptic ulcer. He needed surgery—a gastric resection—but had to wait until his insurance company could arrange for it. In order to give him immediate relief, the doctor suggested he drink a quart of fresh cabbage juice (4 glasses) daily. The patient returned 2 weeks later with his insurance papers; but he felt fine, cancelled the surgery, and went home.

The same doctor tells of a man who had been diagnosed at a famous clinic as suffering from a serious brain tumor and peptic ulcer. He was told to drink 4 glasses of raw cabbage juice a day for his chronic peptic ulcer, to stop smoking, and to cut out white sugar, white flour, and pastry from his diet. In a short time, he was free of peptic ulcer pain, and all symptoms of brain tumor left him and he was able to return to work.

A startling case was that of a woman with hundreds of ugly black warts covering her face, neck, and chest. She also had a paralyzed eyelid. Her doctor, making no promises, told her about a raw juice therapy involving cabbage juice. In a few weeks, the ugly mess cleared almost completely and the paralysis disappeared!

The Sun God's Elixir

In *Plants in the Bible* by Harold and Alma Moldenke, there is reference to Palestinian chamomile, which was used by the early Christians. The Egyptians revered chamomile for its power to cure fevers, particularly the recurrent fevers of malaria. Its daisylike flowers reminded them of the sun, so they dedicated it to Ra, the sun god, one of the most important gods of the pantheon. From the sixth dynasty all pharaohs claimed descent from Ra. The body of Ramses II was anointed with chamomile oil. Common chamomile is agreeably aromatic, with a distinct scent of apples, hence its name from the Greek *kamai,* meaning "on the ground" and *melon,* meaning "apple." When walked on, its strong, fragrant scent will often reveal its presence before it is seen. In fact, walking over the plant seems beneficial to it:

Like a chamomile bed
The more it is trodden on
The more it will spread . . .

Chamomile used to be called the "plant's physician" because nothing seems to contribute so much to the health of a garden as a number of chamomile herbs dispersed about it. If another plant is drooping and sickly, in nine cases out of ten it will recover if you place an herb of chamomile near it.

Its active principles are a volatile oil, anthemic acid (the bitter principle), tannic acid, and a glucoside. Boiling dissipates the oil. Chamomile tea should be prepared in a covered vessel, in order to prevent the escape of steam, as the medicinal value of the flowers is largely lost by evaporation. To make a tea, the flowers should be allowed to steep in extremely hot, but not boiling water for at least 10 minutes, strain, and sweeten to taste.

Relief for Stomach Ulcers, Gallstones, and Diverticulitis

Herbalists regard chamomile as the first-choice herb for heartburn and stomach distress. Rudolf Fritz Weiss, M.D., called the dean of German medical herbalists, author of *Herbal Medicine,* writes that for stomach ulcers, "The remedy of choice is chamomile. . . . There can be no other remedy more tailor-made, including all synthetic products." It's uniquely suited to treating digestive ailments, including ulcers, because it combines anti-inflammatory, antiseptic, antispasmodic, and stomach-soothing properties.

Chamomile tea has long been known to dissolve gallstones. Nicholas Culpepper wrote: "That it is excellent for the stone appears in this which I have tried—that a stone that hath been taken out of the body of a man, being wrapped in chamomile, will in time dissolve, and in a little time, too." In one reported case, two gallstones were placed in a glass of chamomile tea. The next day the stones were in four pieces. In 5 days they were like gravel. In 10 days they were completely dissolved.

Chamomile tea is particularly valuable in treating diverticulitis because its anti-inflammatory action soothes the entire digestive system. A suggested dose is 2 teaspoons of dried chamomile per cup of boiling water. Steep 5–10 minutes. Sip throughout the day.

Swelling, Inflammation, Neuralgia, Abscess Relieved

Apart from their uses internally, chamomile flowers are also extensively used as a poultice and fomentation for external swellings, inflammatory pain, or neuralgia and will relieve where other remedies have failed, proving invaluable for reducing swellings of the face caused through abscesses. Bags may be loosely stuffed with flowers and steeped well in boiling water before being applied as a fomentation. The antiseptic powers of chamomile are said to be 120 times stronger than sea water.

One woman, having cut her finger on a rusty nail, soaked her hand in a chamomile infusion. "My hand was healed in a few days, and in the years that have followed I have found these blossoms infallible wherever I have used them," she wrote. "In recent months it cured my foot when badly poisoned by lye. Soaking in a warm infusion [made like tea but covered and steeped longer—10–20 minutes] is very restful for tired feet, and takes the soreness from calluses. It is also an excellent remedy for poison ivy."

The whole herb is used for external applications in toothache, earache, and neuralgia. One ounce of the dried herb is infused (soaked) in 2 pints of boiling hot water and allowed to cool.

Claims Migraine Cured

French Herbalist Maurice Messegue says: "My grandmother Sophie always gave me a good infusion of chamomile when she suspected that I had worms, and I later learned that she used to recommend it to women in the village who suffered from painful periods. My father prescribed it for bowels and for stomach cramps, colic and spasms. . . . to speed up the healing of . . . wounds and to stop the pus. I myself have made use of its virtues in treating facial neuralgia and migraine. . . . I like to quote the case of a man who came to consult me about his migraine, which was resistant to all the 'classical' pharmaceutic products that he had been taking and that were destroying his stomach and his kidneys. But after 14 days of intensive treatment with chamomile he was cured."[9]

For migraine and neuralgia, Messegue made a decoction by putting a handful of dried chamomile flowers into a liter (1-3/4 pints) of water. (See instructions for making infusions and decoctions in Appendix A.)

"Soothing Sedative Effect Absolutely Harmless"

Herbalist Maude Grieve writes: "The [chamomile] infusion, made from 1 oz. of the flowers to 1 pint of boiling water and taken in doses of a tablespoonful to a wineglass . . . is an old-fashioned but extremely efficacious remedy for hysterical and nervous affections in women and is used also as an emmenogogue [stimulates menstruation]. It has a wonderfully soothing, sedative and absolutely harmless effect. It is considered a preventive and the sole certain remedy for nightmare. It will cut short an attack of delirium tremens in the early stage. It has sometimes been employed in intermittent fevers."

Caution: Chamomile is a member of the ragweed family. If you have hay fever, there is a remote possibility that drinking chamomile tea might trigger a reaction. At one time, the *Journal of Allergy and Clinical Immunology* claimed chamomile tea might cause a potentially fatal allergic reaction—anaphylactic shock—in people allergic to ragweed. Further research of the entire world literature for the 95-year period from 1887 to 1982 revealed no deaths, and a grand total of 50 cases of a histamine-like reaction—45 from common (or Roman) chamomile and five from the German variety (German chamomile is most common in the United States).

---

[9]From *Health Secrets of Plants and Herbs* by Maurice Messegue. Copyright © 1975 by Opera Mundi. Copyright © 1979 by William Collins & Co., Ltd. By permission of William Morrow & Company, Inc.

Moses' Toothache Remedy

Moses included cloves in the holy incense of the Tabernacle. All translations of the Bible use a word *onycha,* which has its origin in the Greek word *onux,* which is the same basic derivation of the word "clove," from the Latin *clavus.* Since onycha in the Bible is always one of several sweet spices, the evidence points strongly to cloves:

> And the Lord said unto Moses: "Take unto thee sweet spices,
>
> stacte, and *onycha,* and galbanum . . ." *Exodus 30:34*

India's traditional healers have used clove since ancient times, and it is believed that it became a prized—and exceedingly rare and expensive—possession of the Israelites through trade.

Clove oil is 60 to 90 percent eugenol, which gives it antiseptic and anesthetic power. Dentists use it as an oral anesthetic—a few drops are placed in a cavity—and to disinfect root canals. It is also the active ingredient in such over-the-counter toothache remedies as Benzodent and Numzident.

A scientific committee reporting to the Food and Drug Administration commented that oil of clove was the only one of 12 ingredients commonly found in toothache preparations that was "safe and effective for temporary use on a tooth with throbbing pain." The oil is placed directly on the tooth, not ingested.

Reported uses:

One way to use clove oil is to squirt a few drops of it on a cotton ball and then dab it on a sore tooth. This can bring you an hour's worth of relief. Keep doing this until you can get to a dentist. The same technique works after an extraction. Clove oil is available at most health-food stores, and is a good thing to keep on hand for emergencies.

If a filling falls out, you can relieve the pain by packing a tiny piece of cotton soaked in clove oil in the cavity, according to my dentist. Then fill the hole with a temporary filling material—like Dent Temp—available at most drug stores. Chewed sugarless gum can also be used as a temporary filling. That should protect it and relieve your pain until you can get to a dentist.

Cloves are one of a number of spices that can help the body use insulin more efficiently. The others are bay leaf, cinnamon, and turmeric.

Helps Preserve Vision in Old Age

Clove oil is a powerful antioxidant. Studies show it helps prevent the breakdown in the retina of a substance called docosahexaenoic acid. This action helps preserve vision in old age. One scientist suggests adding 1 or 2 drops of clove oil to mint teas and drinking up to 4 cups a day.

Medicinal Powers of the Holy Bark Used for the Cross of Calvary

No discussion of plants of the Bible would be complete without black elder, thought by many to be the tree from which the Cross of Calvary was made, as stated in this ancient verse:

> "Bour tree—Bour tree: crooked rong
> Never straight and never strong;
> Ever bush and never tree
> Since our Lord was nailed on thee."

Legend identifies elder as the famed Judas tree. Sir John Mandeville, writing of his travels, tells us that near the Pool of Siloam, he was shown the actual "Tree of Eldre that Judas hanged himself upon, in despair, having sold and betrayed our Lord."

Medicinally, black elder is an extremely valuable plant. The whole tree has a narcotic smell. No plant will grow under the shadow of it, being affected by its volatile aromatic oils. Sleeping under the elder supposedly produces a drugged, dream-filled sleep. Due to their diuretic and detoxifying properties, people eat elderberries to lose weight. Strong elder-flower tea is very good mixed with peppermint and yarrow for colds, flu, and asthma.

Nerve Spasms, Sciatica, and Rheumatic Pains Banished

In 1899, an American sailor told his doctor that getting drunk on genuine old dark-red port was a sure remedy for painful sciatica. By trial and error, the doctor discovered that while genuine port wine has practically no nerve-soothing properties, the cheap stuff faked to resemble tawny port by the addition of elderberry juice often banishes nerve spasms. In his book *Miracle Medicine Foods,* Rex Adams says:

> Spasms of the face, with pain of a stabbing or throbbing nature, and twitching, is known as tic douloureaux or trigeminal neuralgia. Many drugs have been used to treat this condition. Surgery may relieve it. In 1914, a Prague doctor cured 48 cases with pure elderberry juice!

"Patients took 20 grams daily for five days. Some were cured with only one dose! Others after a few days. It was discovered that adding 20% alcohol speeded the healing. Two years later a Norwegian doctor combined 10 grams of port wine with 30 grams of elderberry juice, and discovered that acute cases of sciatica were cured in as little as one day! No case lasted longer than two or three weeks."

A Powerful Bible Plant that Eliminated Arthritis Pain

Ginger is mentioned several times in the Talmud—the 39 books of biblical commentary dating back to the first century—as a powerful plant medicine that is, along with pepper and wine, beneficial to the whole body.

Ginger is an anti-inflammatory agent that has been used to relieve rheumatoid arthritis for thousands of years. It works by blocking the formation of inflammatory chemicals in the body.

Many anti-inflammatory drugs do this, too, but have side effects such as stomach ulcers that prevent long-term use. Ginger also appears to neutralize inflammatory acids in the joint fluids.

Dr. Krishna C. Srivastava of Odense University in Denmark reports the following uses of ginger for rheumatoid arthritis:

A 50-year-old auto mechanic, who had been diagnosed as having rheumatoid arthritis, was told to eat about 1-3/4 ounces of fresh ginger daily, mixed with lightly cooked vegetables and meats. His symptoms began subsiding within a month. In 3 months, he was "completely free of pain, inflammation or swelling" and has remained so for 10 years.

Fifty patients obtained relief from rheumatoid arthritis by taking either 1/6 ounce of fresh ginger or 1/3 teaspoonful of ground ginger with food or dissolved with liquid, three times daily, during a 2-year study. No side effects were noted, in small therapeutic doses.

Dr. Srivastava also says that powdered ginger is effective in relieving pain and inflammation of osteoarthritis. He says that 75 percent of patients tested who took 1/3 teaspoon of powdered ginger three times daily for up to 2-1/2 years got significant relief.

Relief for Nausea, Dizziness, Morning Sickness

Ginger has a long-standing reputation for relieving motion sickness, morning sickness, dizziness, vertigo, and the nausea of stomach flu. It does this better than the standard drug, Dramamine, according to a study published in the British medical journal *Lancet*.

Researchers gave volunteers with a history of motion sickness either 100 mg of Dramamine or 940 mg of ginger powder capsules. Then they were seated in a rocking chair that simulated the kind of motion that produces sea sickness. As soon as they felt nauseated they could stop the chair. Those taking ginger lasted 57 percent longer than those on Dramamine.

In an 8-year study conducted by one researcher, ginger worked for over 90 percent of the people who tried it. People who suffered from dizziness or vertigo were able to leave their homes for the first time in years, without feeling sick or dizzy. A suggested dose is 1,500 mg about 30 minutes before travel. In pregnancy, morning sickness can be relieved by taking ginger before getting out of bed, staying in bed until symptoms are gone. In the study published in *Lancet,* less than 1,000 mg was used to prevent nausea. Ginger can stimulate menstruation at very high levels (in Chinese studies, 20 to 28 grams). No miscarriages have been reported. Ginger is on the Food and Drug Administration list of herbs generally regarded as safe.

"Completely Safe"

One researcher says he has not observed even the slightest toxic symptoms in lab animals at doses of ginger root ten times higher than what a human would normally ingest. "Lethal dosage levels have been established," he says, "but are so high that the herb has been accepted as completely safe by the FDA. . . . I know people who use [ginger] on a daily basis, to treat chronic problems, without the slightest indication of a side effect."

Male Fertility

In an article titled "Studies in Herbal Aphrodisiacs Used in the Arab System of Medicine" published in the *American Journal of Chinese Medicine,* some Saudi scientists asserted that ginger extracts significantly increase sperm motility and quantity.

Hair Growth

I am told by an acquaintance that ginger root can grow new hair. My hairless friend claimed that his nightly ritual of grating some fresh ginger root, squeezing it through a piece of cheesecloth to get some juice, mixing this juice with alcohol (ten parts alcohol to one part juice), and applying it to the bald area, rinsing a half hour later with lukewarm water, actually caused a balding area that bothered him to fill in, over a period of 6 months.

Humble Bible Plant Called One of the Most Valuable and Important Items in Medicine

References to heath in the Bible, in the Book of Jeremiah (17:6 and 48:6) are thought by experts to refer to juniper, which grows in the mountains of Sinai and is a common shrub in desert places in the Holy Land. Medicinally, juniper leaves and berries were used to cause the bowels to move, to eliminate tapeworms, to relieve asthma, to cure headache, to induce menstruation, and much more. At the dawn of the twentieth century, juniper was known as "one of the most valuable, important and universal articles of the Materia Medica." In his book, *The Way of Herbs,* Michael Tierra, N.D., says that 4–6 drops of juniper-berry oil taken with honey three or four times a day has been a successful home remedy for stones and gravel, lumbar pains, gout, and rheumatic problems.

Asthma Cured with Simple Plant Medicine from the Bible

In *Folk Remedies of the Low Country,* Dr. Julia F. Morton presents a treasury of plant remedies used by natives of the Charleston, South Carolina, coastal area—the Gullah folk.

She tells of an elderly woman who, years earlier, had suffered from asthma. When she was 18, a black woman told her to soak the berries of the white cedar (juniper) in whisky and take 1 teaspoonful at a time when she felt an asthma attack coming on. This remedy not only prevented attacks, it seems to have cured her. For the rest of her long life—another 60 years—she never had any further trouble with asthma.

Experts warn, however, that juniper should not be taken internally by pregnant women, small children, those with kidney problems or hay fever. "The rule," says famed German herbalist Rudolph Fritz Weiss, M.D., "is never take juniper for more than 6 weeks." The main active ingredient in juniper is its volatile oil. A constituent of the oil, terpinen-4-ol, works on the kidneys and is responsible for its diuretic action. But prolonged use of it can irritate and possibly damage the kidneys. Overdose symptoms include diarrhea, intestinal or kidney pain, blood in the urine, rapid heartbeat, or elevated blood pressure. If any of these occur, stop using it. Always consult a doctor before attempting to self-medicate.

Bible Food Remedy for Kidney, Bladder, Urinary Problems

For centuries, juniper has been used as a diuretic, to increase urine. English herbalist Nicholas Culpepper wrote that juniper "is so powerful a remedy against dropsy [congestive heart failure], it cures the disease." It has also been used for bladder infections, and as a deodorizer in cases of incontinence because it gives the urine the fragrance of violets.

Reported cases:

"My mother had a bladder affection and she made tea of Juniper Berries and Scouring Rush, and took it off and on for 6 years, but she was cured. She made the tea and drank it just whenever she noticed her troubles and did not take it continually."—G. C.

"Juniper Berries made into a tea given to my old mother 3 times daily, a small cup each time, has cured her of a very unpleasant smelling discharge caused by pus on the kidneys (according to a urinalysis)."—F. S.

"I got some Juniper Berries for my son for his kidney and bladder trouble. He had tried all kinds of medicines without doing him any good. The Juniper Berries helped him very much, and now I am getting more of them."—Mrs. M. H.

Medicinally, juniper berries are prepared as a tea. A table-spoonful of crushed berries is placed in a pot, and covered with 4 cups of water. The pot is covered, and the water is boiled down to 2 cups, and strained. One cup is taken twice a day, once at midday, once before bed, for no more than 6 weeks. It has a pleasant aromatic taste.

Relief Claimed for Emphysema, Sinusitis, Head Cold, and Flu

It is said that a cupful of juniper berry tea, once every couple of hours, can chase away the flu in a hurry. And vaporized juniper berry oil (15 drops with 3/4 cup of water in a vaporizer near your bed, inhaled for an hour) is a Native American remedy that can bring hours of relief from emphysema, sinusitis, head cold, and flu. Juniper berry tea (1/2 cup sipped slowly every couple of hours) is also said to stop internal bleeding quickly.

"They Said the Diabetes Was Gone"

A remarkable use for juniper berries is cited in part of an interview with Mathew King, spokesman for the Lakota (Sioux) Nation of the Pine Ridge Reservation of South Dakota:[10]

"Once, while I was up on the mountain, I prayed to God to give us a cure for diabetes. And while I was there, somebody said, 'Turn around!' So I turned around and there was the most beautiful Indian woman I'd ever seen. She had long black hair and the most wonderful face. She was holding something out to me in her hand. It was those little berries of the [juniper], the dark blue berries on [juniper] trees. She held them out, but before I could reach out my hand she disappeared.

---

[10]From *Wisdomkeepers: Meetings with Native American Spiritual Elders* by Harvey Arden and Steve Wall © 1990. Published by Beyond Words Publishing, Inc., Hillsboro, Oregon. Reprinted by permission.

"I know who she was. She's the one who brought the sacred pipe to our people. We call her White Buffalo Calf Woman. God sent her to save the Indian people. That was long ago. . . . So I knew when I saw her up on the mountain that this was the same woman. But she disappeared before I could take those blue berries from her hand.

"Later on, when I got diabetes, I forgot about the berries. They sent me to White Man's doctors. They gave me pills. Every morning I had to take insulin. I spent a lot of time in the hospital. Then I remembered White Buffalo Calf Woman and those little blue [juniper] berries. I picked some, boiled them, strained the juice and drank it. It's so bitter it took the sugar right out of my body. The doctors checked me and were amazed. They said the diabetes was gone. I didn't have to take insulin anymore. They asked me how I did it, but I didn't say. God gave us medicine to share with people, but if the White Man gets his hands on it he'll charge you a great price and will let you die if you don't have it. God's medicine is free. God doesn't charge a fee. We don't give money to God. We give Him our prayers, our thanks."

It should be stressed that juniper berries should not be regarded as a cure for diabetes, but rather as a way of controlling it, a supplement to existing treatment if your doctor approves.

How the Oil Used to Bless Jesus Heals

When the bridegroom in the Song of Songs compares his bride with all kinds of lovely plants, he repeatedly mentions spikenard (*Lavendula spica*), which is closely related to common Lavender (*Lavendula vera*). Common lavender oil is virtually identical to the oil used to anoint Jesus.

And being in Bethany in the house of Simon the leper, as He sat at meat, there came a woman having an alabaster box of ointment of spikenard very precious; and she brake the box, and poured it on his head. *Mark 14:3*

Then took Mary a pound of ointment of spikenard, very costly,

and anointed the feet of Jesus, and wiped his feet with her hair;

and the house was filled with the odour of the ointment.

John 12:3

Famed herbalist Maurice Messegue calls lavender "God's gift to earth." No scent could be sweeter, he says. His father would gather it in the fields, and bring it home. "It was as if a little bit of Paradise had come down to earth." He recalls a patient who was suffering from dizziness, headaches, nausea, and hot flushes who quickly recovered when he was given lavender tea. Another of his patients suffered from distension of the stomach and intestine, with indigestion and loss of appetite. Lavender brought him welcome relief.

Another patient "was very nervous, with bouts of neurasthenia, palpitations, and uncontrollable trembling, and he too became a new man after a cure [with lavender].

"Lavender is also effective in cases of asthma, general weakness, influenza, infections of the liver and the spleen, jaundice, congestion, vaginal discharge and for weakness of the eyes. . . .

"It works wonders for gout and rheumatism, and children can be kept in good health by being given full baths of lavender. It is worth mentioning, too, that this plant helps in cases of skin trouble such as eczema, acne and so on; that it can be used for burns and for venereal disease not, in this latter case, as a cure, of course, but as a help towards healing. And it is helpful for ulcers, superficial inflammation and for infected wounds.

"When inhaled it speeds up the treatment of colds, influenza, tonsillitis and bronchitis. As a gargle it cleans out all the little infected places in the mouth, and it can also treat paralysis of the tongue and stuttering because it has a relaxing effect on the nerves and the muscles.

"Used as a compress for the liver, it helps this vital organ to do its work as the body's 'chemical works.' Used in frictions on the chest, it tones up the lungs and thus helps speed up the treatment of pneumonia, pleurisy and pulmonary congestion."[11]

---

[11]From *Health Secrets of Plants and Herbs* by Maurice Messegue, *op. cit.*

⊙fficially Recognized for over 200 Years

Tincture of red lavender is composed of the oils of lavender and rosemary, with cinnamon bark, nutmeg, and red sandlewood macerated in spirit of wine for 7 days.

This preparation, sold under the name of Lavender drops in England, has been officially recognized in the British Pharmacopia for over 200 years. The popularity of this remedy may be understood by looking at its claimed uses against stroke, palsy, convulsions, vertigo, amnesia, dimness of vision, depression, and female infertility.

It was taken in blackberry juice, or in wine. Also in milk or water sweetened with sugar. As an infusion (tea), if taken too freely, lavender can cause griping and colic, and lavender oil in too large doses is a narcotic poison and causes death by convulsion.

"Lavender oil," says herbalist Maude Grieve, "is found of service when rubbed externally for stimulating paralysed limbs. . . . The oil is successfully used in the treatment of sores, varicose ulcers, burns and scalds. . . ."

Spike lavender oil, made from *Lavendula spica* (spikenard) "is said to admirably promote the growth of the hair when weakly or falling off. A decoction—Spike Water—can be made from the plant.

"Lavender Water can easily be made at home," says Grieve. "Into a quart bottle are put 1 oz. essential oil of Lavender, one drop of Musk and 1-1/2 pint spirits of wine. These three ingredients are well mixed together by shaking. The mixture is left to settle, shaken again in a few days, then poured into little perfume bottles fitted with air-tight stoppers."

Lions and Tigers Become Docile under Its Influence

Lavender has been found to be an extremely effective insect repellent. Surprisingly, not only are insects averse to the smell of lavender, says Grieve, "but it is said on good authority that the lions and tigers in our Zoological Gardens [in England] are powerfully affected by the scent of Lavender Water, and will become docile under its influence."

The Ultimate Aphrodisiac

In 1995, scientists at the Smell and Taste Research Institute in Chicago reported that certain smells dramatically increased the penile blood flow in healthy male volunteers more than other aromas did. Lavender flowers and pumpkin-seed oils gave 40 percent more erections in men between the ages of 20 and 39 when they were told to sniff small swatches of material containing tiny amounts of each of these oils.

Instant Cough Relief

"If you ever have one of those coughing spells that sounds like the barking of a dog, then here is something to quell it in minutes," says medical anthropologist Dr. John Heinerman: "Add one-half cup dried lavender flowers to two cups boiling water. Cover, remove from heat, and steep for 30 minutes. Strain and sip a cup of the warm tea through a plastic straw, if necessary, every 3 hours."[12]

Infantile Colic Relief

Dr. Heinerman quotes an Amtrak train conductor whose infant son had been keeping him up every night. They'd been to five pediatricians. The child had what doctors called "infantile colic." But nothing they prescribed seemed to help.

"I went to work one night as usual in a grouchy mood 'cause the kid had kept me up. . . . Our train engineer asked me what the matter was and I told him all about my kid's colic. He told me that his mom used lavender flower tea on the kids for this same complaint and he had used it on his own kids successfully. So sometime later . . . we gave some of it warm in a bottle to our kid. I swear that

---

[12]John Heinerman, *Heinerman's Encyclopedia of Healing Herbs and Spices,* West Nyack, NY: Parker Publishing Company, Inc., 1996.

the minute my kid started drinking this stuff, he began looking and feeling much better. In two days, what the doctors couldn't cure, the lavender did—his colic disappeared and never came back."[13]

Healing Miracles from a Tiny Seed

Mustard is mentioned in two of Jesus' parables. In one of these (Matthew 13:31, 32), he says: "The kingdom of Heaven is like a mustard-seed, which a man took and sowed in his field. As a seed, Mustard is smaller than any other; but when it has grown it is bigger than any garden plant . . ." In the other parable, he says:

> Your faith is too small. I tell you this: if you have faith no bigger than a mustard-seed, you will say to this mountain, "Move from here to there!" and it will move; nothing will prove impossible for you. *Matthew 17:20*

As medicine, mustard seeds can be a true life saver. Crushed and mixed with water, two substances within the seeds—sinigrin and myrosin—combine to form a volatile oil that generates intense heat. When placed on the skin, this relieves congestion in various organs by drawing blood to the surface.

For this reason, mustard is of considerable value in treating a wide variety of disorders: asthma, bronchitis, pneumonia, fever and chills, sciatica, neuralgia, gout, sprains, tendinitis, cold and flu, suppurating sores and boils, and irritation of the kidneys.

In many cases, a simple mustard plaster—the kind Grandma use to fix—can bring amazing relief: Spread a little Vaseline or lard on the skin over the affected area. Measure one part mustard powder (from crushed mustard seeds) and mix with four parts wholewheat flour. Add water till a paste forms thick enough to spread nicely on a piece of cloth or gauze and apply directly to affected area, holding it in place with adhesive tape. This can be kept on for several hours, or overnight, if desired.

---

[13]Heinerman, *op. cit.*

Vaseline protects the skin. Otherwise blisters might form. Herbalist Jethro Kloss claimed that mixing ground mustard seeds and flour with the whites of eggs instead of water prevented blistering. He wrote that mustard plaster is excellent when applied over the kidneys in cases of kidney irritation.

A stronger plaster can be made by omitting the wheat flour and mixing 4 ounces of fresh-ground mustard seed with warm water to make a thick paste, which can then be applied as described previously.

A world-renowned European herbalist has remarked that "a poultice or a mustard bath (made using mustard powder) has saved the life of many a child who had already turned blue from a severe case of bronchiolitis (inflammation and gradual blockage of the tiniest air tubes in the lungs) and who was frantically gasping for air."

But, he says, care must be taken that the skin is not exposed to the active ingredients of the mustard for too long at a time. An intense reddening of the skin is desirable, he says, but blisters should never be allowed to form. If cases of whooping cough are treated in this manner, children can be protected from serious complications, he adds.

More Surprising Facts

AIDS—We are told of an AIDS victim[14] surviving in glowing good health after doctors gave him up for dead 4 years earlier. His secret? Spices. Every 2 days he eats some kind of hot food, including hot Chinese mustard, Japanese green mustard (wasabe), ginger, horseradish, or spicy pickled cabbage—all Bible foods, by the way.

He says he knows several other long-term survivors who have very low T4 levels but who appear to be in robust health, who are energetic, working full time, putting on weight—and most of these long-term survivors are also eating spicy food at least once a week, particularly the Korean *kim-chi jige,* which has been described as liquid fire.

---

[14]John Heinerman, *Double the Power of Your Immune System,* West Nyack, NY: Parker Publishing Company, Inc., 1991.

He says that since he conscientiously started eating spicy food, he has been consistently more alert, and able to work better than at any other time in the past 10 years. He tries to dine at restaurants that feature many different kinds of hot spicy food, Mexican, Brazilian, Chinese, Korean. His theory is that different spices affect different micro-organisms in different ways.

Asthma—One researcher points out that hot, pungent foods such as mustard and garlic can bring "immediate relief from asthma" due to their "mucokinetic" (mucus-moving) power to thin out thick secretions, thereby opening up passageways and making breathing easier for asthmatics.

Hypothyroidism—Thyroid hormones are made up of iodine and tyrosine. Mustard greens are the richest food source of tyrosine. They top a list of foods high in tyrosine that includes carob, bean sprouts, soybeans, oats, peanuts, spinach, watercress, and cabbage. Kelp—described in Jonah 2:5 as "weeds" or "seaweeds"—is the richest food source of iodine. These foods have the potential of boosting thyroid hormone output and reversing hypothyroidism.

Raynaud's Disease—In Raynaud's disease, constriction and spasms of the small arteries that bring blood to the fingers cause the fingers to become cold, painful, and turn white or bluish. Sometimes this also occurs in the nose and toes. It's a fairly common condition in women. It may occasionally be a symptom of scleroderma, a rare disease that involves hardening of the skin and damage to the internal organs.

If you suffer from Raynaud's disease, you can apply a mustard plaster to increase the circulation in your fingers. You can also try vegetable or minestrone soup spiced liberally with "hot" spices such as mustard powder, cayenne, garlic, or ginger that will rev up your circulation.

One of the Wise Men's Gifts to Baby Jesus Helps Chronic Lung Conditions, Arthritis, Blood Clots, and More

"The ancient Hebrews," writes Richard Lucas, " regarded myrrh as one of the earth's most precious and versatile products, for as a medicine it healed their bodies, as an incense it lifted their spirits, and as a perfume it pleased their hearts. . . .

"One of its most important uses was as an ingredient in the holy oils with which they anointed the Tabernacle, the Ark, the altar and the sacred vessels."[15]

Myrrh was used for purification rituals. The maidens who were led before King Ahaseurus, who would choose a new queen from among them, were purified for 12 months, according to the law for women: 6 months with oil of myrrh and 6 with balsams and other means of beautification. (Esther 2:12).

Myrrh was one of the Wise Men's gifts to the baby Jesus and was also used for the burial of Jesus:

> He was joined by Nicodemus [the man who had first visited
> Jesus by night], who brought with him a mixture of myrrh and
> aloes, more than half a hundredweight. They took the body of
> Jesus and wrapped it, with the spices, in strips of linen cloth
> according to Jewish burial customs. *John 19:39–40*

The ancient Hebrews attached great value to the disinfectant power of volatile oils, and myrrh gum contains several. Myrrh is one of the best antiseptics and disinfectants known.

Myrrh gum's three great actions are on digestion, infection, and women's reproductive organs. For centuries it has been used to treat vaginitis, menstrual difficulties, leukorrhea, and other forms of bleeding, including hemorrhoids and ulcerated sores.

Myrrh is one of the best antiseptics known. When combined with goldenseal, it can be made into a healing, antiseptic salve useful for the treatment of hemorrhoids, bedsores, and wounds. Or in tea form it can be used as a wash. After thoroughly washing sores, ulcers, and the like, with the tea, sprinkle a little of the powder on the sore. Charcoal moistened with this tea and applied to old ulcers and sores is healing. It is also effective for gangrene.

---

[15]Richard Lucas, *Nature's Medicines,* West Nyack, NY: Parker Publishing Company, Inc., 1966.

Myrrh can help chronic lung conditions, particularly where there is thick white mucus. Because it is antimicrobial, it helps any gut infection. It is also very good for stomach flu and excellent for any infection or inflammation of the mouth or throat. For use as a gargle or mouthwash, steep a teaspoonful of myrrh and one of boric acid to a pint of water. Let stand one-half hour, pour off clear liquid, and use. This is also an excellent remedy for diphtheria, ulcerated throat, and sores in the mouth. Use for cough, asthma, tuberculosis, and all chest affections, as it diminishes the mucus discharge. To use as a tea, use 2 teaspoonsful of myrrh gum per cup of boiling water. Take three times a day. Myrrh oil can be used in inhalations for respiratory complaints. Do not swallow the oil. Just dab a few drops on a clean cloth and sniff periodically.

In India, myrrh is purified by cooking it in *triphala* (a mixture of fruits). This is cooked down into a thick black substance called *guggal*. It is taken for hardening of the arteries, arthritis and rheumatism, and to improve circulation and nerve health.

For a drink that might help prevent heart disease and prevent the internal blood clots that trigger heart attacks, brew a teaspoon of powdered myrrh per cup of boiling water. Steep 10 minutes. Drink up to 2 cups a day. Myrrh tastes bitter and unpleasant, so you might want to add honey and lemon, or mix it into another beverage to improve the flavor.

Myrrh is excellent for pyorrhea. Brush the teeth with the powder, thoroughly rinse your mouth with the tea, and bathe the gums. It eliminates halitosis or bad breath when taken internally. Use 1 teaspoonful of gum per cup of boiling water. Take three times a day. The taste is bitter yet refreshing and may help relieve gingivitis.

Because it stimulates uterine contractions, myrrh should not be taken during pregnancy. Also, because it is a resin, it can be hard on the kidneys if taken over a prolonged period—longer than a couple of weeks.

An Ancient Vegetable Medicine Proves Its Worth

Herodotus records an ancient inscription in the Great Pyramid of Cheops stating that the sum of 1,600 talents of silver—equivalent to $30 million U.S. dollars today—had been paid to supply the workers with onions, garlic, and radishes while the pyramid was being built. In the days of the Pharaohs, the radish was extensively cultivated in Egypt, and the roots were remarkably sweet. Radishes were also used for medicinal purposes. Radish oil was used to treat skin diseases. Early Christians used radish seeds to treat internal complaints, and the oil for cooking and anointing.

Radishes are an excellent food remedy for gallstones and kidney stones. They have long been used in Russia for treating both Grave's disease (overactive thyroid) and hypothyroidism (underactive thyroid). Strong radish-seed tea has been used for reducing stomach cancer and externally as a heated poultice for treating breast cancer.

In cases of Grave's disease, radishes gently suppress thyroid hormone production. All vegetables of the cabbage and mustard family do this, but apparently radishes do it best. The reason radishes also help in cases of hypothyroidism—low hormone production—is that they contain a chemical (raphanin) that helps keep levels of thyroid hormones in balance.

To prevent and relieve gallstones, according to herbalist Maude Grieve, the expressed juice of white or black Spanish radishes is given in increasing doses of from 1/2 to 2 cupsful daily. The 2 cupsful are continued for 2 or 3 weeks, then the dose is decreased until 1/2 cupful is taken three times a week for 3 or 4 more weeks. The treatment may be repeated by taking 1 cupful at the beginning, then one-half daily, and later one-half every second day.

Reportedly, a good method for managing kidney stones, or to prevent their occurrence, is to combine 2 chopped red radishes and 1/2 cup of red wine in a blender and drink this every day—twice a day in cases of difficult urination.

Hard-fat deposits in the body can be removed, using a radish remedy developed by doctors in Japan. Grated carrot and grated white Daikon radish, 1 teaspoon each, are added to 2 cups of water with 7 drops of soy sauce, 1 teaspoon of lemon, and a pinch of kelp. Boil for 5 minutes. The broth is then strained and 1 cup prescribed twice daily, morning and night.

"Fresh radishes and radish seeds have been employed in the treatment of cancer around the world," says Dr. John Heinerman. "Such success has been carefully documented in a variety of scientific publications. Lily M. Perry's *Medicinal Plants of East and*

Southeast Asia, published by the Massachusetts Institute of Technology Press in Cambridge, describes the use of the seeds made into a strong tea for reducing stomach cancer and their external application as a heated poultice for treating breast cancer in women."[16]

The Seven-Candle Plant that Saves Lives

The ancient Hebrews took many of their symbols from plants. The waterlily was the inspiration for the lily work in Solomon's temple. The pomegranate flower was the inspiration for ornamental bells, and its fruit suggested the form of royal crowns from the time of Solomon to the present day.

The 7-branched candlestick, which has come down to us through the ages as an important Jewish symbol representing the 7 days of creation, had its origin in the lowly sage plant growing on the mountains and hills of Palestine.

When pressed flat, the plant has almost exactly the shape and form of the 7-branched candlestick—the *menorah*—with its central spike and 3 pairs of lateral branches, each bending upward and inward symmetrically; on each branch were the whorls of buds (the "knops" or "knobs") of the Biblical golden candlestick, exactly as described 3,000 years ago in Exodus 37:17.

Sage's botanical name, *Salvia,* comes from the Latin salvere, "to be saved." This plant once enjoyed such a strong reputation as an age-retarding, life-lengthening herb that a fourteenth-century writer asked, "Why should a man die whilst sage grows in his garden?"

Heart-Healing Power

Modern-day discoveries about this Bible plant read like a litany of miracles. In China, a species called purple sage (*Salvia miltiorrhiza*)

---

[16]John Heinerman, *Heinerman's Encyclopedia of Fruits, Vegetables and Herbs, op. cit.*

is widely used as a popular medicine for treating heart blockages (myocardial infarctions), heart pains, cardiac edema (excess fluid around the heart), and high blood pressure. It also has a tranquilizing effect on the central nervous system. Only the bitter root is used. In the body, the oleoresins in this root are strongly invigorating to the heart, liver, kidney, bladder, and blood circulation.

As an example of sage's life-saving power, the case is reported of a scientist who, while visiting China, suffered a major heart attack. The diagnosis, made with an electrocardiogram, was myocardial infarction (heart blockage). After being sedated for excruciating pain, he suffered another major attack a few hours later, requiring cardiac massage. To restore blood circulation to his heart, the doctors gave him an injection of an extract of purple-sage root. In a short time, circulation was restored in the small blood vessels of his heart. The man recovered, regained his health, and a month later was leading an active, normal life, back home in the United States.[17]

Japanese scientists have reported that certain chemical compounds in Chinese-sage root seem to prevent blood clotting in laboratory animals, which may explain why Chinese-sage root is so useful in treating heart blockages and heart pains. Also, certain acids in sage kill bacteria harmful to the heart. In China, sage is a widely used popular medicine for treating staph infections.

If you can find purple-sage root, otherwise known as Chinese-sage root, then make a simple tea out of it. Medical anthropologist Dr. John Heinerman says, "Bring a pint of water to a boil; add 1 level tablespoon of the dried root. Cover and reduce heat to simmer for *no longer than 3 minutes*. Remove from stove and permit to steep for half an hour. Strain and drink 1 cup *warm* on an empty stomach twice daily where myocardial and angina problems are likely to occur."[18]

If you are unable to obtain purple-sage root or Chinese-sage root, then ordinary garden sage leaves (*Salvia officinalis*) can be substituted.

---

[17]John Heinerman, *Double the Power of Your Immune System, op. cit.*
[18]Heinerman, *ibid.*

A Remedy for Shaking Palsy

When John Wesley, an eighteenth-century English clergyman, noticed that his hands had begun to tremble, he searched a book of herbal remedies and discovered these words:

> "Sage soothes the nerves and by its powerful might
> Pagets and palsies often puts to flight."

He resolved to drink sage tea daily, and in a short time was able to record the following in his diary: "My hand is as steady as it was at fifteen."

Dangerous Throat Swelling Disappears

Quinsy is a severe inflammation of the throat with swelling and fever. During his travels through Africa, the French explorer Francois Le Vaillent fell ill with this condition. Due to severe swelling of the throat and tongue, he could communicate only by hand gestures. For almost a week he could hardly breathe and expected to suffocate at any moment.

Some natives then suggested that he use a plant medicine they had prepared. Some hot, wet leaves were placed against his throat, repeatedly. They also used the leaves to brew a tea for him to use as a gargle. By morning, his throat was so much better that he could breathe freely. He kept using this remedy until he felt completely cured.

When he asked the natives what they had used to save his life, he was astonished to discover that it was nothing more than common sage, growing wildly right outside his tent.

A Remedy for Alzheimer's?

In his journal, John Gerard (1545–1612) wrote: "Sage is effective for quickening the senses and memory."

British researchers, 450 years later, report that sage inhibits the enzyme that breaks down acetylcholine, thus preserving the compound that seems to help prevent and treat Alzheimer's disease.

"Sage has been found to have an action on the cortex of the brain which is said to be beneficial in mental exhaustion, strengthening the ability to concentrate," says researcher Richard Lucas.

According to Lucas, a society of school teachers tried drinking sage tea, and many members declared it wonderfully strengthened the memory and seemed to clear the brain when tired.[19]

To prepare such a beverage, place an ounce of powdered sage into a container and pour a pint of boiling water over it. Let it stand for 10 minutes. Then strain, sweeten to taste, and drink two or three times throughout the day.

Useful for Halting Milk Flow, Relieving Intestinal Spasms, Relieving Fevers

Sage contains a volatile oil that inhibits the release of fluid from the body. This makes sage tea a valuable remedy for women who wish to halt their milk flow after the breast feeding of a baby has ended. The flow ceases in just a few days.

Sage tea also relieves intestinal spasms and lowers body temperature, thereby making it valuable for relieving fevers.

To Darken Gray Hair or Grow New Hair

To darken gray hair, 2 heaping teaspoonfuls of sage and 2 of ordinary tea are placed in a pint container and filled with boiling water. This is covered and placed in an oven on low heat for 2 hours. The longer it remains in the oven the darker the solution will become. The liquid is then strained and allowed to cool. When cool, some of

---

[19]Richard Lucas, *The Magic of Herbs in Daily Living*, West Nyack, NY: Parker Publishing Company, Inc., 1972.

the liquid is rubbed into the roots of the hair every night. If this mixture is to be kept more than a few days, a tablespoon of brandy or vodka is added to preserve its strength.

To stimulate new hair growth, one-half ounce of sage and one-half ounce of rosemary are placed in a container. A pint of boiling water is poured over this. The container is covered and the solution is allowed to stand for 15 to 20 minutes, stirring occasionally. Do not boil. Then the liquid is strained and stored in a bottle. Used externally, this mixture is said to stimulate new hair growth.

Reduces Blood Sugar in Type II Diabetes

My father used to drink sage tea to help bring his blood sugar back to normal. After suffering for 3 years from Type II diabetes—the kind that can be managed without insulin injections—he read about the benefits of sage tea in reducing blood sugar and decided to give it a try.

He would brew enough tea for a day by placing 3 tablespoons of dried, powdered sage leaves into a container and adding 3 cups of hot water. The amount he drank depended on his blood-sugar level. If it was high, he'd have 3 cups that day. If medium, he'd drink just one. If normal, he'd skip the tea altogether.

Some Type II diabetics have been able to cut their daily medication in half since drinking sage tea. If you have diabetes, make sure you are under a doctor's care. Tell him about sage tea, and ask if it's okay for you to try it. "You still have to eat right," said my father, "but that sage tea will bring your blood sugar down."

Kidney Infection Gone

One woman reports that she suffered from a kidney infection for more than a year. She says: "My doctor treated me with antibiotics, which helped for a while, but the infections returned. I finally had so many treatments with antibiotics that they no longer worked at all.

"Then one night my son brought home [a] friend whose father was an herbalist. The young man . . . told me to try a tea of sage and peppermint. The next day I bought the herbs and began drinking the tea. I took two cups a day for three months, and my kidney infection is all gone."[20]

To make such a tea, 1/2 ounce of powdered sage leaves and 1/2 ounce of powdered peppermint leaves are placed into a container. A pint of boiling water is poured over these herbs, the container is covered and allowed to stand until cold. One cupful is taken three times a day.

"Fantastic Liver Regeneration"

Medical herbalist John Heinerman says that when the liver breaks down or is partially removed through surgery, it has the ability to regrow or regenerate the parts lost, to a certain extent. He says there are three plants that will definitely assist the liver to regenerate itself—sage, beet, and tomato.

He cites a number of experiments in China in which lab animals regenerated lost liver tissue when fed sage tea or tomato juice.

To make a health cocktail for liver regeneration, he recommends combining 1/2 cup of fresh sage tea with 1/4 cup of fresh beet juice and 2/3 cup of fresh tomato juice. Drink this at least once or twice a day between or with meals, he says.[21]

A Remedy for Bleeding Gums, Laryngitis, Tongue Sores, Tonsillitis

Sage is widely used in European countries in gargles and mouthwashes. It is used to reduce excessive flow of saliva and also to treat bleeding gums.

---

[20]Richard Lucas, *Secrets of the Chinese Herbalists, op. cit.*
[21]John Heinerman, *Heinerman's Encyclopedia of Fruits, Vegetables and Herbs, op. cit.*

An infusion of sage made by steeping a handful of the leaves in a pint of boiling water and covering until cool is a folk remedy for laryngitis and pharyngitis. One wineglassful of the strained infusion three times a day between meals has been suggested. This is said to be especially valuable for sores of the tongue or mouth (buccal ulcers), and tonsillitis.

Another formula that may be used as a gargle for tonsillitis consists of pouring 1 quart of boiling water over 2 ounces of sage. This is allowed to stand for 2 hours, then strained and a small bit of pulverized alum added.

One woman who tried the sage-alum gargle wrote: "My oldest boy woke up with tonsillitis one morning, so I prepared a tea of sage and alum and had him gargle with it several times a day. The next day he was rid of the tonsillitis, where other times he would suffer for weeks and could not eat or sleep."[22]

A Word of Caution

One expert warns that sage contains a fair amount of thujone, a compound that in very high doses may cause convulsions. Although sage is an excellent healing herb, he says, don't overdo it.

An Aphrodisiac from the Bible

Savory is believed to have been one of the spices mentioned in the Bible several times, in the Song of Solomon. Experts think it was included, along with lavender, rosemary, sage, and thyme—all members of the mint family—in Solomon's gardens at Etham.

Savory is famous for its aphrodisiac effects. Renowned French herbalist Maurice Messegue says: "My father used to have a high regard for this herb. 'Son,' he would say when we went looking for it in the hills, 'this is the herb of happiness!' I was in fact perfectly happy to be scouring the country for it and to be learning from him

---

[22]Richard Lucas, *Herbal Health Secrets from Europe and Around the World,* West Nyack, NY: Parker Publishing Company, Inc., 1983.

the secrets of plants, but it was not till later that I understood what sort of happiness he meant. The monks of former times were not allowed to plant savory in their gardens because it was an herb of love! . . .

"When I make up a 'love potion' it does not contain things like Spanish flies and horns of rhinocerous. . . . No. It is very much more simple and very much more agreeable. . . . I just advise couples who want to retrieve their married bliss to sprinkle powdered savory on their meat. Or I advise impotent men and frigid women to take the osmosis treatment that my father used to advise: to rub the base of the spine with a decoction of savory and fenugreek."[23]

Savory has been known since the very earliest times as an aphrodisiac, but it has other properties. It has also been recommended for gout, paralysis, rheumatism, kidney stones, diarrhea (acute and chronic), vaginal discharge, and stopped periods. It is reportedly good for asthma and blockages of the respiratory tract. It contains an expectorant (cineole). It relieves stomach cramps and stomach and intestinal gas. In Europe, diabetics drink savory tea to alleviate excessive thirst. It is a vermifuge, useful for getting rid of parasites such as roundworm and tapeworm. There are no reported ill effects from using savory. It's on the FDA list of herbs generally regarded as safe.

To use it as an aphrodisiac, Messegue recommends putting a small handful of fresh or dried savory leaves into a liter (1-3/4 pints) of boiled (not boiling) water. Strain, sweeten to taste, and drink 2–3 cupfuls a day and 1 before bed "if you have ideas."

To make a decoction of savory and fenugreek to use externally, simmer 3-1/2 teaspoons of fenugreek seeds for 5 minutes in 1 quart of boiling water. Remove from heat and add 2 handsful of dried savory leaves. Steep an additional 50 minutes. Apply to base of spine at bedtime. Medical anthropologist Dr. John Heinerman recommends drinking 2 cups of this brew as well, before going to bed. To do so, strain and sweeten to taste.

For an infusion to treat a cough, cold, or stomach upset, put 4 teaspoons of savory into a cup of boiling water (for child use 1 to 2 teaspoons per cup). Steep 10 minutes. Strain, sweeten to taste. Drink up to 3 cups a day.

---

[23]From *Health Secrets of Plants and Herbs* by Maurice Messegue, *op. cit.*

A Plant from Solomon's Garden that Acts as an Antibiotic

It is believed that Solomon had thyme in his gardens at Etham, among all the sweet-smelling plants—all rare and expensive, all known for their volatile oils. In the Talmud, the 39 books of Biblical commentary dating from the first century that interpret Biblical law, we find thyme listed as part of a remedy for puerperal illness that included cumin, caraway, and ammi (mint). Thyme was found in the tomb of Tutankhamun and grows in Egypt today. The *Assyrian Herbal* quotes thyme in treatment of lung and stomach ailments. Thyme was sprinkled on sacrificial animals to make them more acceptable to the gods.

Thyme contains thymol—a volatile oil—whose smell destroys viruses and bacteria in the atmosphere and infectious germs in the body. French herbalist Maurice Messegue says: "From boils to typhoid fever, from whitlows to tuberculosis, I do not know any infection that cannot be mitigated if treated with this precious herb."[24]

Everyone should grow thyme "because it is an excellent weapon against epidemics and much cheaper than other means of controlling them," he says. "It is antispasmodic, which makes it effective in cases of whooping cough, palpitations, coughs, stomach cramps, asthma and insomnia. It is also diuretic, useful for weakness in the kidneys and the bladder, for retention of urine, for rheumatism and for gout . . .

"It regulates women's periods, and works well in cases of respiratory disease such as colds, tonsillitis, bronchitis, pneumonia, pleurisy. Above all, from my long years of experience as an herbalist, I can appreciate thyme because of its antiseptic qualities . . .

"Used externally, it disinfects wounds, abscesses and burns, and is also useful for bruises, gout, rheumatism and toothache in the form of a compress, a dressing, a lotion, and so on, as the case may be . . . local baths soothe sore breasts in women and sore eyes in children."[25]

---

[24]*Health Secrets of Plants and Herbs, op. cit.*
[25]Messegue, *ibid.*

The druggist of today may dispense prescriptions containing fluid extract of thyme or may sell the well-known over-the-counter remedy Pertussin and yet know little or nothing of its ingredients. The label on a bottle of Pertussin will declare that it is composed of a "saccharated extract of thyme" whereby the alcoholic extract (thyme leaves steeped in grain alcohol) is mixed with sugar and water to form syrup. This syrup is of benefit in whooping and bronchial cough. *But a reasonable facsimile can be made right in your own kitchen merely by steeping or simmering wild thyme herb in warm water, the standard remedy for centuries.*

Messegue recommends several ways of using Thyme. As an infusion or tea, put 10 sprigs into a liter (1-3/4 pints) of water. Boil for several minutes. Take 3 or 4 cupsful a day. For a footbath, handbath, or vaginal douche, mix a handful of wild thyme into a liter (1-3/4) pints) of water. For a bad liver, put a pinch of wild thyme and a pinch of anise into a cupful of water and drink before bedtime.[26]

A Bible Healing Plant for Facial Neuralgia and Epileptic Fits

Medical herbalist Maria Treben recommends thyme for facial neuralgia. Her treatment consists of making an herbal pillow, consisting of thyme, chamomile (see page 271), and yarrow, picked fresh, dried, and placed on the affected area. Also, 2 cups of thyme tea are sipped throughout the day, she says.

She cites the case of a 79-year-old farmer who had suffered from facial neuralgia for 27 years. He'd had a couple of operations, but it got worse. In the last couple of months, his mouth was pulled almost to his ear and this caused great pain. Only after using thyme, as described above, was he able to obtain relief.

He kept drinking the tea long after the neuralgia was gone. For epileptic fits, Treben recommends 2 cups of thyme tea daily, for 2–3 weeks, alternating with a 10-day rest period, all year long.

---

[26]Messegue, *op. cit.*

An Extraordinary Bible Food Medicine for Water Retention, Urinary Infection, Migraines, and Poison Ivy

We remember . . . the cucumbers, and the melons . . . which we did eat freely in Egypt. *Numbers 11:5*

Watermelon, its seeds, and its relatives—cucumber and other melons—contain a chemical called cucurbocitrin that increases the permeability of the capillaries, the small blood vessels, in the kidneys, allowing increased amounts of water to escape into the urine. This can rid your body of swelling (edema) due to excess retained water.

Watermelon is also a good source of potassium, which pulls excess water out of your system, counteracting the fluid-retaining tendency of sodium (salt), present in excessive amounts in many processed foods.

One doctor describes watermelon as "by far the best and most dependable natural diuretic." He says it quickly washes retained poisons and debris out of the bladder, without any side effects. He says that watermelon should always be eaten between meals, or at least 1 hour after meals, never with your meal, in small bites, equivalent to sipping rather than guzzling. "It can open the urinary system like a hydrant," he says.

The seeds are used to prepare a tea, as follows: Boil 2 tablespoonsful of watermelon seeds in a pint of water for 5 minutes, steep (allow to stand) until cold, and strain. Drink 1 teacupful three or four times a day, sweetened.

Another way of using the seeds is to grind them into a powder and use about 1 heaping teaspoon per cup of boiling water.

Reported cases:

"Watermelon-seed tea is better than anything," says Stephanie, 54, a physiotherapist from Portland, Maine, who says that sipping 2 or 3 cups of watermelon seed tea throughout the day helps relieve her fluid retention.

"For about ten years I suffered from a bladder infection," says Mrs. J. R. "During this time I cooperated fully with my family physician, and we tried many antibiotics, drugs, and sulfas. In spite of this I would suffer a recurring bladder infection about four or five times a year. Then a neighbor told me about watermelon-seed tea. Since I felt it was a perfectly harmless remedy and I had nothing to lose. . . I gave it a try. What a surprise to find that it worked! I take the tea about three times a week, and I have not had a recurrence of the bladder infection in 16 months. I also eat plenty of watermelon itself when it's in season and have the seeds for year-round use."[27]

For a migraine headache, take a slice of watermelon, eat the meat, and place the rind against your forehead, making sure it stretches to your temples.

For poison ivy, glide the meat or rind of a watermelon over the rash area of your skin and let it dry naturally. Within a day, the condition should improve greatly.

Cucumbers (related to watermelon) contain plant hormones beneficial to the prostate; they also contain a hormone needed by the pancreas to produce insulin; they have been recommended as an anti-nausea remedy; and they can be used to deodorize your body (just wash some cucumber slices over the perspired areas and let the skin dry naturally—cucumbers are rich in magnesium, which is said to be a natural deodorant).

The drawback of watermelon, cantaloupe, honeydew, and cucumbers is that they contain certain proteins similar to ragweed, which make them good foods to avoid if you have hayfever due to ragweed sensitivity.

Cantaloupe, incidentally, is an anticoagulant. Researchers mixed blood platelets with "the sweet watery flesh of melon homogenized in a blender." Their conclusion was that "the melon contains an agent [adenosine] that strongly inhibits human-platelet aggregation." Thus, cantaloupe helps prevent heart disease and stroke.

---

[27]Richard Lucas, *Secrets of the Chinese Herbalists, op. cit.*

☉verpowering Relief for Pain

Wormwood is one of the oldest remedies and was known as such in ancient Egypt, where it was a sacred plant carried in religious processions. It is mentioned in the Bible many times. Its chief constituent is a volatile oil,* usually dark green, sometimes blue in color, with a strong odor and bitter taste—next to rue, the bitterest in the plant kingdom. A drink called absinthe was made from a species of wormwood known as *Artemisia absinthium*. It was a green-colored liqueur, now illegal in most countries. It first produces pleasant sensations and inspires the mind with grandiose ideas, well illustrating the Biblical phrase "he hath made me drunken with wormwood." The habitual use of it, however, brings on a stupor and a gradual diminution of the intellect, ending in delirium, seizures, and sometimes death. Impressionist painter Vincent van Gogh is said to have been drinking absinthe when he thought it would be a good idea to whack off his ear and send it to a lady friend.

Used externally, however, wormwood is a valuable remedy which, in the words of one researcher, can bring "overpowering relief from pain."

Researcher John Heinerman says: "An alcoholic tincture of [wormwood], applied externally, often has a profound effect in relieving the soreness of aching muscles, the hurt accompanying swollen, arthritic joints, and the terrific pain felt with a bad sprain, dislocated shoulder/knee or fractured bone."[28]

He cites the following episode, related by the eldest son of Mormon prophet, Joseph Smith, Jr.:

> Our carriage had stopped by the roadside for lunch and to rest the horses. Upon getting back into my seat after the brief interval, I thoughtlessly put my hand around one of the carriage posts, and as the driver closed the door, two of my fingers were pretty badly crushed.

---

*The active principle of wormwood is thujone, which in large amounts is a convulsant, poison, and narcotic, somewhat similar to marijuana.

[28]John Heinerman, *Heinerman's Encyclopedia of Healing Herbs and Spices*, West Nyack, NY: Parker Publishing Company, Inc., 1996.

The wounds bled freely and Mother bound them up with some cloths from her bag, and we traveled on. My fingers became very painful, and after a while we stopped at a farmhouse. Mother unwrapped them, soaking the temporary dressing off with warm water and rewrapped them with fresh cloths. Taking from her trunk a little bottle of whiskey and wormwood, she turned the tips of my fingers upward, and poured the liquid upon them, into the dressings—at which, for the first time in my life I promptly fainted! It seemed as if she had poured the strong medicine directly upon my heart, so sharply it stung and so quick was its circulatory effect.

When I returned to consciousness I was lying on a lounge against the wall and Mother was bathing my face most solicitously. I soon recovered and we proceeded on our journey, reaching home in good time and without further mishap.

To make an effective tincture for relieving excruciating pain, Dr. Heinerman says: "Combine 1-1/2 cups of finely cut herb or else 8 tbsps. of the powdered herb in 2 cups of Jim Beam whiskey. Shake the jar daily, allowing the wormwood to extract for 11 days. Let the herbs settle and then pour off the tincture, straining out the powder through a fine cloth or paper coffee filter. Rebottle and seal with a tight lid until needed. Store in a cool, dry place. When using this tincture to relieve external pain, remember that because of its *strong potency* a little bit goes a long way! Wormwood oil used externally can relieve pain, too."[29]

Another example of the anesthetic and analgesic power of wormwood can be found in *The Autobiography of Benvenuto Cellini,* in which the writer recalls an injury he received during the seige of Rome in 1527, on the battlement of the fortress of St. Angelo, while fighting in the service of Pope Clement VII:

A cannon shot reached me, which hit the angle of a battlement . . .the whole mass struck me in the chest and took my breath away. I lay stretched upon the ground like a dead man and

[29]*Heinerman's Encyclopedia of Healing Herbs and Spices, op. cit.*

could hear what the bystanders were saying. . . . Attracted by the uproar, one of my comrades ran up. . . . On the spot he flew off for a stoop of the very best Greek wine. Then he made a tile red hot, and cast upon it a good handful of Wormwood; after which he sprinkled the Greek wine, and when the Wormwood was well soaked, he laid it upon my breast, just where the bruise was visible to all. Such was the virtue of the Wormwood that I immediately regained my scattered faculties.

Fallen Arches Cured

Village healers in some parts of the world treat fallen arches with a liniment made of wormwood steeped in rum. Richard Lucas recounts the case of a man who was unable to walk for 3 months due to fallen arches. Doctors prescribed special shoes, massages, and physiotherapy, to no avail. Finally, an old-fashioned folk healer told him to prepare a liniment by placing 1 ounce of powdered wormwood in a pint of rum and let it steep for a week, shaking the bottle vigorously every night. At the end of a week, the clear liquid was to be strained, placed in a clean bottle and capped tightly. He was advised to rub this herbal liniment on his feet twice a day, once in the morning, once at night, and keep his feet bound with gauze during the day. Within 3 weeks he was able to return to work. Since using the liniment over 20 years ago, there has been no recurrence of fallen arches.[30]

R̢x for Athlete's Foot

A truck driver from San Diego reports using an over-the-counter remedy containing wormwood to get relief from athlete's foot. The product is called Absorbine, Jr. "I just follow the directions on the bottle," he says. "It smarts a bit, but it works pretty well."

---

[30]Richard Lucas, *Common and Uncommon Uses of Herbs for Healthful Living*, West Nyack, NY: Parker Publishing Company, Inc., 1969.

Anorexia Cured

French herbalist Maurice Messegue says, "Wormwood is an excellent tonic, stimulating the appetite and the whole digestive system. On one occasion I used it to treat a young girl who was suffering from anorexia nervosa and refusing to eat. The wormwood quite literally restored her taste for life."[31]

For Liver and Jaundice, Viral Hepatitis

Wormwood is also good for malfunction of the liver and for jaundice, according to Messegue. "I like to use it for convalescents who are suffering from viral hepatitis," he says. "Another of its virtues is its fever-reducing quality. . . . I also prescribe it for regularising periods or bringing on late periods, and it is a useful antiseptic, as well as being effective for diarrhea."

But he warns that for internal use, you should keep very strictly to the recommended dose. If you exceed it, then you lay yourself open to serious trouble: headache, vertigo, conjunctivitis, and more. Pregnant women should never use it, nor should nursing mothers, nor anyone suffering from hemorrhage of the stomach or intestine.

To make an infusion (tea), Messegue says to put 5–20 pinches of wormwood leaves into 1-3/4 pints of hot or cold water, sweeten generously, and drink 2 cupsful a day.

As an aid to digestion, or as a vermifuge (to get rid of intestinal worms), he recommends a syrup made by putting 2 handfuls of dried wormwood flowers, half a handful of dried red-rose petals, 6 pinches of cinnamon, and 14 ounces of honey into a liter (1-3/4 pints) of white wine; let it stand for 24 hours in the warm or let it stand for a week at room temperature; strain. Take a liqueur glassful before meals.[32]

---

[31]Messegue, *op. cit.*
[32]Messegue, *op. cit.*

CHAPTER 15
DIRECT FROM THE BIBLE: THE WORLD'S MOST POWERFUL NATURAL ANTIBIOTIC

We remember the fish, which we did eat in Egypt freely; the
cucumbers, and the melons, and the leeks, and the onions, and
the *garlic* . . . *Numbers 11:5*

Is there a Bible food so powerful that it can protect you from bubonic plague? So powerful that scientists are testing it against AIDS? So powerful that it could heal a short, withered, paralyzed arm? So powerful that the aged, the sick, and those afflicted with all types of infirmities have been transformed from hopeless invalids, some barely able to shuffle a few feet, to hearty, robust men and women able to run, kick, jump, and keep stride with anybody? Incredibly, there *IS* and you'll find it—not in your medicine chest—but in your vegetable garden.

There are about 67 kinds of garlic in the Holy Land, so it is not at all strange that the Hebrews should have developed a liking for this plant. The once-famous city of Escalom in Palestine is literally named after a species of garlic, the shallot, or *Allium ascalonicum,* in Latin.

In Biblical times, garlic was used medicinally for a wide range of ailments. Records brought to light by German archeologists digging south of the ancient sites of Babylon and Nippur show that garlic was widely employed:

309

1. As an infusion (tea) for reducing fevers.
2. As a decoction for loose bowels.
3. As a fomentation for painful swellings.
4. As a liniment for strained muscles or pulled ligaments.
5. As a tincture for intestinal parasites.
6. As a general tonic for improving the heart and strengthening digestion.

The Talmud—the 39 books of Biblical commentary that interpret Biblical law, dating from the first century—directs that many kinds of food are regularly to be seasoned with garlic to ward off the sickness that arises from the spoilage of food. They also hung it at doorposts to ward off evil influences. Such thinking may seem antiquated, but it just so happens, as modern science has shown, that the strong sulfurous fumes emitted by garlic kill bacteria and viruses and disinfect the air, the body, and whatever else they come in contact with.

In ancient Egyptian medicine, one Hesy Re, Chief of Dentists and Physicians around 2600 B.C., plugged cavities with crushed garlic. The idea at that time was to preserve a bad tooth at all costs rather than pull it.

Ancient Toothache Remedy Still Works

Dr. John Heinerman tells of using this 4,500-year-old remedy himself with good success, when one of his fillings fell out. A throbbing pain soon ensued. He couldn't find a dentist over the weekend, so he went to a local grocery store and purchased several cloves of garlic and a small jar of peanut butter. He then peeled a garlic clove, pounded it flat with the bottom of a heavy ashtray, mixed it with a little peanut butter, and stuck it into the gaping hole. "Within minutes, the pain ceased," he says, "and I managed very nicely," until he could get to a dentist to have the tooth refilled.[1]

---

[1]John Heinerman, *The Healing Benefits of Garlic,* New Canaan, CT: Keats Publishing, Inc., 1994.

The Wisdom of King Solomon

King Solomon is said to have written a book containing plant cures for all diseases known to man. For those afflicted with epileptic seizures (regarded then as a form of madness), he prescribed valerian root or garlic clove. He inserted a small portion of either of these herbs into the top of a large ring he wore on one of his fingers. This was placed directly beneath the nostrils of the afflicted person, apparently with a great degree of success. Valerian is now known to be a natural sedative and tranquilizer. And the sulfur compounds in garlic may have acted in much the same way that smelling salts do in bringing someone out of a temporary stupor, as one scientist speculates.

Angels Tell of Plant's Curative Powers in a Vision

As mentioned in Chapter 12, Hildegarde von Bingen was a German mystic and herbalist who lived in the twelfth century. She was the abbess of a Benedictine convent, who was regarded as a saint in her time, a true prophetess of the Lord.

She claimed to have received a series of visions showing new ways to use medicinal herbs, which she recorded in a book called *Physica,* the earliest work on natural history in Germany. These visions were recorded on rolls of parchment that can still be viewed by scholars in various European museums.

In one of these visions, an angel appeared to her and told her that a mixture of two herbs—garlic and hyssop—would cure asthma. The angel instructed her to brew a plain tea from a handful of green hyssop tops and two garlic cloves, cleaned, chopped, and placed in a pot of water, simmered on low heat.

For bloody coughs, the angel told her to add a plant called all-heal to the mixture, saying that this would dramatically stop the bloody coughing within minutes. For consumption—now known as tuberculosis—the angel told her to add lavender blossoms and comfrey leaf to the garlic-hyssop brew.

Protection from Bubonic Plague

Perhaps the greatest proof of garlic's germ fighting power is its ability to protect humans against the bubonic plague, which swept through Europe several times in bygone days, wiping out entire populations. Once, in Marseilles, France, for example, 80 percent of the population was dead within months.

Historical records show that when the plague swept the town of Chester, England, in 1665, the only residents of the town that survived lived in a storehouse with a cellar full of garlic; no one living in the house died.

During the great plague of 1722 in Marseilles, there were some clever thieves who went about robbing money and jewels from the homes and bodies of the dying and the dead—yet were themselves immune from infection. They were arrested, charged with the offense, and sentenced to death, but were offered clemency in return for the secret of their survival amidst the plague. They were immune, they said, because they had rubbed their faces, necks, hands, arms, bodies, and even their clothes with a liquid made by soaking 50 cloves of peeled garlic in 3 pints of strong wine vinegar for 2 weeks. They also drank some of the solution and gargled with it. The authorities then posted these instructions in public places, and the remaining citizens of Marseilles were able to resist the plague.

Spread by rodents and fleas, the airborne form of this disease—from the coughing of sufferers—is so virulent that it kills virtually everyone who contracts it within 3 days. Infected patients must be treated with powerful antibiotics within 15 hours in order to survive. But common garlic, a gift from God, can prevent it from ever happening in the first place.

The World's Most Powerful Natural Antibiotic

Garlic is the most powerful natural antibiotic known in the form of pure food. Against its juice, cold, flu and virus germs don't stand a chance. It cuts phlegm, fights infections, and clears sinuses, bronchial tubes, and lungs. It kills the most horrible germs—even leprosy, gonorrhea, and gangrene—in 5 minutes flat.

In lab tests, these germs were actually hurled to the side of a culture dish! One tiny milligram of garlic had the same power as 25 units of penicillin.

It is such a powerful herb that when rubbed on one's feet, it quickly passes into the bloodstream and can have a beneficial effect in the lungs. A garlic plaster placed on the soles of the feet is very good for stopping coughs and relieving colds. It is made by mincing several cloves of garlic, mixing them with a little olive oil, and applying this to the bottom of the feet.

Lung patients—near death's door—suffering all manner of respiratory ailments (asthma, emphysema, and horrible lung abscesses, allergies, and bronchitis), have revived and walked away completely cured, praising this miraculous plant.

Fights Germs Penicillin Won't Touch

In 1948, after years of research, scientists firmly established garlic's "penicillin power," by isolating various substances in it.

Alliin, the first substance isolated, was effective against the germs that cause salmonella poisoning, dysentery, and the staphylococci germs that cause skin boils and running sores. It was also effective against the streptococci germs that cause scarlet fever, sepsis, diphtheria, erysipelas, and inflammation of the lining of the heart (rheumatic fever). *Allicin,* another ingredient, fights conjunctivitis (eye infection), putrefaction (food decay in stomach and intestines), typhoid, cholera, and TB.

Since then, many other important substances have been found in garlic. The proven anti-cancer nutrient *germanium* is one of them. In fact, garlic is one of the richest sources of organic germanium and *selenium* (vital in the prevention of heart disease and many forms of cancer, see page 153). *Ajoene* is a chemical substance that "thins" the blood, thereby warding off potentially dangerous clots. When lab animals were fed a single dose of this garlic ingredient, blood clotting was reduced 100 percent for 24 hours. Ajoene also works against two types of fungi: one that is often present in the outer ear canal and another that causes Candida and vaginitis. Ajoene also "is toxic to Burkitt's lymphoma cells when they are grown in tissue culture," according to the August 1991 *Harvard Health Letter.*

Other sulfur compounds within garlic "will block the development of colon, esophageal, and skin cancers in rodents exposed to specific chemical carcinogens that produce these malignancies," the report continues. Garlic has over 100 known sulfur compounds. Some scientists believe there may be as many as 500 or more.

It is these sulfur compounds that give garlic its disease-fighting power, help reduce blood pressure and blood sugar, relieve asthma and bronchitis, improve circulation and heart function, prevent cancer, and assist the body in getting rid of dangerous toxins.

Asthma, Bronchitis, Emphysema, and Other Respiratory Problems Relieved

One medical doctor prescribes garlic as a "mucus regulator" for chronic bronchitis. He thinks garlic works by stimulating the same reflexes that cause the nose and eyes to water. These reflexes cause the lungs to release fluids that thin the mucus, enabling the body to expel it. He says that regular use of garlic may keep some susceptible persons from developing chronic bronchitis.

Garlic, says this doctor, may help prevent lung damage from bronchitis and emphysema. There is increasing evidence, he says, that emphysema may be partly due to free radicals in the system that destroy lung cells, free radicals that may be neutralized by sulfhydryl agents in garlic.

The major flavoring agent in garlic, alliin, is closely related, chemically, to Mucodyne, a popular European drug for relieving excess mucus. The alliin in garlic escapes when a clove is cut or crushed. For that reason, he advises using whole peeled cloves in soups. He suggests using one bulb of garlic (about 15 cloves) with 28 ounces of chicken broth and various other herbs and spices, boil (inhaling the fumes), simmer for 30 minutes, filter out the solids, and drink in equal portions before each meal, one to three times a day. Chewing a little parsley makes garlic odors vanish.

Reported uses:

One woman states: "It was from an herb book that I learned about the wonders of garlic, and cleared up pneumonia congestion in my lungs when antibiotics failed."

Speaking of garlic for respiratory ailments, one expert says: "Garlic is an effective preventive or treatment for the flu, whereas conventional medicine has no treatment."

If you feel a sore throat or cold coming on, eat some garlic or onions, says James North, chief of microbiology at Brigham Young University. "If you do it early enough, you might not get sick." Studies show that garlic extract is almost 100 percent effective in destroying the rhinovirus that causes colds; parainfluenza 3, a common respiratory and flu virus; and herpes simplex 1, which causes fever blisters. Garlic kills these germs on contact, says North.

Effective against Tuberculosis, Brain Infection

Garlic's antibiotic power has been proven in literally hundreds of tests, documented at the National Library of Medicine in Bethesda, Maryland. About 125 scientific papers on garlic have been published since 1983 alone. A recent report listed its effectiveness against 72 different types of infectious agents, the broadest range of any antimicrobial substance known, says one expert.

Dr. M. W. McDuffie used garlic to cure practically hopeless TB cases brought in on stretchers and wheelchairs, expecting to die. In the *North American Journal of Homeopathy,* May 1914, he calls it "the best individual treatment found to get rid of germs," and says, "we believe the same to be a specific for tubercle bacillus and for tubercular processes no matter what part of the body is affected."

Similar results were reported by an English physician, Dr. Minchin, in charge of a large TB ward at Kells Hospital, in Dublin. He found that garlic has a specific destructive effect on the tubercle bacillus.

Garlic combats fungal infections such as tuberculosis, by killing the organism. It also stimulates the patient's own immune system.

Chinese doctors have, for centuries, administered garlic to patients to fight infections. In 1980, an article appeared in *The Chinese Medical Journal* on the use of garlic in cases of meningitis. Doctors in the province of Changsha, unable to afford amphotericin, an antibiotic, fed and injected garlic into patients with a serious infection called cryptococcal meningitis. Out of 16 who got garlic, 11 survived, a cure rate of 68 percent. *This means that chemicals in garlic were able to cure a brain infection, which even certain powerful antibiotics cannot do, with no serious side effects, unlike many drugs.*

Anti-cancer Properties

Garlic even appears to have anti-cancer properties. It has long been known to be effective against various types of tumors in laboratory animals. In 1942, Russian scientists successfully used garlic extracts against human tumors.

In China, a comparison was made between two counties in Shandong province, one where garlic was popular and one where it was rarely eaten. It was found that non-garlic eaters were 12 times more likely to develop cancer. Specifically, it was noticed that the residents of Cangshan County enjoyed the lowest death rate due to stomach cancer (3 per 100,000), whereas the county of Qixia had a thirteen-fold higher death rate due to the same cancer (40 per 100,000). A look at the diets of both counties showed that Cangshan residents regularly ate more than half an ounce of garlic, onions, leeks, and similar vegetables every day, while residents of Qixia ate almost none.

In Shanghai, China, around the same time (1990), 200 people with cancer of the larynx (the "voice box" in the throat) were compared with 414 control patients who did not have the disease. It was found that garlic, along with fruits and dark green and yellow vegetables, seemed to prevent that form of cancer.

In 1987, researchers at the Akbar Clinic and Research Center in Panama City, Florida, found that when volunteers ate raw garlic in large quantities, and samples of their blood were mixed with live cancer cells, it destroyed 140 to 150 percent more cancer cells than in the blood of non-garlic eaters. Specifically, they had people eat two to three bulbs of garlic daily (that's bulbs, not cloves). After 3 weeks he placed natural killer cells from their blood in a lab dish containing a variety of cancerous tissues. The garlic-eaters' killer cells killed more than two-and-a-half times more cancer cells than killer cells from people who had not eaten garlic. Patients do not need to eat such large amounts to gain some benefit. An amount as small as half a clove results in an increase in natural killer cell activity.

In "Plant Remedies for Cancer," in *Cancer Therapy Reports* (7:19–20, May 1960), Dr. Jonathan Hartwell tells of a Victoria, British Columbia, physician who successfully treated several different malignancies (unnamed) by having his patients just eat garlic. We are reminded that Hippocrates prescribed the eating of garlic for uterine tumors somewhere between the fourth and fifth centuries B.C. Folk literature from India (circa 450 A.D.) speaks about garlic as a cure for abdominal tumors. France is supposed to have one of the lowest incidences of cancer due to the large amount of garlic consumed there. Garlic eaters in Bulgaria are virtually free from any kind of cancer.

In 1986, researchers asked 41,837 women aged 55 to 69, selected randomly in Iowa, about their diet. They were asked to pick out, from a list of 127 foods, those they regularly ate. Then they were watched over a period of time to see what diseases they developed. Researchers were especially on the look-out for colon cancer, a major killer in the United States. Of all the foods they ate, none stood out as a cancer preventive except garlic. The study showed that garlic seemed particularly effective in preventing colon cancer.

Garlic appears to prevent cells from turning cancerous by stimulating the body's own anti-cancer defense mechanisms. For example, it invigorates the liver, which produces anti-cancer enzymes and filters poisons out of the bloodstream. Garlic also protects the liver itself from damage.

Not just one but many factors in garlic seem to fight cancer. One factor is garlic's high sulfur content, which seems to confuse certain types of tumors, preventing them from reproducing. Another cancer-fighter in garlic is selenium (see page 153), which even in tiny amounts—as low as five parts per million—exhibits anti-cancer effects.

Garlic also seems to protect against radiation-induced cancer, which is prevalent in areas surrounding some nuclear power plants. It also prevents some of the symptoms and side effects of chemotherapy. In one study in Japan, garlic was given to a group of women who received chemotherapy and radiation: nearly 70 percent of the women taking garlic reported no side effects at all.

AIDS Research

Garlic as a possible treatment for AIDS was discussed at the Fifth International AIDS Conference in Montreal, in June 1989, where Dr. Tariq Abdullah, director of the Ak Bar Clinic of Panama City, Florida, presented the results of a 12-week study which showed that seven AIDS patients in Jacksonville and New Orleans improved after taking a special garlic extract called Kyolic® Special Garlic Preparation (SPG), manufactured by Wakunaga Pharmaceutical Company of Japan. The patients took 10 capsules, equivalent to two cloves, daily for the first 6 weeks; then 20 capsules, equivalent to four cloves, for another 6 weeks.

All the patients had severely low natural killer cell activity and abnormal helper-to-suppressor T-cell ratios—both of which are blood measurements that often show advanced AIDS, and a short life expectancy. All the patients also had opportunistic infections such as cryptosporidial diarrhea or herpes infections.

The results were dramatic, and as one expert observed "had a pharmaceutical drug been involved instead of garlic, no doubt the news would have spread rapidly in the media." Six of the seven who completed the trial had normal natural killer cell activity within 6 weeks, and all seven had normal activity by the end of 12 weeks. The helper-to-suppressor T-cell ratios returned to normal in three of the patients, improved in two, remained the same in one, and lowered in one.

At the end of the test, these AIDS patients' sores, diarrhea, and genital herpes disappeared. Among conditions that improved was a chronic sinus infection, in a patient who had gotten no relief from antibiotics during more than a year of treatment before the garlic study began.

News of the results spread rapidly, and many AIDS patients now take garlic regularly, in addition to the other medications they may be taking.

Effect of Garlic on AIDS-Related Infections

Various trials have shown garlic to be effective against cryptococcus, cryptosporidia, herpes, mycobactria, and pneumocystitis, all common infectious agents in AIDS. Researchers have also recently found evidence that the garlic constituent *ajoene* may directly interfere with the spread of the HIV virus in AIDS patients.

The Immune Enhancement Project in Portland, Oregon, uses garlic as their main agent for prevention and treatment of the opportunistic infections that accompany AIDS. They offer a full range of natural services, including office visits, herbal treatments, and more for about $100 a month to clients. "Compare this to the cost of some AIDS drugs, which are more than $1,000 a month just for the medication," says one expert, "and which are no more effective than the natural treatments."

Cerebrospinal Disorders, Convulsions, Pneumonia

Garlic has been applied to the feet as a poultice for brain and cerebrospinal disorders of children and for convulsions. As odd as it may seem that something applied to the feet might affect the brain, garlic foot poultices—due to the heat they generate—draw blood away from the top of the body. The effect is strong enough to stop a nosebleed. The antibiotic chemicals in garlic are also absorbed into the bloodstream through the feet.

One herbalist used garlic foot poultices to treat her own case of pneumonia. She was 8 months pregnant at the time, and her case was further complicated by severe pleurisy, which caused pain with each breath or cough. Her doctor offered her antibiotics, but she refused to take them in late pregnancy. Instead, she ate six to ten chopped raw garlic cloves a day, swallowed with water. She applied poultices of ginger and garlic directly over the spot that hurt her from the pleurisy, and applied garlic to her feet. She was out of the crisis in 2 days and had a full recovery in 2 weeks.

Preventing Clogged Arteries

Eating garlic may help prevent diseased arteries. Medical tests have shown that the pungent root has a "very significant protective action" in limiting the effects of fat blood coagulation, according to Drs. Arun Bordia and H. C. Bansal of R.N.T. Medical College, Udaipur, India. Reporting in the December 29, 1973, issue of the British medical journal *Lancet,* the doctors said the blood of ten patients clotted more slowly when they ate garlic with fatty food than when they ate it without garlic. They said this meant garlic could slow down the buildup of fatty deposits on artery walls and help prevent the arteries from clogging.

Specifically, 100 grams of butter (nearly a quarter of a pound) were added to a regular meal that the test patients ate. Three hours later, they averaged a blood cholesterol count of 237.4 milligrams percent.

When the juice or oil extracted from 50 grams of garlic was added to the identical meal, after 3 hours the blood cholesterol count was only 212.7 milligrams percent. It was found that garlic oil alone has the full effect, whether taken as pure oil, as garlic juice, or as whole garlic.

In addition, garlic oil reduced the level of fibrogen (a clotting factor in the blood). A meal containing butter resulted in a fibrogen level of 320.9 milligrams percent—in 3 hours. When garlic was added to the same meal, the blood level of fibrogen 3 hours later was 256.4.

Garlic in both cases actually brought the levels of cholesterol and fibrogen below their fasting levels.

Lowers High Blood Pressure

Reportedly, hundreds of physicians have found garlic to be the safest, most dependable way to relieve high blood pressure. No one knows exactly why this is so. Some doctors think it dilates (opens) arteries, relieving pressure. Others cite its germicidal power to relieve infections of various kinds and thereby reduce elevated blood pressure.

Blood pressure is definitely reduced, however. Doctors report— in case after case—such symptoms as weakness, dizziness, throbbing headaches, ringing in the ears, angina-like chest pains, shortness of breath, backaches, numbness, or tingling sensations— all relieved quickly and easily.

In fact, garlic seems to fulfill all the requirements of a perfect therapeutic agent to reduce blood pressure:

1. It is absolutely safe.
2. No bad after-effects, no limit to dosage have been found.
3. Blood pressure is reduced gradually—over a period of time— without a sudden drop that could shock the system.
4. It will not interfere with any other medication you may be taking, under a doctor's care.
5. In almost every case tested, it has relieved weakness, dizziness, headaches, ringing ears, chest pain, and annoying gas pains.
6. Good results may be obtained regardless of age or condition.
7. It is easy to take in odor-free tablet form.

In experiments at the University of Geneva in 1948, symptoms such as headaches, dizziness, ringing in the ears, angina-like pains, and pains between the shoulder blades began to disappear in 3–5 days after garlic treatment began. In cases of headaches, especially, 80 percent of those treated reported relief. Patients found that they could think much more clearly and concentrate on their jobs.

One thing should be clear, however: Garlic is not a cure for high blood pressure; it merely relieves the symptoms, which may return when garlic therapy is stopped. However, prolonged use of garlic in many cases has tended to permanently lower high blood pressure.

Cheats Death with Bible Food

"My father-in-law lay waiting—yes, just waiting—to pass on," says Mrs. R. E. "He could raise his voice only to a whisper. The doctors gave him two days to live. Then we heard that garlic juice would cure high blood pressure. [This was long before beta blockers.] We put it on his food, and fed him cooked garlic as well.

"In a remarkably short time he felt better, so we kept giving it to him as a main part of his diet for a day or two. In six days, he went downtown to his locksmith shop.

"It was all so remarkable that the news spread like wildfire—so much so that for a long time he was receiving letters from all over the United States, wanting to know what he could say about it."

Dangerously High Blood Pressure Normalized

One man writes, "Six months ago, I had my yearly physical and was told I had high blood pressure of 190 over 90. I was told to go on a diet and lose weight, and that would bring the blood pressure down. Somehow I never got around to counting calories. But a friend advised me that garlic could get my blood pressure down in a hurry. So I started taking 1 garlic oil capsule daily.

"A couple of weeks later I bought one of those home blood pressure machines and guess what. My blood pressure was down to 130/75. I have not lost one ounce of weight, so it must be the garlic. I've been taking one capsule a day without fail."

A Bible Food Remedy for Diabetes

The use of garlic has reduced blood sugar in diabetes. In one case, a man with advanced diabetes was told by doctors his condition was hopeless, and was sent home to die at age 60.

At age 90, he was still alive, in excellent health. He had started eating a combination of garlic, parsley, and watercress. His blood sugar dropped from over 200 to 110. And he went on happily using this remedy for many years.

Garlic is not a cure for diabetes and should not be used without your doctor's permission. But it may be a helpful way to lower blood sugar and thereby control the disease. It is a startling and interesting fact, however, which has been recorded several times, that garlic can reduce blood sugar in diabetes.

Bible Food Tested against Diabetic Medication

The use of garlic reduced the blood sugar in a case of diabetes reported by Dr. Madaus in the German publication *Lehrbuch der Biologischen Heilmittle,* volume 1, page 479. In the December 29, 1973, issue of *Lancet,* the British medical journal, two Indian doctors point out that garlic—though a little slower in action—is as effective as tolbutamide (an oral drug for diabetics) in clearing the bloodstream of excess glucose.

Mrs. S. L., a garlic user, says: "Recently, I was diagnosed as having mild diabetes. The doctor told me I would have to take an oral drug if my blood sugar didn't drop. I had read how garlic can lower blood sugar. So I immediately began taking a five-grain garlic capsule along with my vitamins and brewer's yeast after each meal. The result—my blood sugar fell to normal and no drug was needed or prescribed."

Bible Food Stimulates Sexual Powers

In his book, *Garlic Therapy* (Japan Publications, Inc., Tokyo, 1974), Tadashi Watanabi, D.Sc., says, "The infamous powder made from the beetle known as Spanish fly or the poisonous yohimbine obtained from the bark of a West African tree have the immediate effect of causing erection of the penis, but they provide no nourishment for the body and may in fact do harm. The allicin in garlic stimulates the central nerve of the penis and helps cause erection, but garlic [also] has a nourishing effect and stimulates the hormone glands, which in the long run strengthen long-term sexual powers by strengthening the entire body."

Rejuvenates Liver

Garlic's major value in liver disorders is its power to detoxify putre-factive bacteria in the intestines and thereby give the liver a rest. It is a proven stimulator of gastric juices, which help digestion, and an aid to increased and vigorous blood circulation through the liver.

It is claimed that a teaspoonful of garlic mixed with a table-spoon of olive oil or soybean oil, taken at night, will liven the liver and so rejuvenate it that the skin of the body will glow with renewed activity. Users say it is indeed a miracle vegetable.

A Bible-Food Remedy for Cystitis

Urinary infections can be painful and debilitating. Mrs. N. Q. tells how garlic was used to relieve a persistent bladder infection:

"For those of you who may be suffering from cystitis, garlic may be the answer. After having it several times, I decided to try my own remedy. I chopped up three large cloves of garlic three times a day, put them on a teaspoon and into my mouth and washed them down with water. After five days, the cystitis was gone."

A Bible-Food Cure for Stomach Ailments

Taken regularly, garlic can cure stomach and intestinal ailments, says a leading scientist and expert on garlic therapy. Reportedly, the allicin in garlic stimulates the walls of the stomach and intestines to secrete digestive enzymes. But garlic taken by people suffering from such conditions must be diluted or mixed with other foods, says this expert. An excellent way to tame garlic is to cook it or mix it with egg and milk.

Garlic need not even be eaten, however. Garlic may be used in poultices or foot- and handbaths to soothe the stomach. Its penetra-tive powers are so strong that it absorbs right through the skin. Used in this manner it has been reported 95 percent effective.

From ancient times to the present, garlic has been praised the world over for relief of gas, cramps, and catarrhal (inflammation) symptoms. The classic work in this area that finally established a firm scientific basis for use of garlic in stomach and digestive disorders was done by Damrau and Ferguson, and reported in the *Review of Gastroenterology* for May 1949. Each of the 54 patients treated was given two garlic tablets twice daily, after lunch and dinner, for a period of 2 weeks:

Heaviness after eating was completely relieved in 15 cases, and partially relieved in six out of 25—for a total of 84 percent effectiveness.

Belching was completely relieved in 13 cases, partially in nine—out of 25—a total of 88 percent effectiveness.

Flatulence was completely relieved in 20 cases out of 25—a total of 80 percent effectiveness.

Gas colic was completely relieved in 13 cases, and partially relieved in eight—a total of 84 percent effectiveness.

Nausea was completely relieved in six out of eight cases—for a total of 75 percent effectiveness.

It is reported that garlic brought not just temporary relief, but permanent freedom from these gastric disorders. The researchers concluded that garlic is a carminative that, used for flatulence and colic, expels gas from stomach and intestines and diminishes the gripping pains.

A Bible Food that Brings Speedy Relief for Intestinal Ailments

E. E. Marcovici, M.D., in an article entitled, "Garlic Therapy in Diseases of the Digestive Tract Based on 25 Years' Experience" in

Practical Therapeutics, January 15, 1941, reports that he first became interested in garlic in 1915 when, as an army physician, he had the opportunity of studying and treating innumerable cases of gastrointestinal infections, including dysentery and cholera.

Dr. Marcovici found that garlic brought speedy relief from the extreme diarrhea of dysentery. Some patients objected to the strong and pungent taste of the plant, so garlic tablets were used with equally good results. Results were so remarkable that garlic was later introduced as a routine treatment and cleansing measure in hundreds of cases of digestive disorders.

In chronic hypertension of the aged, Dr. Marcovici believes that garlic brings good results because of its cleansing effect on intestinal germs that cause putrefaction. It thereby prevents these poisons from being absorbed by the bloodstream.

"These patients are known to suffer frequently from chronic constipation, cecal stasis (intestinal blockage) or chronic appendicitis," he explains. "As a result of these disorders, foodstuffs incompletely predigested in the stomach on account of subacidity or hyperacidity, reach the cecal region where they undergo pathological putrefaction. As a consequence, toxins are absorbed and carried into the bloodstream. This toxemia is responsible for the varying symptoms from which these patients suffer: headaches (migraine), dizziness, fatigue, capillary spasms, etc." Garlic kills germs of putrefaction to cleanse and purify the system.

A Bible-Food Cure for Diarrhea

Dr. E. Roos, writing in *Münchener Medizinische Wochenschrift,* a German medical magazine, tells how he used a garlic preparation with success in treating many intestinal ailments, mostly involving diarrhea. He states that garlic is effective in three ways: it soothes, cleanses, and reduces inflammation. Garlic he says, has an almost narcotic effect. Like a narcotic, it seems to make stomach aches, diarrhea, and other intestinal ailments disappear within a short time. Unlike narcotics, garlic rarely causes constipation.

"It makes little difference," says Dr. Roos, "what kind of diarrhea you are dealing with or where it principally has its origin. A favorable result has been obtained in the great majority of cases treated, even in stubborn, chronic cases with recurrence."

Although results cannot be guaranteed, he says, in cases of serious organic disorder such as cancer or tuberculosis, he goes on to give several examples of seemingly hopeless cases treated with success.

Reported cases:

M. F., a college professor, had suffered from gas, dyspepsia, and colitis for 17 years. Occasionally, the diarrhea alternated with spells of constipation. He was given 2 grams of the garlic preparation two to three times daily. In 2-1/2 months the patient considered himself cured.

Mrs. O. S., 59, suffered from diarrhea for almost 9 months. Before that she had always been constipated, with a very sensitive and delicate digestive system. At the end of a month, with garlic treatment, she gained weight, appeared healthy, and her stools were completely normal. Evidence of large deposits of harmful bacteria in her intestines completely disappeared.

Mr. L. R., 33, a churchman, suffered from chronic colitis, involving much pain and abdominal discomfort. He began by taking 2 grams of garlic twice a day for 14 days, then once daily. Within the first few days he felt better. In less than month, he was having two normal bowel movements daily.

Ms. L. H., 24, suddenly experienced terrific body pain, nausea, chills and fever, along with persistent diarrhea. Her condition was diagnosed as acute enterocolitis. She took 2 grams of garlic three times a day, and by the fifth day her condition was perfectly normal.

C. R., 48, a baker, suffered from intense pressure pains in his upper abdomen. The pain had bothered him for more than a year, sometimes all day long, and yet he did not suffer from gas. He was given two tablets of garlic three times a day, and in a matter of days he experienced great improvement. In about a month, he declared himself in perfect health.

I. W., a scholar, troubled with abdominal pains, stomach trouble, hyperacidity, and diarrhea, was scheduled for an appendectomy. As luck would have it, the surgeon was not available. In the meantime, he was given the garlic preparation, 2 grams twice daily. After a few days, he claimed he felt perfectly well and the operation was canceled. (Dr. Roos gives this example just to show garlic's soothing influence, not recommending it as a substitute for needed surgery.)

"Often, after a very short time," notes Dr. Roos, "the difficulties improve, the patients feel relieved and look better. . . . So far as our patients could later tell, the effect also seems to last." He recommends two tablets of garlic three times daily as the best possible daily dose for intestinal complaints; in severe cases, three tablets five times daily, and in light cases, two tablets once or twice daily. Most important, he notes, these tablets can be taken without any fear of disagreeable side effects.

Diarrhea Ceased Almost Immediately

Mrs. H. L. of Bethesda, Maryland, says: "I have at times been subject to persistent diarrhea. The various medications given me by my doctor did nothing for it and made me feel sicker. I finally tried taking raw garlic after each meal, and the diarrhea ceased immediately. I don't like chewing garlic so I chopped it fine and swallowed it with fruit juice."

Mrs. K. V. reports: "I had diarrhea for a long time, and was so weak I could hardly move. I felt exhausted, and my weight dropped alarmingly. Every time I stopped taking the doctor's prescription, the diarrhea came back, worse than ever. Then I was told to try garlic, by taking a teaspoonful of the diced pieces with milk or honey, two or three times a day. The amazing thing is, my diarrhea ceased almost immediately."

How to Use this Bible-Food Remedy for Diarrhea

Used correctly, garlic is gentle, delicious, and has no odor. The way to tame garlic is to cook it. This gives it a smooth, buttery texture and a delicious nut-flavored taste. And the finished dish has no garlic odor at all.

This is true even in certain exotic cooked dishes calling for as many as 60 cloves. The reason is that the essence (or odor) of garlic is a volatile oil that rapidly escapes in heat.

Cooked garlic, says one expert, is safe and flavorful—as are small amounts of fresh garlic, diced in salads or meat—and he recommends these for people in poor health, or with allergies or stomach ailments. It is in large, raw doses that some people find garlic most upsetting. For such people it should always be diluted in some way, as in soup or with milk and crackers.

A Bible Food Cure for Constipation

A leading scientist and expert on garlic therapy states that people who suffer from constipation can find relief by regularly eating moderate amounts of garlic mixed with onions and milk or yogurt. The allicin in garlic, he says, stimulates peristaltic motion of the intestinal walls and in this way produces bowel movement. Kristine Nolfi, M.D., a Danish naturopathic physician, also states that "garlic has a strengthening and laxative effect."

Bible-Food Remedy for
Immediate Relief of Earache and Burns

Mrs. L. C. says: "For one year I have used garlic oil for earaches. I have seen it work wonders within 10 to 15 minutes of puncturing a garlic oil capsule, pouring it into the ear, and stopping it with a little cotton. I have told friends and relatives about how the pain stops soon after, and they all swear by it!

"Also, I found quite by accident that burns are helped by garlic oil rubbed into the burn. The pain goes away almost immediately upon application and rubbing it into the burn. My nephew burned his hand quite badly on top of the electric stove. When garlic oil was applied, he was very much relieved and slept through the night without crying."

Bible-Food Cure Relieved Ringing Ears

Mrs. S. A. says, "I have discovered a very simple and cheap remedy for bad hearing and ringing in the ears. . . . My ears would ring so much and my hearing was very cloudy. Three years ago I read, 'It is said that a drop of onion juice in the ear is good for bad hearing.' I tried it with wonderful results. Start about three times a week and as your condition improves you may cut down. I now use it about every week or ten days and maintain good results."

A Bible-Food Cure for Nose and Throat Problems

Garlic has long been known as a miracle antiseptic in cases involving eye, ear, nose, and throat infection. As Kristine Nolfi, M.D., says in *My Experiences with Living Food:* "If one puts a piece of garlic in his mouth, at the onset of a cold, on both sides between cheek and teeth, the cold will disappear within a few hours or, at most, within a day."

Garlic also has a curative effect on chronic diseases in the upper respiratory organs, the doctor says, absorbing the poisons - and this is true for "chronic inflammation of the tonsils, salivary glands and neighboring lymph glands, empyema of the maxillary sinus, severe pharyngitis and laryngitis" and other conditions. For example:

+ This miracle healing plant, says the doctor, "makes loose teeth take root again, removes tartar."

+ It has a curative effect on eye catarrh and inflammation of the lacrymal (tear) duct.

+ Got an earache? Just wrap the plant in some gauze, says the doctor, and place it in the outer-ear canal.

+ Got a headache? Garlic is nature's aspirin, dilating the veins and arteries to relieve congestion. Just squeeze some garlic juice into a teaspoon of honey (it's an old American Indian remedy).

+ Sneezing, stuffy nose, or allergy got you down? Try a little diced garlic downed in water. Garlic reportedly works miracles in such cases.

A Bible-Food Cure Brings Immediate Relief from Colds

Dr. J. Klosa experimented with garlic and reported his findings in an issue of the German magazine *Medical Monthly,* March 1950. Dr. Klosa experimented with a specially prepared solution of garlic oil and water (2 grams of garlic oil to 1 kilogram of water).

In 71 cases, clogged and running noses completely cleared up in 13 to 20 minutes. Burning and tickling in the throat could be stopped immediately by administering 30 drops of the oil-of-garlic solution, if symptoms were caught in the first stage. Otherwise, they abated to the point of disappearance in 24 hours.

Dr. Klosa reports the results with grippe, sore throat, and rhinitis (clogged and running nose) patients. The fever and catarrhal symptoms of 13 cases of grippe were cut short in every case. Cough symptoms were suppressed. Not one of the patients suffered from the usual post-grippe complaints, such as swelling of the lymph glands, jaundice, pains in muscles or joints, or chronic inflammation of the lungs. All patients showed a definite lessening of the required period of convalescence. The usual dosage was 10 to 25 drops taken partly by mouth and partly by being administered directly into the nostrils every 4 hours.

A Bible-Food Cure for Sore Throat

"Garlic works faster than vitamin C in curing colds," says researcher Rex Adams. "If one keeps a clove of garlic in the mouth, the cold will disappear within a few hours, or at most half a day, in my experience. It will not burn at all unless you chew it. Just score it with your teeth, every so often, to release a little juice. (If garlic is too strong, try one of its milder cousins such as rocambole or sand leek.)

"In this manner, a sore throat can be stopped in minutes (it even works for dreaded sore-throat symptoms of diphtheria)! I have found it to work every time—and to be much more reliable than vitamin C, which may or may not work, and often only forestalls the inevitable. Garlic gives permanent, not just temporary relief.

"It's a lot simpler than vitamin C, which must be taken in large doses, 500 mg. every two hours (according to F. Klenner, M.D.) or up to 1,000 mg. an hour (according to Dr. Linus Pauling), and takes up to 48 hours to work."

Bible-Food Cure Clears Sinus Congestion

Mrs. L. E. says, "I wish to let you know what wonderful results I had with garlic to clear up an attack of sinus. Normally, when my little daughter begins to have a fever (about twice a year), headaches and dizziness, I rush her off to the doctor [who prescribes a drug] of some sort. This last time she began to get sick, I had just read about how good garlic is for infections and colds, so I decided to try it. I bought garlic (with chlorophyll) and gave her two tablets about every four hours. After about six tablets, she woke up the next morning with a clear head and felt fine. All signs of sinus congestion were gone."

A Bible-Food Cure for Allergies

The story is told of a European houseworker, Klara Y., who amazed her employers by rarely catching cold and resisting contagious diseases when others had serious bronchial disorders and winter ailments.

She said that it was a folklore remedy to chew and eat garlic daily to help build resistance to infections and act as a natural healer for respiratory or bronchial disorders. Other members of the household began taking this folklore healer and were able to heal their allergic symptoms.

As reported by Carlson Wade in *Magic Enzymes:* "The harmful effects of the virus organisms are inactivated and a healing power is experienced. For many Europeans, eating garlic is a natural way to help fight allergic disorders ranging from the common cold to bronchial spasms and attacks."

Claims Allergy Relief Like a New Religious Experience

Mrs. A. S. says, "The greatest thing ever to happen to me healthwise was . . . garlic! For years I have been plagued with stomach and respiratory problems. 'Allergies,' the doctors would say and drop the matter.

"I grew steadily worse, until 11:00 P.M. became the most dreaded time of the day. When sleep would finally come I soon awakened almost drowning. I coughed, wheezed, and gasped for air. At 56, I threatened an early retirement. . . . I became an important customer of the drug companies who made antacids. These created other problems. Then I heard about garlic oil for allergies. I began taking 20 drops a day.

"The results are like a new religious experience. I was one who felt the difference in seven days. The comfort and ease I feel now is beyond description. All things being equal, I'll go to the full route to retirement."

Bible-Food Remedy Claimed Effective for Viruses

Reportedly, an effective remedy for treating virus and other infections is six cloves of garlic. These can be chopped and added to green salad, or crushed and blended with butter and spread on bread (or toast). In addition, one should drink a glassful of hot water in which has been stirred 4 tablespoons of cider vinegar and 2 tablespoons of honey.

Bible-Food Cures Near Fatal Attack of Sneezing

The story is told of a young man from Reno, Nevada, who had been sneezing for 4 days. Doctors tried everything, but nothing stopped the spasms.

Finally, a doctor who had read of the case in his local newspaper suggested feeding the patient lots of garlic. This was tried. Almost immediately, the patient stopped sneezing and fell into a restful sleep—his first since the attack.

"I believe the garlic cured him," said his physician. In another case, Carmella J., 21, of Oak Ridge, Tennessee, experienced an attack of almost continuous sneezing for 6 days. A diet of garlic halted the seizure. Her sneezing, which had been as rapid as 14 per minute, gradually subsided and finally stopped when the garlic was eaten.

A Bible-Food Cure for Hay Fever and Chronic Allergies

Phyllis S. suffered from hay fever and a whole raft of allergies that kept her sneezing, sniffling, and miserable the year round. She could hardly breathe. She complained of a stuffed-up feeling that even prevented her from sleeping. She'd have to prop herself up with pillows; sitting bolt upright was the only way she could get any rest.

Phyllis was allergic to practically everything, including dogs, cats, grass, dust, pollen, ragweed, mold, and spores. One doctor told her to avoid chills and drafts and keep her neck warm. Another doctor said she had nasal polyps and removed them in a painful operation; they promptly grew back. Another doctor wanted to give her a series of allergy shots in a special 3-year program, which she refused. "What I really need," she said, "is a new body."

Then she discovered garlic, the miracle rejuvenation plant, and herbs such as nettle, horseradish, and elderberry—all Bible foods famous for their ability to ease allergy symptoms.

Within 2 weeks, Phyllis felt better than she had in years. Within a month an allergy specialist gave her a clean bill of health. No more allergies!

Elderberry, for example, contains two compounds active against flu viruses. A patented Israeli drug (Sambucol) that contains elderberry is active against various strains of viruses. Of those who used it during a flu epidemic, 93 percent felt better, some in as little as 1 day, with significant relief of fever, aches, and pains, and were completely cured in 3 days. In a group that received a placebo, only 26 percent were improved in 2 days, and it took most of them 6 days to feel well. This Israeli drug also stimulates the immune system and is being tested against other viruses, such as Epstein-Barr, herpes, and even HIV. Sambucol is now available in the United States at pharmacies and health-food stores. If you can't find it, you can make a tea from the herb itself.

Stinging nettle tea—see Chapter 18—has a long history as a treatment for coughs (including whooping cough) and colds, runny nose, chest congestion, and bronchitis. Over 400 years ago, British herbalist Nicholas Culpepper claimed that nettle roots or leaves, used in juice or tea, were "safe and sure medicines to open the pipes and passages of the lungs." Recent scientific studies have shown that nettle is a potent antihistamine. There is nothing as dramatic as the allergy and hay-fever relief afforded by freeze-dried nettle leaves, according to Andrew Weil, M.D., author of *Natural Health, Natural Medicine*. Try 2 teaspoons of this herb per cup of boiling water. Steep until cool. Sweeten to taste.

Horseradish—used by Jews for centuries to symbolize the seven bitter herbs of Passover (see Chapter 2)—has a long-standing reputation for being mucokinetic, that is, for its ability to thin phlegm or mucus, thereby making it easy to move the mucus out of the system. As medical botanist Dr. James Duke and medical anthropologist Dr. John Heinerman point out, there is nothing like a teaspoonful of fresh horseradish to clear the sinuses. Another endorsement comes from Glenn W. Geelhoed, M.D., and Robert D. Wilix M.D., both surgeons, who recommend a Japanese horseradish called wasabi in their book, *Natural Health Secrets from Around the World*. They say, "A daily dosage is necessary only until the symptoms of your allergy subside. Thereafter, you only need a few teaspoons of horseradish each month to prevent another allergy attack."

Bible-Food Cure for Vaginal Infection

One woman says, "I'm only 23 years old, but for five years I suffered from an agonizing vaginal yeast infection. I saw a total of four doctors, the last one being a specialist. They gave me every remedy from purple dye to strong antibiotics, and at the same time, believe it or not, the good doctors told me antibiotics can cause yeast infection by killing off the good bacteria as well as the bad. . . . After reading that garlic acts like an antibiotic, I began to take fresh garlic cut up, and later on, manufactured garlic pills. I have found that, like an antibiotic, when I discontinue the garlic, the infection starts again. But there are two distinct advantages to taking the garlic (combined with vinegar douches) over the doctor-prescribed antibiotics. It is much cheaper and there are no side effects."

Bible-Food Cure for Anemia

One woman claimed that garlic cured her anemia. She says that eating this vegetable completely relieved her symptoms of weak digestion, numbness, tingling, fatigue, shortness of breath after slight exertion, pallor, lack of appetite, diarrhea, weight loss, and fever. With no complications, these symptoms are usually relieved with liver and vitamin B-12. But this woman says that garlic did it. She just couldn't seem to get enough of it and was never sick again after that "garlic binge."

A Bible-Food Cure for Women's Problems

Mild depression, irritability, anxiety, nausea, headache, tiredness, agitation, abdominal bloating, swelling of the extremities, dizziness, blurred vision, swelling and tenderness of the breasts, cramps, anemia, thyroid problems—all have been relieved by garlic or substances that garlic contains. A proven emmenagogic, it stimulates the menstrual flow. It is an age-old remedy for women's problems.

Reported cases:

Mrs. L. D. writes: "I've always had menstrual cramps constantly the first two days of my period. But ever since taking garlic (about three months) I have hardly any. It's hard to believe, but it is the only thing I'm taking that I didn't take before that time. Now on each day of menstruation I take four or five garlic pills. I take two or three every day and, as said before, four or five on those difficult days."

Harriet D., a 35-year-old housewife, suffered extreme weakness during her period, so extreme she could hardly do anything except lie still and not talk. She felt very shaky on her feet, with nervousness and trembling. She suffered cold sweats, extreme thirst, a feeling of faintness, and sometimes violent nausea and diarrhea. A friend suggested that she build up her resistance with garlic in her diet. To her surprise, each month she felt better and stronger. The trembling and nervousness disappeared, and she no longer dreads her period time.

Garlic, of course, comes in powder, pill, or capsule form, available at most health-food stores and herbal pharmacies. A tea is made simply by stirring a teaspoon of the powder in a cup of hot water, adding honey to taste. Or a small amount diced in a teaspoon of honey may be swallowed with water before meals.

Bible-Food Cure for Impetigo

Miss L. D. reports: "Within a year's time, infectious impetigo has victimized me twice. The first time, not knowing what it was and fearing its rapid spread and the unbearable itching, I went to the doctor. After two weeks of sticky medication, agonizing self-denial of scratching, and a medical bill, I was finally relieved. I was satisfied to pay anything just to be relieved of the constant itching and the spreading of more itching that always followed.

"But this second time it has all happened quite differently. One day, when my hands and face were to the point where I felt I had to see a doctor for medication . . . all of a sudden I realized that garlic might relieve the itching, if not cure the impetigo altogether. So I took one of my friend's pills, opened it, spread some garlic on the irritated areas and swallowed the remaining garlic. In half an hour, the itching was gone completely! I was able to sleep at night. I continued to rub fresh garlic on these areas and to eat garlic as long as it was necessary (three days)."

Bible-Food Cure for Blisters

Mr. R. F. states: "I am a letter carrier and had suffered in pain from blisters that had developed from ill-fitting shoes. I had tried every pharmaceutical product on the market with absolutely no lessening in pain or size of the blisters.

"I then remembered the antiseptic properties of garlic and immediately rushed to the health food store and purchased a bottle of natural garlic perles. I broke open a few capsules and massaged the oil into my blistered feet. The next day the swellings were practically gone and no more pain!

"When I told this to my doctor he was dumbfounded! He could not believe that all the sophisticated medicines I had purchased from the drugstore had no effect on my blisters, while nature's simple garlic had ended my misery. I then threw all the unnatural drugs down my sink and vowed to trust Mother Nature first."

Bible-Food Cure for Bedsores

"Garlic is a sure cure for bedsores," say Mr. and Mrs. C.R.G. "It is a miracle. I've tried everything that was recommended by nurses, hospitals, and others, but nothing helped for nearly a year. . . . I read that garlic was good for boils and suppurating sores. So I tried it.

"I grated some garlic on a very fine grater, mixed it with oil, made a poultice to put over the bedsore, and left it on for two days. My husband said it burned. I was afraid to look at it. When I took the pad off, I couldn't believe my eyes. The scab was off, the swelling was down, and there was no bleeding. Then I kept putting a pad with comfrey salve on it for over a week. All of the dead skin from around where the opening was peeled off. It was all smooth."

Bible-Food Remedy for Painful Growths and Spastic Colon

M. V., a dentist, reports that for 10 years he underwent X-ray and radium treatments to eradicate ugly skin growths that kept reappearing, even though a doctor said they were nonmalignant. On applying the oil of this amazing plant, garlic, which had relieved his spastic colon, the painful growths on his face completely disappeared.

The first time he tried this was for a growth near his eye. He applied garlic oil, from capsules, regularly, and in about a month it disappeared. The next time he tried it was for a growth just inside his hairline that grew rapidly; in fact, it was about the size of a nickel before he realized it was there.

Again, apparently, garlic oil healed it.

These growths, he says, were caused by a severe sunburn, and the radiologist who diagnosed them advised him to use alcohol to dry them up, which he tried for 2 or 3 months without success. "Can you wonder," he says, "that we are interested in statements about garlic and cancer? Whether or not these growths were malignant, they certainly could have so developed, with my past history. And they were definitely not healing until we applied the garlic. Furthermore, they were unsightly and painful. We hope this experience of ours may prove helpful to others. The treatment is harmless and in our case proved most beneficial."

Bible-Food Cure for Athlete's Foot

For years, James T. suffered in silent misery from a "galloping case of athlete's foot," as he described it. He moaned that it was all due to a ringworm or fungus he picked up on a wet locker-room floor. His toes were red, peeling, and painful. The heel and ball of his feet were rough with a million little dry pockmarks.

He tried everything to get rid of it: frequent soaking with soap and water, fresh dry stockings, powders, A&D ointment, antifungal creams. Some made it worse. Some actually did clear it up temporarily, but it would always come back, and the redness or peeling of the toes never really subsided. It was endless. His feet had an offensive odor, and he was embarrassed to take off his shoes. There was burning, itching, and soreness.

When all medicines have failed, garlic is a sure cure for athlete's foot. The method here is to spread some freshly crushed garlic over the affected area. It will feel warm for about 5 minutes. This should remain on the skin for a half hour. Then wash the foot with plain water. Do this once a day for a week and good-bye athlete's foot. (If the skin burns, remove the garlic immediately, wash with plain water, and try again later with diluted garlic juice mixed with water, until you find a mixture that doesn't burn, since too much garlic can worsen this condition.) To prevent reinfection, boil your stockings.

A Bible-Food Remedy for Arthritis, Rheumatism, and Neuralgia

Garlic remedies for arthritis include using it as a tonic or liniment (ordinary vegetable oil in which garlic has been fried is used as a liniment). Reportedly, a simple tonic made of diced garlic in a tablespoon of honey, taken with meals over a period of time, can do wonders to relieve pain and suffering, especially in cases of sciatica and gout.

An Indian scientist states that the oil extract from garlic, used as a liniment, has always been used with great success in paralytic and rheumatic afflictions. Another doctor says that the pain of rheumatic parts may be much relieved by rubbing them with garlic. "It gives excellent results," he says. Another leading scientist and expert on garlic therapy states that, taken internally, garlic quickly calms rheumatic and neuralgic pains.

How Bible Foods Healed a Withered Arm

In his book, *Of Men and Plants,* renowned French herbalist Maurice Messegue describes a patient, Anne-Marie M., 19, who had been born with a short, withered arm that never grew much, was useless, and remained bent back across her chest. She had no feeling in the arm (except during rainy weather, when the bones hurt) and could not move it. She had been to many doctors, none of whom were able to help the paralysis and stunted growth.

This was a new problem for Messegue, who diagnosed the atrophy as a kind of rickets. The most important ingredient in his remedy, he states, was a simple Bible healing food—garlic's nearly identical milder cousin, onion ("its sulfur content makes it very effective against rheumatism"). Other ingredients included wild thyme, stinging nettle, great burdock, and parsley—all Bible healing foods used as diuretics to eliminate the poisons (onion, too, he says, is "a powerful enough diuretic for one to have seen it clear the kidneys of patients with uremia"). Hawthorn, a Bible healing food, and linden blossom were prescribed as mild sedatives. Common chamomile, another Bible healing food, was used to calm the nerves. For the atrophy, he used field horsetail in a poultice of cabbage, and watercress, one of the bitter herbs of the Last Supper. This type of poultice has worked miraculously on animals who could barely stand on their feet. These she was to use in external applications only, in poultices and foot- and handbaths.

Three months later, she returned miraculously cured. She held out her hand. "Look!" she said, and she picked up a sheet of paper off the table with it. "I am so happy!" she cried. "It's so marvelous, I can hardly believe it . . ."

A skeptical witness said, "You mean you couldn't previously move your arm and hand? And now you can?"

"Exactly," she said, and to prove it she pinched him several times. The story appeared in all the Paris newspapers. Anne-Marie's parents said it was like a miracle. Only the doctors who had treated her unsuccessfully refused to believe it. "Nothing can be done," said one. "It is beyond the power of any doctor to correct congenital deformities."

CHAPTER · 16

THE NECTAR OF HEAVEN THAT WORKS HEALING MIRACLES ON EARTH

Palestine and Arabia abound in honey, which was well-known to the ancient Israelites—so much so that anything sweet, such as the syrup made from pressed figs or dates, sweet fruit juices, and the sap of trees, was called honey, leading to some confusion. However, beehive honey is clearly in the Bible

Bees frequently build their hives in trees, and so we read of Jonathan entering a forest on Mount Ephraim and finding honey literally flowing from the trees and spilling on the ground:

> And all the people came to the forest; and there was honey
>
> upon the ground . . . Jonathan . . . put forth the end of the rod
>
> that was in his hand, and dipped it in the honeycomb, and put
>
> his hand to his mouth; and his eyes brightened . . . *I Samuel*
>
> *14:23–30*

The Bible clearly spells out "bees and honey" in this well-known account of Samson in the Book of Judges:

> ". . . he turned aside to see the carcase of the lion: and behold there was a swarm of bees and honey in the carcase. . . . And he took thereof in his hands and went on eating . . ."

343

The Promised Land of the Bible is referred to 21 times as a land overflowing with milk and honey. Laurie Croft, M.D., a noted expert on honey, says: "[for bees to allow honey to overflow from the honeycombs] does occasionally occur, particularly during a heavy nectar flow, as any beekeeper will verify. Indeed, travelers to Israel in more recent times have recorded seeing enormous honeycombs hanging from trees with honey actually dripping from them."

What is the Bible trying to tell us with all these many references to honey? (The word is used 64 times.) I believe the message is clear: This is a Bible healing food—use it, and many of your problems will disappear.

The ancients used honey as a remedy for everything from arthritis and asthma, to burns, constipation, and hangovers, from hay fever to hemorrhoids, migraine, and shingles, from varicose ulcers to battle wounds. The magic of honey was that it could ward off infections and speed healing.

Because of its sheer versatility, honey was considered a divine creation—a nectar from heaven. True to that ancient belief, its miracle healing powers have never been surpassed to this very day.

A Nectar of Heaven with Spectacular Germ Fighting Power

Honey has a fatal effect on germs, which is mainly due to its moisture-absorbing ability. Its power to do this is phenomenal. Honey can withdraw moisture from a *rock,* or even from a metal or glass container. When germs come in contact with honey, all their moisture is withdrawn—they shrivel and die. It has killed the most harmful bacteria imaginable, with actual penicillin power.

When various disease germs were placed in a pure honey medium, the results were astounding. Typhoid germs were destroyed in as little as 24 hours. Germs that cause bronchopneumonia, peritonitis, pleuritis, running pus, and dysentery were all history in a few hours' time, or at most a few days.

Since antiquity it has been known that honey is able to prevent bacterial decay. A jar of honey that was placed in an Egyptian tomb some 3,300 years ago was so well-preserved when it was unearthed after so many centuries that it had only partially solidified—it was still semi-liquid and as aromatic, delicious, and wholesome as when it was put in the tomb.

Startling Emergency Relief[1]

Because of its hygroscopic or water-attracting properties, honey has been found to be a good healer of wounds and burns. Disease-producing germs cannot live without water, and honey sucks it out of them, causing them to shrivel and die. This wards off infections and speeds healing.

One man wrote: "In the winter of 1933 I heated a boiler of about 35 gallons of water. When I opened the cover, it flew with great force against the ceiling. The vapor and hot water poured forth over my unprotected head, over my hands and feet. Some minutes afterward I had violent pains, and I believe I would have gone mad if my wife and daughter had not helped immediately.

"They took large pieces of linen, daubed them thickly with honey and put them on my head, neck, hands, and feet. Instantly the pain ceased. I slept well all night and did not lose a single hair on my head. When the physician came to see me he shook his head and said, 'How can such a thing be possible?' "

Other reported cases:

An elderly woman was admitted to a hospital with gangrene of the foot, but after examining her the doctors decided she could not survive an amputation. It was decided to try honey.

---

[1]From *Miracle Medicine Foods* by Rex Adams, West Nyack, NY: Parker Publishing Company, Inc., 1977.

Her foot was literally tied in a bag of honey. To everyone's amazement, the foot soon healed, and she walked out of the hospital on her own power! She remained well.

Another woman had a horrible case of chickenpox. She was covered from head to foot with spots. Remembering the healing power of honey, she smeared some over her entire body, covered herself with toweling, and went to bed. In 3 days, she felt perfectly well, the chickenpox was gone, and her skin was completely smooth and clear!

One man had a large carbuncle on his back. It was operated on by a surgeon and left a deep, ugly scar. Then he developed another. This he treated with honey. Although enormous in size, the second carbuncle rapidly disappeared, leaving only a tiny dot.

A lady reports that while brewing some coffee for guests, she accidentally spilled the entire pot of boiling water on her thigh. Without telling anyone, she managed to get to the kitchen, in agony. There, she covered the burned area with lots of honey and wrapped a clean towel around her leg. In a few seconds, the pain was gone. She returned to the party in a clean skirt as if nothing had happened. The pain had gone away so completely that she forgot about it and slept soundly that night. Next morning, removing the dressing, she found a huge blister—bigger than two hands—but repeated applications of honey soon healed it.

It is reported that ulcerated legs from varicose veins do not heal easily, particularly in the elderly, but that regular daily application of honey can soon reduce the infection and bring a complete healing. It is said that an amazingly effective remedy for erysipelas is to cover the area—and a little beyond—with lots of honey, dress with cotton, and allow it to remain for 24 hours, repeating as necessary. In the jungles of South America, doctors smear honey over raw, open wounds after surgery, with excellent results. Honey is truly a miracle medicine food—a nectar from heaven.

Medical Science Discovers This Bible Healing Food

The most celebrated physician of antiquity, Hippocrates (460–377 B.C.) , wrote of honey: "It causes heat, cleans sores, and ulcers, softens hard ulcers of the lips, heals carbuncles and running sores." Over 2,000 years later, we find that:

In 1959, in Russia, a 63-year-old patient was treated with honey after resection of his larynx for removal of a malignant tumor. His wound healed quickly, and 10 years later he was still well, active and working.

In 1955, an English surgeon wrote: "All those who have seen the effects of honey dressings have become convinced of their value. . . . The advantages claimed for it are that it is non-irritating, non-toxic, self-sterile, bactericidal, nutritive, cheap and, above all, effective."

In 1970, doctors applied pure honey directly to the wounds of 12 patients recovering from radical surgery for carcinoma of the vulva. Rapid healing was observed. The doctors concluded that honey treatment was far more efficacious than conventional treatment with expensive antibiotics.

In 1973, an American surgeon wrote: "I have found that [honey] when applied every two or three days, under a dry dressing, promotes the healing of ulcers and burns better than any other local application I have used."

A 25-year-old woman had a massive bedsore that exposed the bone. A thin layer of pure honey was applied and covered with a dry dressing. Although surgical closure of the wound was planned, this was subsequently found to be unnecessary as the wound closed of its own accord. The patient recovered completely.

A 20-year-old woman had a grossly infected laparotomy wound that failed to respond to antibiotic therapy. Pus was running from the wound and vagina. Honey on clean dressings was applied and within 2 weeks the wound had completely healed without recourse to antibiotics.

ℿiracle Medicine for Lung Victims

In his book *Miracle Medicine Foods,* author Rex Adams tells of a man who became ill and consulted several doctors who said he had active tuberculosis. After a few months the doctors gave him up, and said his only hope was to go to Arizona, which he could not afford to do. Later, they told him flatly he had only a few weeks to live. He began using honey daily. Five years later, the same doctors examined him and found only a few spots on his lungs. Forty years later, the man was still alive and well.

In another case, a young girl was given up by her physicians as a hopeless consumptive (TB). Someone prescribed a diet of honey and goat's milk, with the result that she was free of illness the rest of her life and still spry and healthy at 90.

A Bible-Food Cure for Allergic Asthma

In 1969, Dr. William Peterson, an allergist, found that he could successfully treat patients suffering from allergic asthma with pure honey. His treatment consisted of small daily doses of honey, which he specified must be pure, unprocessed, and unheated.

Dr. Peterson's treatment of bronchial asthma using unheated honey was nothing new. Sir John Hill, in his book *The Virtues of Honey,* published in 1759, recommended honey for asthmatic patients. Dr. Donald Monro in his *Treatise on Medical and Pharmaceutical Chymistry* and the *Materia Medica,* published in London in 1788, gave the following remarkable account of the curative properties of honey:

> The late Dr. John Hume, of the Commissioners of the Sick and Hurt of the Royal Navy, was for many years violently afflicted

with asthma. Having taken many medicines without receiving any relief, he at last resolved to try the effects of honey. For 2 or 3 years he ate some ounces of it daily and got entirely free of his asthma and likewise of a gravelly complaint which he had long been afflicted with. About 2 years after he had recovered his health, when he was sitting one day in the Office for the Sick and Hurt, a person labouring under a great difficulty of breathing, who looked as if he could not live many days came to him, and asked him by what means he had found relief. For 2 years after he heard nothing of this person, who was a stranger to him, and had seemed so bad that he did not imagine that he could have lived many days, and therefore had not even asked him who he was; but at the end of that period, a man seemingly in good health, and decently dressed, came to the Sick and Hurt Office and returned him thanks for his cure, which he assured him had been entirely brought about by the free use of honey.

A Cure for Hay Fever

The use of honey in the treatment of hay fever has a long and successful record and has resulted in "complete cures" which have been described as nothing less than sensational. According to Laurie Croft, M.D., an English researcher, unlike allergy shots, which can result in shock and death, the honey treatment is "completely harmless with no possible side effects."

It seems to work by building up a person's immunity to the offending substance, pollen. The pollen in the honey seems to be the active ingredient.

Although this treatment had been known to people living in rural areas for a long time, it was first popularized in 1958, in an explosive best-seller called *Folk Medicine* by D. C. Jarvis, M.D. Dr. Jarvis recommended chewing 1 teaspoonful of honeycomb, one to three times a day—or taking 2 teaspoonfuls of liquid honey at each meal—starting about a month before the hayfever season begins. This will keep the nose open and dry. He claimed a 90 percent success rate.

Honey seems to create an immunity to breathing problems, and acts as a kind of desensitizing agent.

A cousin of mine, who had the worst case of hay fever I've ever seen, claims that it works. He took more than the recommended dose. He says he chewed it about five times a day for a couple of days, and then leveled off to three times, but that his watery eyes were dry in 2–3 minutes, his stopped-up nose was open in 3–5 minutes, and he could breathe through his mouth. His sneezing stopped. He could pet the dog, sleep on a feather pillow. He could work in the garden, and smell the roses. All his symptoms vanished over a 2–3 day period.

Reported cases:

Back in the 1950s, I used to stay with friends who had a farm in upstate New York. They had a 15-year-old boy about my age who said that whenever he emptied bags of grain, his nose would run and his eyes would tear. His mother, having heard about honeycomb for hay fever on a radio program, gave him some to chew. In less than a week, he felt fine, and remained free of hay fever, even in the dust of haying.

For 25 years, one man reports he suffered from hay fever every June. Attacks started in the first week of June and ended in the first week of July. Upon hearing that honeycomb was recommended for hay fever, he purchased some and chewed on a teaspoonful during a severe attack. The hay fever vanished in seconds, and each time it recurred the same simple remedy banished it.

Mrs. F. O. reports: "My husband used to have bad hay fever. [Then a friend suggested honey], two tablespoons a day, starting one month before hay fever time, and on through. It really worked. He took shots and was in air conditioning. This is his second year without shots. Our daughter got it too. She would not try it at first. She did not like honey at all but takes it now. No shots now. It's wonderful."

A Fine Heart Stimulant

Honey is a fine heart stimulant, better than brandy or whisky, which pep up the heart temporarily and then wear off. Honey has a long-lasting effect because of its slow-absorbing sugar, levulose. Many doctors have used honey in heart cases. Dr. G.N.W. Thomas, of Edinburgh, Scotland, in an article in *Lancet* remarked, "in heart weakness I have found honey to have a marked effect in reviving the heart action in keeping patients alive. I had further evidence of this in a recent case of pneumonia. The patient consumed two pounds of honey during the illness; there was an early crisis with no subsequent rise of temperature and an exceptionally good pulse."

Diabetes

Honey is largely a combination of various sugars, and contains a rare type of sugar known as levulose, which has the advantage of being absorbed so slowly that it does not have the "shock" effect of other sugars, which are difficult for people with high or low blood sugar to handle. One medical doctor, an expert on honey therapy, suggests there is more than a possibility of using honey for these sufferers.

Another medical doctor states: ". . . the employment of honey in the treatment of diabetics may look anti-scientific, anti-medical, even rather silly to the theoretical mind, to the uninitiated, or to a superficial observer. Just at this writing, my bee flock . . . is busy gathering honey from a plant now in bloom here. . . . We make tincture and fluid extract of this plant . . . and I give it to diabetic patients in drop doses (with decidedly good effect)."

If the plant is good for his patients, he reasons, why not the honey derived from it? Dr. A. Y. Davidov of Russia has found honey to be a good substitute for sugar in diabetes. One of his patients used 1 pound of honey in 10 days without an increase of sugar in the urine. When the honey was stopped, the sugar rose. With 4 teaspoons of honey daily, the sugar rate dropped. He reported six more instances where honey had a beneficial effect on diabetes. Dr. L. R. Emerick of Eaton, Ohio, a specialist, used honey in the diet of more than 250 diabetic patients with success.

Seemingly Hopeless Cases Cured

Some people claim that honey has been used by them in hopeless diabetic conditions with the best success and resulted in cures. One man writes:

"I became a diabetic and had to retire because I felt so weak. Doctors said there was no cure. Then I began a diet of raw vegetables sweetened with honey and lime: spinach, lettuce, cabbage, carrots, fresh tomatoes, and whole wheat bread. I began this diet around 1920, and a year later the doctors could not find a trace of sugar. Now, at 70, I can eat anything on the table, and do more work than any man my age."

Another man writes that he cured many cases of rheumatism and diabetes with honey. He cites the case of a man and his wife who both suffered from diabetes, doctoring with various physicians for a long time without improving. Finally, they went on a diet consisting of large amounts of honey and plenty of fruit and today both are fit as a fiddle.

Caution: **As with all remedies in this book, you are cautioned not to use honey without the approval and strict control of your physician.** You may have a condition, such as juvenile diabetes, which makes this method totally inappropriate for you. It may be incompatible with the medication you are taking, and which your doctor feels you should not stop taking. He may not think it safe for you to depend on this method as the sole means of treating this disease. Only your doctor knows for sure. Discuss it with him or her. For more details on the best treatment for various kinds of diabetes, I recommend *The Best Treatment* by Isadore Rosenfeld, M.D., now a Bantam paperback, which gives an excellent discussion of this and many other ailments from a doctor's point of view. Besides being authoritative, it's easy to understand and fun to read.

Hopeless Ulcer Victims Cured

Dr. Schacht, of Weisbaden, Germany, claims to have cured many hopeless cases of gastric and intestinal ulcers with honey, without operations. Another medical doctor states that "honey will cure gastric and intestinal ulcerations," which he calls a "distressing . . . and most dangerous malady, a precursor for cancer." But he says the news has not yet reached 99 percent of the medical profession, and those who do know it are afraid to say so for fear of being laughed at by their colleagues.

Father Sebastian Kneipp, the great German herbalist of the late 1800s, wrote: "Smaller ulcers of the stomach are quickly contracted broken and healed by (honey)."

One man reports: "I have been a sufferer from ulcerated stomach for several years, part time in the hospital, part time in bed, and nearly all the time in much pain. I noticed (after eating honey) that I was much better and gave no thought to the reason, but kept up eating honey because I relished it. I've had no attacks since."

Horse Cured of Cataracts

One man says: "I had a horse going blind with a white film over his eyes, which seemed to hurt. His eye was shut and watered. I dipped white honey into his eyes with a feather for several nights. In a day or so the film was gone and the eye looked bright and good."

Relieves Migraine Headaches

D. C. Jarvis, M.D., in his book *Folk Medicine,* claims that taking 2 teaspoons of honey will stop any headache—even a migraine—within a half hour.

A woman who suffers from migraine headaches reports that she cures them by taking a tablespoon of honey as soon as she feels one coming on. If the headache returns, she follows with a second dose of honey and 3 glasses of water. Her headache disappears completely and doesn't return.

Bible Food Relieves Hornet Stings

Mrs. A. W. reports: "My husband was mowing the lawn, dressed in shorts, when a swarm of hornets attacked him. He dashed into the house and rolled on the floor to dislodge some hornets that were still biting him, and screamed for a doctor. I frantically started dabbing honey all over his legs and arms. The honey started to relieve his terrible pains almost immediately! (My sister who told me this secret said to alternate honey with ice bags.) And the wonderful part of it is that he had hardly any swelling!" Instant pain relief!

A Strong Bible-Food Sedative that Can Relieve Insomnia

If you find it difficult to fall asleep at night—or you wake up early and can't get back to sleep—add 3 teaspoonfuls of apple-cider vinegar to a cup of honey. Take 2 teaspoonfuls of the mixture just before bedtime. It will enable you to fall asleep within a half hour after getting into bed. Unlike commercial drugs, this Bible-food remedy is harmless and can be taken indefinitely.

How This Nectar of Heaven Lowers Blood Pressure

Honey is a magnet for water. If taken at each meal, it draws excess fluid from the blood, lowering blood pressure. Since it is also a sedative, it relieves any tension in the nervous system.

One woman showed an unusually high blood pressure reading of nearly 300 when it was taken at a clinic. The staff was surprised that she was even alive. But with the help of 2 teaspoons of honey at each meal, she was able to live to the age of 84.

A Bible-Food Cure for Bed-Wetting

Honey's unique power to attract and hold water, combined with its natural sedative effect, makes it an effective cure for bed-wetting.

This moisture-holding ability that honey has can be readily observed in bread and cakes that contain honey and that remain moist and palatable indefinitely.

This same phenomenon can be used to attract and hold the fluid in a child's body during the hours of sleep, so that bed-wetting does not take place. At bedtime, give the child a teaspoonful of honey. It will act like a soothing sedative to help the child fall asleep. And it will attract and hold fluid while the child sleeps.

A Bible-Food Cure for Muscle Cramps

Reportedly, an annoying twitch of the eyelids or at the corner of the mouth can soon be made to disappear by taking 2 teaspoonfuls of honey at each meal. Cramps in the body muscles, especially in the legs and feet during the night, can generally be controlled the same way. Usually, the cramps disappear within a week. The honey should be continued indefinitely.

The Bible Food that Permanently Cured a Paralyzed Drunk in 24 Hours

Michael D. celebrated his fiftieth birthday by going on a drinking binge for 2 weeks. He was paralyzed drunk. He was given 6 teaspoonfuls of honey. Twenty minutes later he was given another 6 teaspoonfuls and 20 minutes later a third dose in the same amount. Treatment was continued for one more hour: 6 teaspoonfuls of honey every 20 minutes.

He had a good night's sleep for the first time in years. When he awoke he took a shot of whiskey, as usual—but was given 6 teaspoonfuls of honey every 20 minutes for the next hour. He then had a light breakfast, followed by another 6 teaspoonfuls of honey.

His lunch consisted of 2–3 teaspoonfuls of honey, followed by a hamburger and coffee. For dessert—you guessed it—he received 4 more teaspoonfuls of honey. After supper, he was offered a drink of liquor. He pushed it away, saying he did not want it anymore. He never took another drink again.

Reportedly honey, being a good source of potassium, counteracts the craving for alcohol and helps cure alcoholism.

CHAPTER · 17
ABRAHAM'S OAK

. . . and he was strong as the oaks . . . *Amos 2:9*

The Lord appeared to Abraham by the terebinths [oaks] of Mamre . . .
Genesis 18:1*

The oak was always respected and even venerated in biblical times for its large size and strength. Abraham's oak was held in especially high regard, not only because it was the place where God and His angels spoke to Abraham, but because under the shade of a holm oak, after His resurrection, Jesus appeared to the saints. It became the tree of Mary, mother of Christ, its branches uplifted to heaven in prayer.

Oaks attain an awesome height, up to 150 feet or more, indeed appearing to soar toward heaven.

. . . I saw, and behold a tree in the midst of the earth, and the
height thereof was great. The tree grew and was strong, and the

---

*The terebinths of Mamre are widely believed by scientists and biblical scholars to have been oaks. The oak is more plentiful in Galilee, and through Palestine as a whole. After visiting the Holy Land in 1860, one scientist stated: "Abraham's celebrated tree at Hebron . . . is now a venerable oak, and I saw no terebinth in the neighborhood."

height thereof reached unto heaven, and the sight thereof to the end of all the earth: the leaves thereof were fair, and the fruit thereof much, and in it was meat for all: the beasts of the field had a shadow under it, and the fowls of the heaven dwelt in the boughs thereof, and all flesh was fed on it. *Daniel 4:10–12*

Oak wood is practically indestructible. Oaken breakwaters built by the Romans still exist. King Arthur's Round Table, made from a single slice of oak cut from an enormous bole, still exists and is on display in Winchester, England. Oak logs buried 1,000 years ago have been recovered, still in good condition for building. It is not unusual for an oak to live 500, 1,000, even 2,000 years.

Medicinal Uses

Since Biblical days, oaks have been used to cure all manner of diseases, not only of human beings, but also of animals.

+ For heart trouble, the inner bark of the bur and red oaks and the aspen were scraped and dried and equal parts of this mixed with equal parts of the root, bud, and blossom of the balsam poplar. The root of the seneca snakeroot, dried and powdered, was added to the others. One swallow was taken as a heart remedy. The healing factor here may have been quercitrin, a pale-yellow glycoside obtained from the bark. Some glycosides have the ability to increase the force and power of the heartbeat without increasing the amount of oxygen needed by the heart muscle.

+ For lung trouble and bronchial infections the root of the blackberry was made into a decoction with the inner bark of the bur oak and drunk. Another method was to boil the inner bark of white oak and drink the steeped, strained decoction. This would cause the patient to throw up phlegm from the lungs and thereby gain relief.

+ "The onset of cataract [in lens of diabetic animals] is effectively delayed when quercitrin [an oak glycoside] is continuously administered," according to an article entitled "Diabetic Cataracts" in *Science,* vol. 195, 1977.

+ For liver injury and to prevent hardening of the arteries, simmer 2/3 cup of coarsely cut dried oak bark in 1 quart of boiling water for 20 minutes, says one expert. Allow to simmer for an additional hour and strain. Drink 1 cup every other day. This solution may also be used, when cool, to wash and dress wounds and major burns. When treating burns, the gauze may be soaked in this solution and changed every few hours.

+ To relieve hemorrhoids, a Native American tribe, the Menominees, would squirt an infusion of the scraped inner bark of oak into the rectum with a syringe made from an animal bladder and the hollow bone of a bird. This type of syringe was commonly made by many tribes. The Iroquois would simply boil the bark of white oak and drink the liquid to cure bleeding piles or diarrhea. Tannin is the ingredient in oak bark that gives such an infusion the power to dry and heal body tissues.

+ For swollen varicose veins, reportedly a tea is made by boiling 1-1/2 pints of water, adding a teaspoon each of crushed acorn and white oak bark. Cover and simmer for 12 minutes, then let it stand for 20 minutes more. Strain, add 1/2 cup to an equal amount of milk. Drink 1 cup of the tea every evening. After drinking a cup of the warm tea, apply external compresses soaked in the tea, alternating between hot- and cold-tea compresses, for about 25 minutes. Do this for up to 10 days.

+ Antidote to poisonous herbs and medicines. For generations, a decoction of acorns and oak bark, made with milk, was considered an antidote to poisonous herbs and medicines, according to Maude Grieve.

An All-Purpose Miracle Remedy

This same combination of acorns and oak bark, made with milk, can help with many other health problems. Whether to take the tea hot or cold depends on the type problem for which it is being used. Herbalist John Heinerman gives the following guidelines:[1]

bloody stool/urine (cold)	fever (hot)
hemorrhoids (cold)	menstruation, excess (cold)
mouth sores (cold)	skin irritations (hot)
sores (hot)	sore throat (hot)

Oak bark has a long history of use in cases of bleeding, diarrhea, colitis, dysentery, fever (as good as quinine), leukorrhea, gonorrhea, ulcers, gangrene, cough, asthma, amenorrhea, rheumatism, growths, venereal diseases, cramps, yeast infections, skin ulcers, ringworm, fungus infections, eczema, hemorrhoids, and varicose veins.

This is due to the fact that it contains large amounts of tannin, which is astringent, antiseptic, and antiviral, with both antitumor and anticarcinogenic activity.

Rudolph Weiss, M.D., in his book *Herbal Medicine,* says that this tannin is well tolerated by the skin, with no risk of causing irritation, and that it is used to treat not only conditions such as dermatitis and wheeping eczema, but also inflammatory eye conditions.

For dermatitis and eczema, Dr. Weiss says the method is simple. One or 2 tablespoons of the chopped bark are boiled for 15 minutes in 1/2 liter of water; the liquid is strained off, left to cool, and used undiluted. It is applied in the form of moist compresses.

It makes no difference what type of eczema or dermatitis you have, says this doctor. Use oak bark compresses. In cases of oozing and acute inflammation, this brings surprisingly rapid relief.

The compresses should be held in place with a bandage, but should be loose enough to allow air to circulate. They should be changed as soon as they get dry and warm, usually every 15 to 20 minutes. The treatment should last about an hour, and should be given three times daily.

---

[1]*Heinerman's Encyclopedia of Healing Herbs & Spices,* West Nyack, NY: Parker Publishing Company, Inc., 1996.

For severe burns, poison ivy, and sumac, one remedy is to split open a couple dozen acorns with a heavy stone or hammer and drop them into a 1/2 gallon pot of boiling water. When this has boiled down halfway, several hours later, strain and save the water, which now contains tannic acid from the acorns. This water can then be applied to any severe burn or rash on the skin in the form of a poultice, or a wash.

Proof of the effectiveness of this treatment is a 17-page report in the July 1926 issue of *Annals of Surgery* by two Cleveland physicians who successfully treated extremely serious burns in children and adults with nothing but tannic acid (which acorns are rich in). Before-and-after pictures show the healings.

Stops diarrhea in minutes. An old Indian remedy for diarrhea calls for four crushed acorns to be boiled in 1 quart of water on low heat for about 40 minutes, then strained. When cool, 1 cupful is consumed. Within minutes even the worst case of diarrhea is known to stop, due to the powerful astringency of the tannic acid in the tea.

Relief for dysentery. A similar decoction made from 1 ounce of oak bark in a quart of water, boiled down to a pint and taken in wineglassful doses, is said to relieve dysentery.

Some people have reported very good results in abolishing conditions of diarrhea and dysentery by using white-oak bark in powdered form in gelatin capsules. Two capsules are swallowed with a glass of warm water three to four times a day.

Relief for colitis. For mild conditions, 1/2 ounce each of oak bark, marshmallow root, comfrey root, slippery-elm bark, sweet-flag root, and bayberry bark are boiled in 3 pints of water for 20 minutes. When cooled, the decoction is strained, bottled, and stored in the refrigerator. Three to 4 teaspoonfuls are taken in a little warm water after meals, until results are obtained.

CHAPTER · 18
THE LOWLY OUTCAST PLANT WITH MIRACLE HEALING POWER

Among the bushes they brayed; under the *nettles* they were
gathered together. *Job 30:7*

The Bible says that outcasts were sheltered under the nettle bushes.
And Job compared inferior people to this lowly plant. But the Bible
also says,

Blessed are the meek, for they shall inherit the earth.
Matthew 5:5

So it should come as no surprise to you that nettle—one of the
lowliest plants in the Bible—has miracle healing power.

Its name, *nettle,* is said to come from the Dutch *netel,* meaning
a needle—a name it definitely lives up to, for it stings intensely when
touched. It needs these protrusions to survive. Yet, when made into
a tea (one ounce of the herb to a pint of boiling water) the needles
wilt, and then the leaves can be eaten safely as delicious greens.

A Bible Plant Juice for the Heart

Rudolf Weiss, M.D., notes, ". . . a pure expressed juice made from
fresh nettles has a definite effect in cases of cardiac edema and

venous insufficiency . . . Here nettle juice is definitely useful. It has the great advantage of being well tolerated and completely safe, as distinct from thiazides that are so widely used.

"Nettle juice can fill a gap in those situations, because it can be given well before the need arises for one of the very powerful synthetic diuretics," he says. It stimulates feeble circulation and relieves edema, including chronic swelling following an injury.

A Bible Food Brings Relief for Kidneys, Bladder, Water Retention, and High Blood Pressure

Nettle tea is considered a safe, gentle diuretic for the kidneys and bladder, and cases of edema (swelling from water retention), nephritis, or cystitis (inflammation of the kidneys or bladder), stopped urine, and gravel may be relieved with it.

One ounce of fresh nettles in a pint of boiling water taken in teacupful doses twice daily is known to be of considerable help in reducing high blood pressure.

Bible Food Relieves Asthma and Bronchitis

Nettle relieves asthma. The juice of the roots or leaves, mixed with honey or sugar, will relieve bronchial and asthmatic troubles, and mucous conditions of the lungs. The dried leaves, burnt and inhaled, have the same effect.

TB Victim Survives

Nettle can be a valuable aid for anyone suffering from tuberculosis. In one case a woman had been seriously ill with tuberculosis of the lung. Her doctor could give her no real hope of a cure. Her husband decided to give her fresh nettle juice or fresh green nettles chopped fine and added to her soup every day. In a year's time, she was a healthy woman.

The seeds have also been used in consumption, the infusion of herb or seeds being taken in wineglassful doses.

Hay Fever Cured

In the late 1980s, a scientist at the National College of Naturopathic Medicine in Portland, Oregon, accidentally discovered that freeze-dried nettles cured his hay fever. Further study revealed that two 300 mg capsules of freeze-dried nettles provided significant relief to hayfever sufferers. As of this writing, these capsules are not available commercially, but nettle tea can be made from the dried herb, available at most health-food stores (1 or 2 teaspoons in a cup of boiling water, steeped for 20 minutes, once or twice a day).

Hailed as a Goiter Cure
and an Amazing Weight Reducer

Nettle seeds, in powdered form, have been considered a cure for goiter, and as an effective weight reducer. It has been reported that those on a semi-diet of cooked stinging nettles have shed up to 32 pounds in 3 months or less.

To get nettles in your diet, young nettles can be finely chopped and sprinkled on soup as a garnish or added to salads. Since the juice (available from health-food stores) is not very tasty it is better to mix it in with whichever soup you prefer—vegetable, potato or oatmeal. A tablespoon per day for an adult and a half to 1 teaspoon for a child has sufficient medicinal properties to take effect. You can also steam young nettles in oil with a little onion. This will give you a tasty spinach-like dish that goes well with mashed or saute potatoes. Or nettle-juice extract may be purchased from a health-food store. For an infant, 5–10 drops of the extract each day, added to different mashed foods should suffice.

A novel treatment for diabetes was reported by a sufferer from that disease in 1926, in the English press. It was reported that a diet of young cooked nettles (following a 2-day fast) and drinking the pot liquor from them had been the means of reducing his weight by 6 stone—84 pounds!—in 3 days, and had vastly improved his condition.

Stimulating Hair Growth

For stimulating hair growth, herbalists recommend combing the hair daily with nettle juice. And to prevent hair from falling out, a tonic is prepared by simmering a handful of young nettles in a quart of water for 2 hours, then straining and bottling when cold. Saturate the scalp with this lotion every other night. In addition to preventing hair loss, it makes the hair soft and glossy. Nettle hair lotion may also be prepared by boiling the entire plant in vinegar and water, straining, and adding Eau de Cologne.

Eating cooked nettles or drinking the tea is also said to make hair brighter, thicker, and shinier, make skin clearer, and help heal eczema and other skin conditions.

A Bible Food Remedy for Impotence

In *Folk Remedies of the Low Country,* Dr. Julia F. Morton says that natives of the Charleston, South Carolina coastal area—the Gullah folk—regard stinging nettle as a powerful aphrodisiac. She says the milky sap of the root is taken internally for "courage" (potency). Nettle roots and "gomo" roots are chopped, steeped in whiskey or gin, and the liquor taken to increase potency. "Men have paid as much as $1 or $2 for a single root," says Dr. Morton.

Burn and Hive Relief

Burns may be cured rapidly by applying linen cloths saturated with a tincture of nettles, rewetting the cloths frequently. Nettle tea is also soothing. The Romans prepared a healing ointment by steeping nettle leaves in oil. Nettle juice has been used to relieve itching hives (a teaspoonful by mouth three times a day, plus some on the hive itself).

Bible Food Stops Bleeding from Nose, Lungs, Stomach, Uterus

Nettles are a powerful hemostatic. That is, they stop bleeding. This is because they contain several astringent components, including nitrate of potash, tannin, and formic and gallic acid. They have been used with good effect in cases of bleeding from the nose, lungs, stomach, or uterus—even in a case of hemophilia. The dose used was 3 ounces of the expressed juice. A syrup was also made by infusing 1/2 pound of nettles in 2-1/2 pints of water for 12 hours. This was filtered, and double its weight in sugar was added. Six ounces were given as a dose and repeated if necessary.

Nettle tea may be used internally for bleeding ulcers or externally as a poultice to stop any major hemorrhaging.

A small piece of cloth, moistened with nettle juice, can be placed in the nostril in bad cases of nosebleeding.

The seventeenth edition of the U.S. Dispensatory stated that nettles had been used particularly to stop uterine bleeding: "The fluid extract may be given in doses of half a fluid drachm [.0625 oz.] or a decoction of an ounce [of dried nettle leaves] to a pint in a teacupful dose."

During the Civil War, the bleeding of a major artery in an animal that was cut was completely stopped, in just minutes, by soaking some gauze in strong nettle tea and applying it directly to the wound. Amazingly, nettle juice was able to make fresh blood coagulate in seconds.

Famous Bible Food Relieves Arthritis, Rheumatism, Gout

Nettles are famous for relieving arthritis, rheumatism, gout, and related disorders. Roman soldiers flailed themselves with nettles in cold European climates to warm their skin and discovered that it relieved joint stiffness and pain.

This evolved into a practice called "urtication," that is, rubbing or striking the affected part with a bundle of fresh nettles. In

Germany in the late 1800s, Father Sebastian Kneipp, the famous "nature healer" said: "Fear of the unaccustomed rod will soon give way to joy at its remarkable healing efficiency."

Reported cases:

"Nettles," says William Thompson, M.D., "always remind me of my old friend, the blacksmith, at Fracombe in Surrey, whom I got to know well during [the Second World War]. In his yard he had a magnificent clump of nettles, and I once asked him why he did not dig them up. . . . 'Doctor,' he said, 'when the rheumatics in my hands get so bad I can't stand them anymore, I plunge them into that bed of nettles, and the pain goes at once.' A drastic but effective, safe and cheap remedy."

A woman who had been suffering for years with rheumatism went blackberry picking and repeatedly brushed her legs against some nettle. To her astonishment, about 3 days later her rheumatic limbs were virtually pain-free and she has been better ever since.

According to Rudolf Weiss, M.D., nettle can be used "to treat neuralgic and rheumatic pain . . . particularly degenerative and chronic arthritic conditions such as lumbago and sciatic pain, chronic tendonitis, sprains, and many other similar conditions."

Painful Muscles, Ligaments, Joints, and Ankles Relieved

But you don't have to rub nettles on you to get their healing effects. According to Dr. Weiss, a good treatment for rheumatism and gout is a teaspoonful of the dried herb boiled for 5 minutes in a cup of water, 3 cupfuls daily; or, nettle juice, available at health-food stores, 1 tablespoonful three times daily, over a 4–6-week period.

Dr. Eric Powell says, "I had a patient who suffered rather badly from rheumatism which affected muscles and joints. He was always straining his ligaments. After several good remedies . . . had failed to bring relief, Urtica [nettle] cured. The dose was 6 drops of [nettle] tincture four times daily.

"In all probability, a tea from the dried plant in larger doses would have had similar results but would have taken longer." Dr. Powell says nettle "has an affinity for the ligaments and should be employed when the sufferer has rheumatism."

Other cases:

Dr. J. Compton Burnett, the famous English homeopathic physician, was so successful in treating cases of gout with a tincture of nettle that his patients called him "Dr. Urtica" after the botanical name of the plant (*Urtica dioica*). He prescribed the tincture of the herb (available from health-food stores) in 10-drop doses in water.

"Some fifty years ago, when I was a boy, my father suffered with gout very badly. A friend [said] . . . 'Get two handfuls of stinging nettles (if they've got the seeds on so much the better). Thinly peel one pound of apples. Put the nettles and the apple peelings into two quarts of boiling water and let it all boil for 20 minutes. Strain, and take it in teacupful doses four times or more daily.' . . . the old lady's advice [worked]. Since then I have given this advice to many gout sufferers, always with excellent results. Recently I have recommended this treatment to people suffering with painful ankles, and in every case they have felt great benefit."—Mr. W.J.G.[1]

Neuralgia and Sciatica Relieved

In Germany, nettle is a favorite remedy for neuralgia. Dose: 4 tablespoonfuls of the decoction three times a day (a decoction is generally an ounce of an herb boiled in a covered pint of water for 30

[1]Richard Lucas, *Magic Herbs for Arthritis, Rheumatism, and Related Ailments,* West Nyack, NY: Parker Publishing Company, Inc., 1981.

minutes, strained and cooled), and at the same time bruise the leaves and apply as a poultice to the affected parts.

Also for neuralgia, a poultice can be prepared by placing a handful of nettles in a muslin bag that is then steeped in hot water for 10 minutes. This is applied to the painful area, as hot as can be comfortably tolerated, several times a day.

Nettle is a good remedy for sciatica. Two ounces of nettles are slowly boiled in 1 quart of water for 20 minutes. The decoction is allowed to stand until cool, then strained. The strained decoction is reheated and taken hot, 1 teacupful every 2 hours. A second decoction of nettles, prepared the same way, is used for hot fomentations, which are applied locally to relieve pain.

Reported cases:[2]

One woman who described the pains of neuralgia as "sickening" reported a complete cure with the use of nettle treatments.

A man who complained that he could hardly get out of bed in the morning due to painful sciatica of the hip began using the nettle treatment. Shortly afterward, the pain was reduced to such a marked degree that he was able to discontinue the fomentations, and to use the tea only. In 3 days he considered himself cured.

Dr. Jon Evans of England writes: "My experience with nettle places it as one of the sovereign remedies in the dispensary of nature. I feel we have by no means exhausted its uses as a medicine and that greater research will put it to further practical account."

A Bible Food That Relieves Enlarged Prostate

If your doctor has determined that you have benign or non-cancerous prostate enlargement, you might consider using nettle tea to obtain relief, if your doctor approves. Researchers gave a few tea-

---

[2]Lucas, *op. cit.*

spoons of nettle extract daily to 67 men over age 60 with this problem, and found that it significantly reduced their need to get up at night and urinate.

When the male hormone testosterone is converted to a related compound, dihydrotestosterone, the cells of the prostate are stimulated to enlarge. Like the prescription drugs Proscar and Hytrin, nettle seems to inhibit the chemical change in testosterone from taking place.

Nettle Beer

Nettle beer is an old English remedy for rheumatism and gout, and a pleasant drink as well. It may be made as follows: Take 2 gallons of cold water and a pailful of washed young nettle tops. Add 3 or 4 large handfuls of dandelion, the same of clivers (goosegrass), and 2 ounces of bruised, whole ginger. Boil gently for 40 minutes, then strain and stir in 2 teacupsful of brown sugar. When lukewarm place on the top a slice of toasted bread, spread with 1 ounce of compressed yeast, stirred till liquid with a teaspoonful of sugar. Keep it fairly warm for 6–7 hours, then remove the scum and stir in a tablespoonful of cream of tartar. Bottle and tie the corks securely. The result is a specially wholesome sort of ginger beer. The juice of two lemons may be substituted for dandelion and clivers. Other herbs are often added to nettles in the making of herb beer, such as burdock, meadowsweet, avens horehound, the combination making a refreshing summer drink.

How to Handle Nettles

When gathering nettles, heavy gloves, a long-sleeved shirt, and long trousers should be worn. When washing and preparing nettles, tongs should be used. It is a strange fact that the juice of nettle is the best antidote for its own sting and brings instant relief when applied. Dock juice has the same soothing effect. The sting of nettle may also be cured by rubbing with rosemary, mint, or sage leaves.

An easier way, of course, is to purchase dried or powdered nettle leaves or roots, which are available at most health-food stores.

HOW TO PREPARE BIBLE PLANT MEDICINES QUICKLY AND EASILY

Natural-food stores sell ready-made pills, capsules, syrups, oils, ointments, tinctures, and lotions. Still, it's far cheaper and more satisfying to make your own Bible-plant medicines with home-grown herbs picked right from your garden. And since they are not grown with any toxic chemicals, their purity is guaranteed.

Tea

Medicinal plants are usually made into tea. To be effective, medicinal tea is much stronger than ordinary tea—more of it is used, and it is steeped longer. It is made by pouring a pint of boiling hot water over 1 ounce (about 2 handfuls) of the dried leaves or flowers and letting it stand for 10 to 15 minutes.

By contrast, nonmedicinal beverage tea bags—the kind you buy in a supermarket—contain only about one-seventh that amount of herbs per pint of water, and it isn't necessary to steep that long. They taste better, too.

That's the trouble with medicinal teas. They don't taste very good, which may be nature's way of keeping you from taking too much. But if you can't get it down, it's not going to do you much good. Therefore, feel free to sweeten it with honey or any sweetener that will enable you to drink it.

Infusion

Some herbalists use the words tea and infusion interchangeably. Infusions are not teas; they are steeped longer and are a lot stronger. Anywhere from 20 minutes to several hours is how long it may take for a plant to release its healing properties into water. Generally, anything brewed for more than 15 minutes is called an infusion.

An infusion is made by placing an ounce of the plant substance (usually the softer parts, such as blossoms, leaves, and so forth) into a container. A pint of boiling hot water is poured over the herb, the container is covered, and the solution is allowed to steep for 15 to 20 minutes, stirring occasionally. Infusions are never allowed to boil. Sweeten to taste. Then the liquid is strained and stored in a bottle. One pint is enough for a day, if you drink 1/2 cup three times daily.

Tisane

Infusions do not have a long shelf life and should be made as needed. To make a smaller amount—for immediate use—a teaspoonful of the plant substance is placed in a cup and boiling water is poured over it. It is then covered with a saucer and allowed to steep for 15 to 20 minutes, after which it is strained and sweetened to taste. This is called a tisane.

Decoction

When a plant chemical is contained in hard material such as roots, barks, or seeds, a decoction is made by placing 1 ounce of the plant substance in 1-1/2 pints of cold water. This is covered and allowed to boil for a half hour; then it is strained and sweetened to taste.

(To allow for some of the water to be boiled down, herbalists use 1-1/2 pints of water, so that when the boiling is finished the decoction measures about 1 pint.)

Tincture

Occasionally, something a little stronger than water is needed to make a plant release its healing ingredient so alcohol is added to dissolve it out, without heating it. In fact, in some cases the value of an herb is lost if heated.

To make a tincture, generally, 4 ounces of water and 12 ounces of spirits (usually brandy or vodka or gin) are mixed with 1 ounce of the powdered herb. This mixture is allowed to steep for 2 weeks and is shaken thoroughly every night. Then the clear liquid is strained out and bottled for use; the sediment is discarded.

Helpful Hints

Use pure water (spring water or distilled water) for making your Bible-plant medicines. Chlorine and other chemicals in public drinking water may keep harmful germs at bay, but they may also interfere or react with healing plant chemicals in undesirable ways. Chlorine, for example, interferes with absorption of iodine from food, which may adversely affect the thyroid gland.

If a recipe calls for a dried herb and you have only a fresh sample of that herb, double the amount called for unless otherwise directed.

If a recipe calls for a fresh herb and you have only a dried sample of that herb, decrease the quantity of that herb by half.

Use a glass or ceramic container for boiled or boiling water. The material in pots and kettles made of aluminum, iron, tin, and other metals can leach into the water with unforeseen effects on its usefulness. Aluminum, for example, has been linked to Alzheimer's disease. An unchipped enameled pot may be an exception and may be okay.

Do not continue to boil water after you pour it over an herb. Remove it from the heat and let it steep with the herb in it.

If you smell an aroma from the brewing tea, it means the herb's essential oils are escaping into the air, rather than being retained in the liquid. To avoid this, cover the pot tightly.

If you are using a fresh herb, it should be rubbed between the palms of your hands or broken up in a mortar and pestle—called "bruising" the herb—to help release its active ingredients.

Syrup

Some recipes call for an herbal syrup to soothe a cough, a sore throat, or a cold. To make an herbal syrup, combine 3 ounces of whatever dried herb the recipe calls for with 1 quart of water in a large pot. Boil down to 1 pint, then add 1 to 2 tablespoons of honey. An herbal syrup can be stored in a refrigerator for up to 1 month.

Compress

Compresses are used to treat congestion, tension, aching muscles, swelling, and sprains. They are made by soaking a towel in a hot herbal brew and laying it on the affected area. Let the towel cool enough so as not to burn the skin. Cover the compress with a dry towel. When the compress no longer feels warm, replace it with another. Continue applying compresses for about 30 minutes. Stop if the area begins to tingle or burn or looks red and inflamed. The herbs used are chosen for their penetrating action and for their ability to either stimulate circulation or cool and dissipate excess heat.

Poultice

Poultices are used to draw out infection and soothe and speed the healing of a wounded or painful area. In a poultice, chopped or crushed fresh leaves, which have also been steeped in boiling water for a short time to soften them, are placed directly on the skin, as hot as can be comfortably borne, and then covered with a dry cloth to retain the heat and keep them in place. This is repeated with fresh leaves, whenever the need is felt.

Using Capsules

Once you have dried and powdered your herbs (crushing them in a mortar and pestle or a coffee grinder), you can pack them in standard gelatin capsules. These premeasured capsules are a convenient way to take herbal medicines that taste unpleasant or to carry them when you travel. These capsules come in different sizes—00 is the standard size—and all you do is measure how much of the powdered herb will fit into a given size, so you won't exceed any recommended dosages. Also, a capsule can later be opened and emptied into a cup of hot water to make a tisane—a small amount for immediate use (see aforementioned instructions).

APPENDIX + B
HOW TO GROW SPROUTS

Growing sprouts in an indoor garden is simple, easy, and enjoyable. You need not be concerned with fertilizers, weeds, or dangerous frosts. It's easy to provide them with just the right amounts of sunlight and water. And the nutritional value of sprouts is much higher than at any other time in a plant's life.

For example, fava beans are our best food source of L-dopa, the drug used for Parkinson's disease, to control trembling and rigidity. While no one is suggesting that fava beans can replace a sufferer's current medication, they might prove helpful in the early mild stages of this disease, if your doctor approves. L-dopa is an expensive drug. But fava beans are cheap. Amazingly, fava bean *sprouts* contain ten times more L-dopa than unsprouted ones.

Many of the Bible foods in this book—such as almonds, cabbage, chick peas, fava beans, fenugreek, kidney beans, lentils, mung beans, and wheat—can be sprouted in an indoor garden. There are several methods. Whatever method you select, the basic steps are so simple that the job can often be given to your kids to do.

You can be eating your first batch of fresh home-grown sprouts in 1 or 2 days, rather than the 3-6 weeks outdoor gardening usually takes. Sprouts are delicious and can be eaten by themselves, added to salads or sandwiches, or they can be juiced.

Getting Started

When choosing seeds for sprouting, look for uniformity of shape and color. Broken, chipped, or damaged seeds may rot, or not sprout at all. A handful of bad seeds can spoil a bunch. Look for absolute colors, like red, or green. Pink or light green means they are probably not ripe. Avoid seeds that are loaded with gravel or dirt. You will only have to separate all this out. Buying seeds in bulk saves you money. Organically grown seeds do make a difference in that they are more resistant to plant diseases.

1. The Jar Method

To start out using the jar method, get seven wide-mouth glass jars, and some pieces of cheesecloth or nylon mesh that can be used to cover the jars yet allow air to circulate. Use a rubber band to secure the cover tightly. Measure the appropriate amount of seed into each jar, using the chart on pages 384–387. Smaller seeds should just cover the bottom of the jar. Bigger beans and seeds should not fill the jar more than 1/8 to 1/4 full. Sprouts expand. For example, 1 pound of alfalfa seeds produces 8 pounds of sprouts. Cover the jar with the cheesecloth or screening. Then fill it halfway with water. Allow the seeds to soak for the required length of time (see chart on pages 384–387). After this, drain off the water. Place jar at 45-degree angle, *mouth down,* in a place where it can drain freely *through* the cheesecloth or nylon mesh cover.

Rinse the sprouts a couple of times a day by placing the jar under the tap, filling it with water, allowing it to overflow. The water should appear a little foamy from waste material produced by the sprouts. Replace the jar of sprouts—*mouth down* (covered with a cheesecloth secured by a rubber band)—at a 45-degree angle so that excess water will drain away. When sprouts mature, follow steps for harvesting and storage on pages 382–383.

2. The Tray Method

Sprouting trays can be purchased from nursery supply stores. Trays about 10" × 14" are good for home use. Smaller sprouting trays are sold at natural-food stores. They come with instructions and a cover. If you buy these, you'll need at least two. The holes in the trays should be a quarter of an inch in diameter or smaller. To sprout seeds in a tray, measure the amount of seed mix needed, from the chart on pages 384–385 (same amounts as for a half-gallon jar). Soak the seeds for the specified time in a jar of water. If the holes in the tray are small enough, you can put the seeds directly on the tray. If the holes are large, it's better to start the seeds in a jar, and even grow them using the jar method for 3 days. When the sprouts are 1/4 to 1/2 inch long, spread them out in the bottom of the tray and place the entire tray in a clear plastic bag. Punch a few holes in the plastic to let air circulate. The plastic bag prevents the sprouts from drying out. Keeping the tray slightly elevated on a rack of some sort will allow air to circulate to the sprout roots. Store-bought sprouters usually have small legs for the tray to stand on.

A couple of times a day, water the sprouts by removing the plastic cover and spraying them with a pump-style mist spray attached to a clean bottle of water. When the leaves turn green the sprouts will be ready to harvest. See harvesting and storage procedure on pages 382–383.

3. The Automatic Sprouter

Automatic sprouters let you sprout seeds with little or no effort. They don't tie up the kitchen countertop and can be placed almost anywhere, as long as there's light, an available water supply, and a drain or bucket to catch the rinse water. The most popular style looks like a miniature chest of drawers. Each drawer is actually a tray set at an angle for proper drainage. Mist sprayers are built in above each drawer. Sprouts that require light are placed in the top drawer, the top of which is clear plastic that lets light in. Sprouts that do not require light, such as beans and grains, are grown in the lower drawers, which remain dark.

To use an automatic sprouter, just hook it up to water and power, according to the instruction sheet. Strew the appropriate amount of seeds into each tray, and turn it on. The sprouts will be misted every couple of hours and the excess water will be drained off. An optional "grow light" bulb can be placed over the top tray for quicker sprouting.

Hints

Cracked or broken seeds should be removed and discarded before sprouting. When preparing seeds for sprouting, if you notice any small insects floating in the water, throw out the entire batch of seeds, not just the ones in the jar but the entire package. Store raw unsprouted seeds in covered glass or plastic containers. If the water supply in your area is of poor quality, try filtering the water used for soaking the seeds, or soak them in bottled spring water.

Harvesting Your Sprouts

When gathering mature sprouts, lentils, peas, and grains can be eaten or stored with their hulls intact. Remove and discard the hulls from cabbage, fenugreek, and mung. They taste better and store longer with their hulls removed, although they can be juiced hulls and all.

To remove the hulls, place them in a sink filled with water. Stir the sprouts gently with your fingers. This causes nearly all the hulls to rise to the surface. Scoop them up and discard them. Then gently scoop the sprouts below out of the water. Place them in a colander to drain before eating or storing them. Spoiled sprouts should be thrown away. They don't taste good and can quickly contaminate healthy sprouts.

Sprouts should be stored in a clean glass jar with a cover, or a sealed plastic bag. They can be kept that way from 7–10 days in a refrigerator.

Sprouting Chart[1]

Variety	Soak (hours)	Dry Measure*	Length at Harvest	Ready in (days)	Sprouting Tips
Adzuki	12	1 cup	1/2"–1"	3–5	Easy sprouter. Try short & long.
Alfalfa	4–6	3–4 table-spoons	1"–1-1/2"	4–6	Place in light to develop chloro-phyll 1–2 days before harvest.
Almond	12	1 cup	0"	1	Swells up, does not sprout.
Cabbage	4–6	1/3 cup	1"	4–5	Develops chloro-phyll when mature.
Chick Pea	12	1 cup	1/2"	2–3	Mixed with lentils & wheat, or use alone.
Clover	4–6	3 table-spoons	1"–1-1/2"	4–5	Mix with other seeds. Develops chlorophyll.
Corn	12	1 cup	1/2"	2–3	Use sweet corn. Try short & long.
Cow Pea	12	1 cup	1/2"–1"	3–6	Grow in dark. Try short & medium.
Fenugreek	8	1/2 cup	1/2"–1"	3–5	Pungent flavor; mix with other seeds.
Green Pea	12	1 cup	1/2"	2–3	Use whole peas.
Lentil	12	1 cup	1/4"–3/4"	3–5	Earthy flavor. Try short & long. Versatile sprout.
Millet	8	1 cup	1/4"	2–3	Use unhulled type.

*per half-gallon jar

[1]From *The Sprouting Book* by Ann Wigmore © 1986. Published by Avery Publishing Group, Inc., Garden City Park, NY. Reprinted by permission.

Nutritional Highlights	Suggested Uses
high-quality protein; iron, vitamin C	casseroles, Oriental dishes, salads, sandwiches, sprout loaves
vitamins A, B, C, E, & K; rich in minerals and trace elements	juices, salads, sandwiches, soups, sprout loaves
rich in protein, fats, minerals, vitamins B & E	breads, cheeses, desserts, dressings, milks
vitamins A, C, & U; trace elements	cole slaw, salads, sandwiches, soups
carbohydrates, fiber, protein, minerals	breads, casseroles, dips, salads spreads, sprout loaves
vitamins A & C; trace elements	breads, salads, sandwiches, soups
carbohydrates, fiber, minerals, vitamins A, B, & E	breads, cereals, grain dishes, granola, snacks
protein, vitamins A & C, minerals	Oriental dishes, salads sprout loaves
rich in iron, phosphorus, trace elements	casseroles, curries, juices, salads, soups, sprout loaves
carbohydrates, fiber, protein, minerals, vitamins A & C	casseroles, dips, dressings, salads, soups, sprout loaves
rich in protein, iron, and other minerals, vitamin C	breads, casseroles, curries, marinated vegetables, salads, soups, spreads, sprout loaves
carbohydrates, fiber, vitamins B & E, protein	breads, casseroles, cereals, salads, soups

Sprouting Chart *(continued)*

Variety	Soak (hours)	Dry Measure*	Length at Harvest	Ready in (days)	Sprouting Tips
Mung	12	1/2 cup	1/2″– 1-1/2″	3–6	Grow in dark. Rinse in cold water for 1 minute.
Mustard	4–6	1/4 cup	1″	4–5	Hot flavor; mix with other seeds.
Oats	12	1 cup	1/4″–1/2″	2–3	Find whole sprouting type.
Pumpkin	8	1 cup	0″	1	Swells up, does not sprout.
Radish	4–6	1/4 cup	1″	4–5	Hot flavor; mix with other seeds. Develops chloro-phyll.
Rye	12	1 cup	1/4″–1/2″	2–3	Try mixing with wheat & lentils.
Sesame	4–6	1 cup	0″	1–2	Tiny sprout, turns bitter if left too long.
Sunflower	8	2 cups	0″–1/2″	1–3	Use hulled seeds. Mix with alfalfa & grow 4–5 days.
Triticale	12	1 cup	1/4″–1/2″	2–3	A grain hybrid like wheat.
Water-cress	4–6	4 table-spoons	1/2″	4–5	Spicy; mix with other seeds.
Wheat	12	1 cup	1/4″–1/2″	2–3	Try short & long. For sweeter taste, mix with other seeds.

*per half-gallon jar

Nutritional Highlights	Suggested Uses
high-quality protein; iron, potassium, vitamin C	juices, Oriental dishes, salads, sandwiches, soups, sprout loaves
mustard oil, vitamins A & C, minerals	juices, salads, sandwiches, soups
vitamins B & E, protein, carbohydrates, fiber, minerals	breads, casseroles, cereals, soups, sprout loaves
protein, fats, vitamin E, phosphorus, iron, zinc	breads, cereals, cheeses, desserts, dressings, milks, snacks, sprout loaves, yogurts
potassium, vitamin C	dressings, juices, Mexican-style food, salads, sandwiches, soups
vitamins B & E, minerals, protein, carbohydrates	breads, cereals, granola, milks, salads, soups
rich in protein, calcium, and other minerals; vitamins B & E, fats, fiber	breads, candies, cereals, cheeses, dressings, milks, salads, yogurts
rich in minerals, fats, protein, vitamins B & E	breads, cereals, cheeses, desserts, dressings, milks, salads, soups, sprout loaves, yogurts
see wheat	*see* wheat
vitamins A & C, minerals	breads, garnishes, salads, sandwiches
carbohydrates, protein, vitamins B & E, phosphorus	breads, cereals, desserts, granola, milks, salads, snacks, soups

INDEX

A

Abdominal cramps, and peppermint/peppermint oil, 13

Abraham's oak, *See* Oak

Abscesses:
and chamomile, 272
and thyme, 300

Acne, 3
and aloe vera, 116
and cabbage, 268
and watercress, 36

Age spots, 3

Aging:
and almonds, 248-49
and olive oil, 229, 233-35
and omega-3 foods, 152

AIDS (Acquired Immune Deficiency Syndrome), 1, 3, 4
and aloe vera, 121-22
and garlic, 318-19
and shark-liver oil, 160-62
and spices/spicy food, 286-87

Ajoene, 313-14

Alkylglycerolds (AKGs), 159

Allergies, 21
and aloe vera, 120
and garlic, 332-35
gluten, and barley, 133-34
and parsley, 56
See also Hay fever

Alliin, 313

Almonds, 247-53
and aging, 248-49
almond salad recipe, 252
and bilary duct disorders, 248
and bladder problems, 248
and cancer, 249-52
and the heart, 249
and intestinal pains, 248
and kidney problems, 248
laetrile, 249-52
and stomach pains, 248
types of, 247-48
and wrinkles, 248-49

Aloe ferox, 108

Aloe succotrina, 108

Aloe vera, 107-25
and acne, 116

and heart problems, 209, 210-11,
    213-14
and hepatitis, 212
raw egg-wine-canned apple
    juice concoction, 214-15
as a tranquilizer, 209
and tumors, 216-17
and viruses, 211-12
See also Grapes; Red wine
Women's problems:
    and garlic, 336-37
    and wheat germ oil, 203-4
Wormwood, 304-6
    and anorexia, 307
    and athlete's foot, 306
    and fallen arches, 306
    infusion, 307
    and jaundice, 307
    and pain, 304-6
    as a vermifuge, 307

and viral hepatitis, 307
Wounds:
    and cabbage, 268
    and chlorophyll, 129-30
    and honey, 345-48
    and myrrh, 289
    and olive oil, 236, 241
    and peppermint, 14
    and thyme, 300
Wrinkles, 4
    and almonds, 248-49
    and olive oil, 245
    and sardines, 157

Y

Youth Restorative X, 157-58

615.85
Dub

Dubin, Reese
 Miracle food cures from the Bible

DATE DUE $15.00

7-8-01			

DEMCO